DIET Watchers Cookbook

By Barbara Gibbons
And The Editors of
Consumer Guide®

Harper & Row, Publishers

New York, Hagerstown, San Francisco, London

Contents

Copyright© 1978 by Publications International, Ltd.
All rights reserved
Printed in the United States of America

Published simultaneously in Canada
by Fitzhenry & Whiteside Limited, Toronto, Canada
Library of Congress Catalog Card Number: 77-90867

ISBN: 0-06-011509-2 (cloth)

ISBN: 0-06-011508-4 (paper)

This book may not be reproduced or quoted in whole or in part by mimeograph or any other printed means or for presentation on radio or television without written permission from:

Louis Weber, President
Publications International, Ltd.
3841 West Oakton Street
Skokie, Illinois 60076

Permission is never granted for commercial purposes.

About the Author

Barbara Gibbons, known as "The Slim Gourmet" in a nationally syndicated newspaper column, also writes the bi-monthly "Creative Low-Calorie Cooking" column in *Family Circle* Magazine. The author of six cookbooks, including the award-winning *Slim Gourmet Cookbook,* Mrs. Gibbons appears frequently on radio and TV.

Mrs. Gibbons weighed over 200 pounds by the age of 12 and remained fat until 10 years ago when she attacked overweight in the kitchen by "decalorizing" her favorite fattening dishes. She lost 80 pounds. Mrs. Gibbons wore a nurse's uniform to her high school graduation because she couldn't find a white dress in size 20½. Now she wears a size 9!

Special thanks to Dorothea Fast, home economist, assistant to the author.

Fighting Fat

The first step in losing weight is to get back into the kitchen. Declare your independence from gooey frozen pastries and TV dinners. Take charge of what goes onto your plate, into your mouth, and onto your hips. Learn to cook all over again, the low-calorie way.

Most lose-weight prescriptions take just the opposite approach, putting a psychological padlock on the kitchen door by telling the reader to forget about food. How can anybody forget about food? Particularly when we are constantly surrounded by food cues. No-work, no-nutrition, high-calorie snacks scream at us constantly from the TV screen, magazine pages, and supermarket ads. Nobody — least of all a person with a weight problem — can remain immune without alternative satisfactions. However, if you can duplicate the taste and texture of the foods you love — without the unneeded extra calories — you can turn a deaf ear!

Become a low-calorie cook. It needn't be time-consuming. With the variety of foods available today — including many convenience foods that are calorie bargains — low-cal cooking is easier than ever. Modern appliances, a well-equipped kitchen, a roomy refrigerator-freezer, and one-stop supermarkets, simplify the job. So do the recipes in this book. Short-cutting preparation time has been considered along with short-cutting calories.

Why Are You Overweight?

You are overweight because you take in more calories than you use up! But so do millions of other Americans, nearly half the population. The fact that so many others are in the same boat is small comfort. The health costs of carrying around your excess burden are just as high no matter how many others share your plight.

The fact that so many people fall beyond the American ideal of slenderness in no way lessens the discrimination overweights are subjected to. Excess pounds cost you money — in terms of lost income and lost opportunity. It has been well documented that fat job applicants lose out to less-qualified slim competitors. Fat executives are passed over for promotion. Fat salesmen, waitresses, and taxi drivers lose commissions and tips, often from fat customers. Even fat people don't like fat people!

In no other society has food been so easily attainable for so little physical effort. Despite inflation and soaring prices, despite occasional shortages, Americans still enjoy the "benefits" of a too bountiful breadbasket — with very little sweat of the brow in payment. You may hate your job, but sitting down at a desk all day doesn't qualify as work, not in the physical sense.

It is ironic that a society that makes the accumulation of fat so easy — almost unavoidable — should profess such an intolerance for obesity. The social pressures to avoid overweight are enormous, but they serve a purpose. Our skinny actresses, flat-gutted athletes, society-page darlings, and other beautiful people do serve a function after all. The standard they set for slimness has made fat unfashionable. And in the long run, vanity is what keeps most of us from eating ourselves into our graves.

Our Most Harmful Food Additive: Calories

Today, family life is increasingly fragmentized, with each individual snacking on the run. Long, late commuter hours between job and home (for Mom as well as Dad), a busy schedule of after-school activities, summers spent at camp, and semesters spent away at college all mean that more Americans of every age are eating outside the home. Even home-cooked meals are less likely to be cooked than thawed and served. The result is that Americans have less control than ever before over what goes into the food they eat.

A good Italian cook would make her homemade ravioli with lots of meat and simmer it with fresh tomatoes. But meat and vegetables are expensive, so a food processing firm that packages frozen ravioli is likely to stuff it with yet more starch, flavor it with a little meat, and freeze it in a tomato-shy sauce that's thickened with syrups and fillers. The second generation Italian-American wife who serves it to her family concedes wistfully that it's not quite like Mama used to make. She's probably not aware that the store-bought product is also more fattening, less nourishing, and less filling because the ravioli is short on appetite-appeasing protein while overly generous with quick-burning carbohydrates. A few hours after their ravioli meal, her family is foraging in the refrigerator for something else to fill their now-empty stomachs.

You might think that the American food industry has purposely set out to make us fat. Just when the technological revolution has entrapped an ever-widening circle of Americans of all ages and both sexes into sit-down jobs (or more years of sit-down schooling), just when our national calorie needs are at their lowest, food manufacturers seem to respond with a bulging cornucopia of nutritionally-neutered junk food, food that requires us to eat more and more calories for less and less nutrition.

But food makers are not intentionally fattening America. It's simply a matter of American business giving the customers what they want. Shoppers want food that's inexpensive, easy to serve and reasonably good tasting. And the food industry has risen to the challenge — hang nutrition and calories!

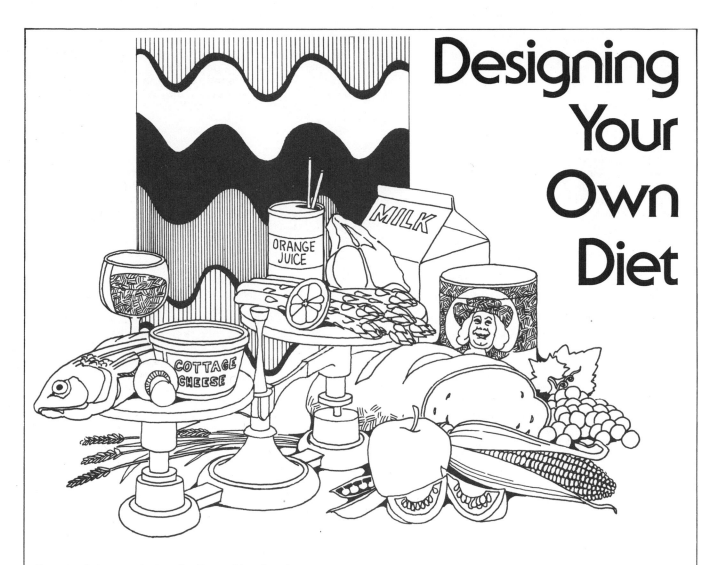

Designing Your Own Diet

Everybody knows that eating lots of food and accumulating extra pounds is no guarantee of adequate nutrition. Many Americans are overfed but undernourished because their tastes run to empty-caloried junk. When a person with a taste for fattening foods attempts to lose weight by simply cutting down, his or her chances of nutritional deficiency are multiplied. So before you become a bookkeeper of calories, it's important to understand that all calories are not alike, and that your calories must come from a variety of food sources for you to remain healthy.

Spending calories is like managing money. The shrewd manager knows that all bills must be paid before the leftovers can be spent on frills. Some people can live comfortably on little, while others spend a great deal and still run into trouble. The undernourished overweight is like a person who buys a car he or she cannot afford, while neglecting to pay the mortgage.

The person who wants to lose weight is in the same situation as somebody who has to live on a reduced income for awhile. Intelligent, imaginative people will find creative ways to do it in reasonable comfort, knowing that the time isn't far off when they can loosen up a little and indulge in a few more luxuries. But the smart dieter knows that a time when basic nutritional needs can be ignored will *never* come.

Protein, Fat, Carbohydrate . . . and Calories

Protein, fat, and carbohydrate are the basic food elements. A balanced diet includes all three. It is nearly impossible to emphasize or eliminate one without causing an unwanted imbalance in another. Therefore, when dieting, it is important to keep each of these elements in a healthy balance without simply cutting out one whole food type.

That's the idea behind the nutritional figures provided with each of the recipes in this book. Once you have computed your daily requirement of calories (see Computing Your Calorie Needs), the carbohydrate, protein, and fat figures given with each recipe will help you determine what percentages of your daily intake are being made up of these vital food elements.

Protein is mainly animal food — meat, poultry, fish, and eggs. But none is pure protein. Each also contains fat, and the more fat, the less protein. Protein is also found in dairy products like milk and cheese, and, along with fat and carbohydrate, in vegetables like beans and nuts. Protein is vital to life because the body needs it to build and repair itself. Protein is also valuable to dieters because it is slowly digested and helps sustain a feeling of fullness.

Approximately 25 percent of the food you eat should be protein; the minimum is 14 percent. But there is no benefit in having more protein than you need because the excess is stored by the body as fat. Too much protein has been linked with calcium deficiency and kidney disorders.

Fat can be either animal (meat fat or butter, for example) or vegetable (margarine, salad oil, or the fat found in nuts). Calorically, it does not matter where it comes from because both animal and vegetable fat have the same calorie count — double the calories of either protein or carbohydrate. Even for very determined dieters, it would be both difficult and undesirable to eliminate fat from the diet altogether because a small amount is needed to help the body absorb nutrients properly. But no more than 30 to 35 percent of the total calories you consume each day should be in the form of fat.

The last columns in the nutritional figures after the recipes in this book tell how much of the fat is saturated fat and how much cholesterol there is. The American Heart Association tells us to keep saturated fats to a minimum because they contain the cholesterol that is believed to be linked with heart disease. Less than 10 percent of your daily total fat intake should be in the form of saturated fats. And the average daily intake of cholesterol should be no more than 300 milligrams.

Carbohydrate is found in the sugars and starches we love so much. A diet plan that attempts to eliminate carbohydrate is a poor idea because fruits and vegetables, which are relatively high in carbohydrate, are the main sources of vital vitamins and minerals, as well as appetite-appeasing fiber.

Approximately 43 percent of a balanced diet should be carbohydrate. A diet that's low in carbohydrate is likely to be too high in fat and protein with possibly serious consequences. To maintain health, at least 60 grams of carbohydrate must be present in any daily diet. What should be avoided in the carbohydrate category are refined sugars and overprocessed starches that have been stripped of everything worthwhile, leaving little but calories.

And calories? A calorie is actually a measure of heat — fuel to power our bodies. If we consume more fuel than we can use up, the excess is stored as unsightly bulges. Calories exist in all foods, otherwise they would not be food. There are roughly four calories in every gram of protein or carbohydrate, and about nine calories in every gram of fat. To lose weight, we need to eat a variety of foods that are high in nutritional value but low in fuel value (calories) so that the body will be forced to use up its excess.

Fiber

Until recently, food fiber was the "forgotten nutrient" because it's not a nutrient at all. Fiber is the non-caloric, non-nutritious, nondigestible part of plant foods — the roughage or bulk in fruits, vegetables, nuts, seeds and whole-grain cereal foods. Since it's not digested but eliminated, it generally doesn't appear on nutrition charts and its importance has been ignored. But current research suggests that our reliance on over-refined processed foods from which much of the fiber has been removed may be related to many diseases, everything from cancer to constipation, from appendicitis to overweight!

Most foods high in fiber are naturally low in calories. They are important to dieters because their bulkiness fills the stomach and minimizes the desire or ability to overeat. Fiber is important to everyone because it speeds food through the system and minimizes constipation. Constipation has been related to diverticulosis, hemorrhoids, varicose veins and colon cancer. Vegetable fiber, particularly the pectin in fresh fruits, has been shown to aid in the elimination of excess fats and cholesterol from the system. So eating more foods that are naturally high in fiber is a good idea for most people, but especially for dieters. On the other hand, the extremes of fiber consumption suggested in some books on the topic, like all extremes, should be avoided.

Dietary Goals

Early in 1977, the U.S. Senate Select Committee on Nutrition issued a significant report: "Dietary Goals for the United States." This report urged sweeping changes in America's eating patterns. The Senate panel noted that Americans have been eating far too much sugar and fatty food, and not enough fruits, vegetables, grains, and other complex carbohydrates. The Senate said that current eating habits may be "as profoundly damaging to the nation's health as the widespread contagious diseases of the early part of the century." Here are those dietary goals:

- Increase carbohydrate consumption to account for 55 to 60 percent of calorie intake.
- Reduce overall fat consumption from approximately 40 to 30 percent of calorie intake.
- Reduce saturated fat consumption to account for about 10 percent of total calorie intake; and balance with polyunsaturated and monounsaturated fats, which should each account for about 10 percent of calorie intake.
- Reduce cholesterol consumption to about 300 milligrams a day.
- Reduce sugar consumption by almost 40 percent.
- Reduce salt consumption by about 50 to 85 percent.

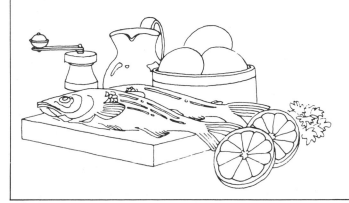

A DIETER'S DAILY DOZEN

Food Group	Suggestions

Dairy products:
Skim and low-fat milk, plain low-fat yogurt, buttermilk, 99% fat-free cottage cheese or other low-fat cheese.

Adults need the equivalent of at least 2 8-oz. glasses of skim or low-fat milk every day. Any of these dairy products may be used as they are or in cooking.

Complete protein main dishes:
Lean meat, poultry, seafood, eggs.

Adults need the equivalent of at least 2 servings a day. The equivalent of 1 serving is 3 oz. of meat after it has been trimmed of all visible fat and bone.

Other protein-rich foods:
Soybeans and soybean products, cheese and other milk products are also sources of complete protein, but individual servings of these generally contain lesser amounts of protein than servings of the main dish protein foods above. Other beans, peas, lentils, and nuts are sources of incomplete protein.

The complete protein foods in this list can occasionally be used in place of the main dish protein foods listed above. The incomplete protein foods can be used to augment complete protein foods.

Green or yellow fruits and vegetables:
Apricots, asparagus, broccoli, cantaloupe, carrots, collards, escarole, green beans, kale, lettuce, mangos, mustard greens, pumpkin, spinach, tomatoes, turnip greens, winter squash.

At least 2 ½-cup servings from this list every day, whether cooked, combined with other foods, included in salads. Raw vegetables also make calorie-safe nibbles.

Fruits and vegetables high in vitamin C:
Broccoli, brussels sprouts, grapefruit, lemons, limes, oranges, papayas, sweet peppers, strawberries, tangerines, tomatoes.

At least 1 serving per day equal to 6 oz. of orange juice in vitamin C.

Other fruits and vegetables:
Apples, bananas, beets, cauliflower, corn, peaches, pears, pineapple, potatoes.

At least 1 apple, banana, peach, or another fresh fruit per day. Or a ½-cup serving of canned or frozen vegetable or unsweetened fruit.

Breads, cereals, and grains:
Bread, rolls, crackers, breakfast cereal, pasta, rice, or other foods of grain origin.

At least 1 serving per day. Examples: 1 slice enriched bread; 1 cup unsweetened ready-to-eat cereal; ½ to ¾ cup cooked cereal, rice, or pasta.

Fats:
Animal fat as found in meat, poultry, fish, butter, or cheese. Vegetable fat as found in shortening, salad oils and dressings, or margarine.

Limit to 2 tbsp. per day. Fat is found in so many foods that no additional fat is needed.

Sugar and other sweeteners:
White and brown sugar, maple sugar, all syrups, honey.

None needed. Limit to 1 tbsp. per day. The only sweetener of value to the body is the natural sugar found in most fruits and vegetables.

Liquids:
Water, milk, fruit juice, coffee, tea, soft drinks, canned soups, bouillon, other beverages.

At least 3 to 4 cups per day. Drink cold water before, during, and between meals. Hot bouillon or fat-skimmed broth drunk before meals is a good way to curb appetite.

Alcoholic beverages:
Beer, wine, scotch, bourbon, gin, vodka, brandy, liqueurs.

Not more than 1 serving per day. These are high in calories but cooking evaporates the alcohol and its calories.

Non-nutritive foods:
Coffee, tea, salt, most herbs, spices, and seasonings.

Since they contain no calories, these may be used freely unless you have a special diet problem. Follow your doctor's advice.

To achieve these goals, the committee suggests the following changes in food selection and preparation:

- Increase consumption of fruits and vegetables and whole grains.
- Decrease consumption of meat and increase consumption of poultry and fish.
- Decrease consumption of foods high in fat, and partially substitute polyunsaturated fat for saturated fat.
- Substitute nonfat milk for whole milk.
- Decrease consumption of butterfat, eggs, and other high-cholesterol sources.
- Decrease consumption of sugar and foods with high sugar content.
- Decrease consumption of salt and foods with high salt content.

All of the recipes in this book reflect the Senate committee's goals and suggestions. The ingredients called for are in all cases the low-fat, low-calorie, unsweetened versions of or substitutions for common cooking ingredients. Cholesterol is also reduced not only by the choice of ingredients but also by special methods of preparation described in the recipes and chapter introductions. Not one recipe calls for sugar or even sugar substitute; naturally sweet fruits and fruit juices provide the desirable sweetness in sauces, desserts, beverages, and other foods. At the end of each recipe, there is also an analysis of the calories, carbohydrate, protein, total fat, saturated fat and cholesterol for the total yield of the recipe and for each serving. CONSUMER GUIDE Magazine's editors used tapes from the U.S. Department of Agriculture, the U.S. Department of Agriculture's *Composition of Foods, Handbook 8,* and *Nutritive Value of Foods, Bulletin No. 72*

to program a computer with every ingredient used in this book's recipes. Food processors and manufacturers provided additional statistics for the computer.

Eating to get thin or stay thin really amounts to healthy eating. So even if you are the only one at your house who is trying to lose weight, your whole family will benefit from the dishes made with the ingredients and methods described in this book.

Computing Your Calorie Needs

If you are an extremely inactive person who eats 3000 calories a day, your weight will eventually stabilize somewhere over the 200 mark. On the other hand, a young active person forced to live on 1500 calories might eventually become a 98-pound weakling. The right combination for you is somewhere between those two extremes.

Most diets expect the lifelong overeater to become an undereater overnight. It is unrealistic to believe that a 3000-calorie-a-day person can summon up the willpower to eat like a 98-pound weakling — unrealistic and unnecessary. If those same overweights simply began eating like the normalweights they want to be, their weight would eventually stabilize at the desired point on the scale. So the first step on your program is determining your proper weight and then computing the calorie intake that can eventually bring you there.

Pick your weight. Shown is a Desirable Weight Chart that you can use as a guide. But it's only a guide. If you are overweight, you might choose a target above the ideal, to make your goal more attainable. However, don't fall into the trap of overestimating your frame. Frame refers to skeleton, which can be small even if it's buried under mounds of fat. Unless you have very

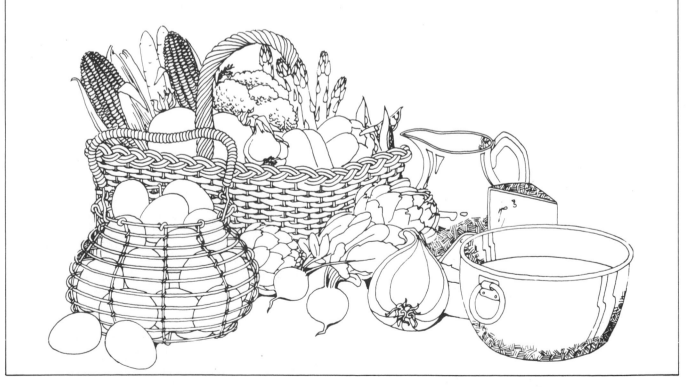

DESIRABLE WEIGHT CHART

	Women				Men		
Height*	Small Frame	Medium Frame	Large Frame	Height†	Small Frame	Medium Frame	Large Frame
4'10"	92-98	96-107	104-119	5'2"	112-120	118-129	126-141
4'11"	94-101	98-110	106-122	5'3"	115-123	121-133	129-144
5'0"	96-104	101-113	109-125	5'4"	118-126	124-136	132-148
5'1"	99-107	104-116	112-128	5'5"	121-129	127-139	135-152
5'2"	102-110	107-119	115-131	5'6"	124-133	130-143	138-156
5'3"	105-113	110-122	118-134	5'7"	128-137	134-147	142-161
5'4"	108-116	113-126	121-138	5'8"	132-141	138-152	147-166
5'5"	111-119	116-130	125-142	5'9"	136-145	142-156	151-170
5'6"	114-123	120-135	129-146	5'10"	140-150	146-160	155-174
5'7"	118-127	124-139	135-150	5'11"	144-154	150-165	159-179
5'8"	121-131	128-143	137-154	6'0"	148-158	154-170	164-184
5'9"	126-135	132-147	141-158	6'1"	152-162	158-175	168-189
5'10"	130-140	136-151	145-163	6'2"	156-167	162-180	173-194
5'11"	134-144	140-155	149-168	6'3"	160-171	167-185	178-199
6'0"	138-148	144-159	153-173				

*With shoes with 2-inch heels

†With shoes with 1-inch heels

broad shoulders and wide wrists (due to bone structure, not accumulated fat or water), it's more likely that your frame is medium or possibly even small. Many heavy people have tiny wrists and narrow shoulders, indications of a small frame.

Multiply by 13. Thirteen is the magic number that can help you assess how many calories a day you can eat to be the weight you want to be. If you should weigh 125, multiply 125 by 13. The result is 1625, and that's about how many calories a day you can eat to weigh 125. If you should weigh only 100, the right answer is 1300.

This is a generalization, of course, but a good enough guide for most overweights. According to general averages, the normal, moderately active person needs 15 calories per pound of body weight a day. For them, the magic number to multiply by is 15. But those who are overweight, underactive, or older need less, so the number 13 instead of 15 is more likely to apply to people with weight problems.

Naturally, cutting your calorie intake even lower will speed you towards your goal. But in no case should you attempt a reducing regimen below 1200 calories a day without medical supervision. You should consume at least 1200 calories a day in order to receive the minimum amounts of protein, fat, and carbohydrate your body needs. Also, a drastic cut in calories may leave you discouraged and defeated, ready to quit far short of your goal.

Designing a Diet to Fit Your Tastes

Weight control researchers have shown that the people most likely to succeed as losers are the ones who have worked out an eating plan that is tailored to their own tastes and life styles, a custom-made diet that takes into account their likes and dislikes, as well as the demands on their day. What good is a printed diet sheet commanding you to eat broiled flounder and two vegetables for lunch when you usually eat at your desk in the office?

Designing a diet to suit yourself may seem like a complicated project, but the results are well worth the effort, like the difference between an exquisitely tailored outfit and an ill-fitting dress off the rack. Here's how:

1. Arm yourself with several calorie guides, including one that lists food by brand names. Have on hand a food scale, measuring cups, and measuring spoons.

2. Keep a record of what you eat every day for a week. Once a day look up and write down the calorie counts for each item and add up the totals. Don't guess at amounts, make use of your scale and measuring tools for more accurate estimates. You may be surprised to learn that your usual calorie intake is nearly double what you should be eating!

3. Go back over your daily food diary and look for ways to pare it down.

- Eliminate any item you can easily do without — bread with dinner, for example.
- Cut down amounts of food where possible — one slice of bread instead of two, for example.
- Substitute a lower-caloried item — diet bread for example, or a slice of melba-thin bread at half the calories.

4. Check your daily food diary for balance. Are you getting enough green vegetables? Too much meat? Not enough milk? Can the items you're short on be added to your diet in place of fattening snacks?

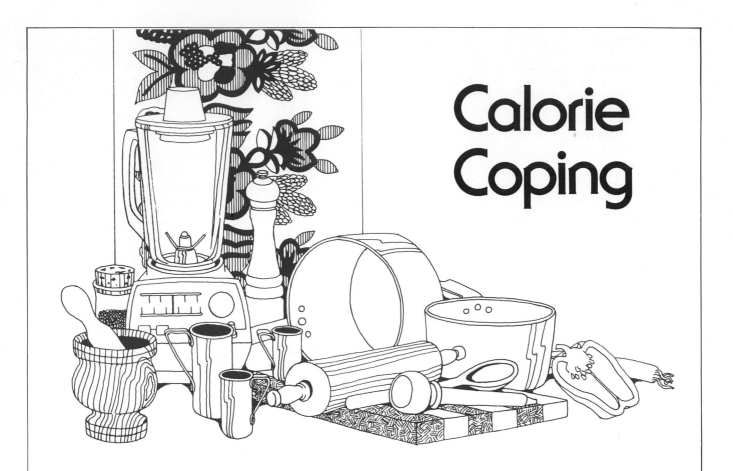

Calorie Coping

By providing yourself with a few special diet utensils and by using some easy cooking, shopping and eating hints, you can slash the calorie content of your favorite foods and daily intake, and lose weight in a painless and delicious way.

Equipment

• Equip yourself with nonstick pots and pans for cooking, baking and frying without fat. Follow the manufacturer's directions for care. Inexpensive utensils can do the job if you keep them well scrubbed. If a skillet loses its ability to cook without added fat, throw it out. You cannot afford to keep it!

• A pressure cooker is a handy gadget for cooks on the go because it cuts cooking time by one-third. The leanest, least fattening, less-expensive cuts of meat profit from pressure cookery. If you buy a new one, choose a model with a nonstick interior.

• A blender makes short work of many kitchen tasks. Dieters can turn a blender into a milkshake maker by combining skim milk powder, ice cubes, water and flavoring. A handful of fresh berries or other fruit can be added for a garden-fresh flavor.

Cooking hints

• Use spray-on vegetable coating for no-fat frying. When used in conjunction with nonstick utensils, the spray eliminates the need for any added fat at all. The base of these products is lecithin, a natural food component much loved by health food fans.

• When making stews and other combination dishes, prepare them a day ahead and store them in the refrigerator — all day or overnight — until serving time. The flavors blend better and all the fat rises to the surface where you can easily lift it off.

• Fat can be removed from the surface of stock, soup, or gravy with a bulb-type baster or by chilling until the fat rises and can be lifted off.

• Keep your crisper well stocked with shredded lettuce, chopped onion and other greenery so that serving a salad at every meal is a snap.

• Keep your refrigerator's fruit compartment well supplied with whatever fresh treats are in season. Fruit makes the perfect dessert. Freeze fruits in season for sugar-free treats during the winter.

• If time is at a premium (and when isn't it?), cook in double or triple quantities. Then package the leftovers into homemade low-calorie frozen dinners. Inexpensive aluminum pie pans can serve this purpose.

• Large roasts, casseroles and other dishes meant for several meals should be packaged away in the freezer right after dinner. Don't keep leftovers around.

• Package meats and other foods for the freezer in serving-size quantities. Four to six ounces of boneless raw meat per person is about right. If you defrost and cook only what you need, you avoid waste.

Calorie-Coping in the Supermarket

• Be a calorie-comparison shopper. Check the nutritional label panel of competing products and choose the one with the lower calorie count. Smart label-readers can save calories the same way a cost-wise shopper saves money.

• Always look for the lowest fat content in dairy products. Cottage cheese that is labeled 99 percent fat-free is only 160 to 180 calories a cup. Regular creamed cottage cheese is 240 to 260.

• Do not pay a premium price for fattening meat. Prime meat, the most expensive, has a higher ratio of fat and calories and less protein than less costly grades.

• In choosing meat, always look for the leanest cuts. Have the butcher trim away all fat, or do it yourself. Trimmable exterior fat is less of a problem than fatty marbling all through the meat.

• Play the substitution game. Look for diet-right versions of fattening products. Experiment with them in recipes.

• Low-calorie cream cheese and part-skim Neufchatel cheese have the same flavor as fattening cream cheese, and perform the same way in recipes.

• Evaporated skim milk can take the place of cream in most sauces, casseroles, souffles, and desserts. It can even be whipped!

• Yogurt or buttermilk can take the place of sour cream in many recipes. Or look for low-fat, nondairy sour cream dressings that can serve the same function. But check the calorie count. Some nondairy dressings contain just as much fat (vegetable instead of animal) as real sour cream.

• Diet margarine has half the calories of regular margarine or butter because it is half water. Unfortunately it cannot replace ordinary margarine in regular recipes. However, many recipes in this book are adjusted to use this low-in-calories spread.

• Low-fat diet dressings and mayonnaise substitute can help keep salads slimming.

• Do not be put off by the word *imitation* on certain low-calorie, low-sugar, or low-fat products. The word doesn't mean that the product is made up of chemicals, but only that the lower sugar or fat content keeps the product from conforming to standard recipes. Often the imitations are more nutritious than the real thing.

• Beware the dietetic product that does not list its calorie count! It may not be diet-wise at all, but simply salt-free. For example, some dietetic candies made for diabetics have just as many calories as regular candy.

• Bottled flavorings and extracts from the supermarket spice shelf are calorie bargains. Some to look for include butter flavoring, rum, brandy, banana, and chocolate. Most spices and seasonings add so few calories to a dish that they do not need to be counted.

• Never go shopping when you are hungry. And leave the kids at home.

Calorie-Coping in the Dining Room

One of the most successful new approaches to weight control is behavior modification. This technique helps overweight people cut calories by forcing them to focus on unconscious eating habits. You can put these methods to work in the dining room by following a few simple rules:

• Never eat standing up. By following this rule, you preclude all nibbling, tasting, testing, and snacking.

• Always eat in the same place, the dining room, for example. Even if you are determined to eat that leftover half-donut, set yourself a place at the dining table, then sit down and eat it. By the time everything is set, you may have changed your mind.

• Always set your place properly. Use a place mat, napkin, water glass, the whole bit. You'll enjoy your meal more in a pleasant setting, and the act of setting a place makes each meal a ceremony.

• Never eat while reading or watching TV. Do not dilute the enjoyment of food by concentrating your attention on something else. Paperwork, crossword puzzles, business negotiations, and family arguments shouldn't cut into your eating pleasure either.

• Never prepare or put out more food than you need, lest you personally clean up the leftovers yourself. Leave the second helpings in the kitchen so you'll have to make a special trip to get them.

• Always compute the number of servings in any dish you make — main course, side dish, or dessert — and apportion it accordingly. If a dish serves six, make it a point to serve yourself one-sixth of the total, and not a tablespoon more.

• Set out at one time everything you plan to eat at a meal, from soup to dessert. With the finale in full view, you'll be less likely to overeat at the main event.

• Equip yourself with smaller plates. Choose a restaurant-style design, with wide rims. A brimming luncheon-size plate is more eye-satisfying than a big expanse of china with lots of white space around modest servings of food. The same strategy applies to wine glasses and dessert dishes.

• Use the other tactic with salads and vegetable dishes. Serve your salad in big soup-size bowls to encourage yourself to fill up on nonfattening fare.

• Do not concentrate on easy-to-eat foods. Foods that take longer to consume are more satisfying than boneless, bite-size swallows. Corn on the cob seems like more than the same amount of cut corn. Lobster in the shell will keep you busy longer than a boneless steak.

• Eat slowly, savor each bite.

. . . and Away from It!

• Once you are finished eating, leave the table. Do not keep others company.

• Do not clean up when you clean the table. If you cannot resist munching on the leftovers, put a piece of gum in your mouth before you start. Or better yet, turn the clean-up job over to somebody else.

• Keep busy. Get out of the house during those crisis hours when you're most inclined to succumb to a peanut butter frenzy. Go window shopping for the new clothes you'll buy when you're slim.

• Take up a hobby, preferably something that keeps your hands busy. It's hard to eat potato chips and refinish furniture at the same time. A good idea is to take up sewing — you'll need seamstress skills to create the new wardrobe in your thin future.

• Make a list of everything you hate about being fat, and post it prominently on the refrigerator. Or take the positive approach and list all the things you'd do if you were trim.

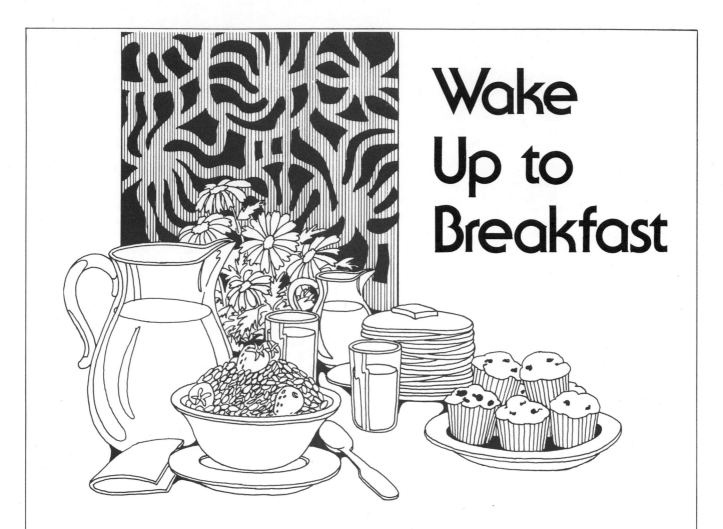

Wake Up to Breakfast

If skipping breakfast is your idea of saving calories, think again. Would-be skinnies who try to subsist without breakfast generally wind up giving into coffee-and-junk breaks at midmorning, or overeating at lunch, or both. The result is more calories consumed than would have been in a decent morning meal.

Breakfast needn't be heavy or elaborate. In fact, if you're dieting, it should be light. But lightness in calories does not mean shortchanging nutrition. Ideally, a dieter's breakfast should include:

- Fresh fruit for vitamins and bulk. Unsugared canned or frozen fruit can be used. High-in-vitamin-C choices like grapefruit, sliced strawberries, or melon are ideal.
- Grain which can be either bread or cereal.
- Protein food. Meat or eggs or egg substitutes are the usual choices. High-protein cereals topped with protein-rich skim milk can also meet your morning protein requirement.
- Milk — preferably nonfat or low-fat, which can be a beverage by itself, poured on cereal or fruit, or used in coffee or tea.

Good Breakfast Combinations

- High-protein cereal with skim milk and sliced berries.

- Grapefruit half, toasted protein bread with low-calorie cream cheese.
- Melon wedge, cottage-cheese-filled omelet, and black coffee. Toast saved for a 10 o'clock snack.
- Pancakes made with high-protein pancake mix, topped with sliced strawberries or crushed pineapple. Add a glass of skim milk.

If you're a confirmed coffee-breaker, there's no harm in saving part of your breakfast menu for a midmorning snack. However, postponing all food until 10 or 11 o'clock is a poor idea since it is likely that more than half a day has passed since your body took in any nourishment.

Bad Breakfast Bets

At the other extreme from breakfast-skippers are those who unwittingly load up on calories without redeeming nutritional value. Many traditional breakfast foods are exceedingly rich in sugar, starch, or fat.

- **Sugar-coated cereals.** Most presweetened cereals contain more sugar than anything else. When choosing cereal, pick a high-protein variety.
- **Bacon** is more than half fat, even after it has been broiled or fried and well drained. Choose lean Canadian bacon instead, only 45 calories an ounce instead of 200.

- **Sausage** is generally 50 percent fat. Instead of buying packaged sausage, make your own home-seasoned patties from lean ground pork.
- **Pastries** are simply empty-caloried concoctions of starch, sugar, and fat. Their low protein means you'll be hungry by midmorning.

Recipes

Country Biscuits

2 cups flour	2 tbsp. diet
3 tsp. baking powder	margarine
1 tsp. salt	¾ cup skim milk

Sift the flour and remeasure to 2 cups. Sift again with the baking powder and salt. Cut in the margarine with a pastry blender. Add the milk. Stir the mixture quickly and lightly with a fork just until the dough clings together into a ball. Then turn the dough out onto a lightly floured board and knead it gently. Roll the dough or pat it out to ½-inch thickness. Cut the dough with a 2-inch biscuit cutter and place the dough circles on an ungreased cookie sheet. Bake 12 to 15 minutes in a preheated 450° oven. *Makes 12 servings*

	Calories	Carbo-hydrate (gm)	Protein (gm)	Total Fat (gm)	Saturated Fat (gm)	Choles-terol (mg)
Total	1084.8	200.8	32.8	14.0	2.0	3.8
Per Serving	90.4	16.7	2.7	1.2	0.2	0.3

Blueberry Cornmeal Muffins

⅔ cup diet margarine	½ cup fresh
2 eggs	blueberries or
1¼ cups cornmeal	unsweetened
¾ cup flour	frozen
2½ tsp. double-acting	blueberries,
baking powder	thawed and
¾ tsp. salt	drained
¾ cup skimmed milk	

Beat the diet margarine and eggs in a medium bowl. Stir in the cornmeal. Sift the flour and remeasure to ¾ cup. Sift again with the baking powder and salt. Stir ⅓ of this mixture into the cornmeal mixture. Then stir in ½ of the milk. Repeat this process. Add the remaining ⅓ of flour mixture. Gently fold in the blueberries. Place a scant ¼ cup of batter in each cup of a muffin tin that has been sprayed with vegetable coating. Bake the muffins in a preheated 350° oven for 20 to 25 minutes until golden brown. *Makes 15 servings*

	Calories	Carbo-hydrate (gm)	Protein (gm)	Total Fat (gm)	Saturated Fat (gm)	Choles-terol (mg)
Total	1194.3	204.8	42.9	23.6	6.0	507.8
Per Serving	79.6	13.7	2.9	1.6	0.4	33.9

Corn Bread

3 cups cornmeal	1½ tsp. salt
2 tsp. baking powder	2 cups buttermilk
1 tsp. baking soda	3 eggs, slightly
	beaten

Mix the cornmeal, baking powder, baking soda, and salt together. Add the buttermilk and eggs. If you want crisp corn bread, bake it in a shallow pan that has been sprayed with vegetable coating. Use a deep pan for thick servings. Bake in a preheated 425° oven for 25 to 30 minutes. *Makes 10 servings*

	Calories	Carbo-hydrate (gm)	Protein (gm)	Total Fat (gm)	Saturated Fat (gm)	Choles-terol (mg)
Total	1727.1	294.5	69.0	33.0	9.0	766.0
Per Serving	172.7	29.5	6.9	3.3	0.9	76.6

Cheese Blintzes

Batter:	Filling:
1 cup flour	3 cups 99% fat-free
1 tsp. salt	cottage cheese
1 cup skim milk	½ tsp. butter-flavored
4 eggs, beaten	salt
	2 tsp. vanilla
	½ tsp. grated lemon
	peel
	1 egg yolk

Combine the flour and salt in a bowl and gradually stir in the milk. Add the eggs and beat mixture. Spray a 6-inch nonstick skillet with vegetable coating for no-fat frying, and heat it for 1 or 2 minutes. Pour about 2 tablespoons batter into the pan. Tip and roll the pan to cover the bottom with batter. Cook the pancake for about 1 minute until the top dries. Then turn it out on a towel, browned side up. Repeat this procedure until all the batter is used. You should have 18 pancakes.

Mix all of the ingredients for the filling in a bowl and blend them well. Put 2 to 3 tablespoons of filling on each pancake. Fold in the sides, and roll the pancake to make an envelope. Place blintzes in a baking pan, and reheat in the oven before serving.

Makes 9 servings

Hint: If you like, the blintzes can be served topped with your favorite low-calorie preserves, with fresh fruit, or with cinnamon.

	Calories	Carbo-hydrate (gm)	Protein (gm)	Total Fat (gm)	Saturated Fat (gm)	Choles-terol (mg)
Total	1489.6	131.2	139.0	36.0	13.6	1323.2
Per Serving	165.5	14.6	15.4	4.0	1.5	147.0

gm = grams; mg = milligrams. Nutritional figures are approximate. Figures are based on findings of U.S. Department of Agriculture.

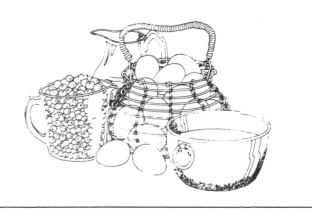

High-Protein Waffles

1 whole egg or 2 egg
  whites
1 tsp. vanilla

½ cup soy-enriched
  pancake mix
½ cup skim milk

Stir the egg, vanilla and pancake mix together and add just enough milk to make a pourable batter. Spray the surface of your nonstick waffle maker with vegetable coating until all surfaces are wet and shiny. Turn on the heat. When a drop of water bounces and sizzles, pour on the batter and close the waffle maker. Don't attempt to open until the waffles stop steaming or the indicator light goes off. When the waffles are done, loosen gently with a fork or knife, being careful not to mar the nonstick surface.

Makes 4 sections (2 servings)

	Calories	Carbo-hydrate (gm)	Protein (gm)	Total Fat (gm)	Saturated Fat (gm)	Choles-terol (mg)
Total	335.0	48.0	20.5	34.0	2.0	254.5
Per Serving	167.5	24.0	10.3	17.0	1.0	127.3

Hotcakes

1 cup flour
1 tsp. baking powder
¼ tsp. salt

1 cup skim milk
1 egg, slightly
  beaten

Sift the flour and remeasure to 1 cup. Sift again with the baking powder and salt. In a mixing bowl, combine the milk with the beaten egg; then add the dry ingredients. Blend the mixture only until the larger lumps disappear. Spray a nonstick skillet with vegetable coating for no-fat frying and preheat the skillet over medium-low heat for 2 to 3 minutes or until a drop of water sizzles on the surface. With a tablespoon, drop the batter to make 4-inch hotcakes in the hot pan, and cook about 1 minute per side. Serve immediately.

Makes 12 hotcakes (6 servings)

	Calories	Carbo-hydrate (gm)	Protein (gm)	Total Fat (gm)	Saturated Fat (gm)	Choles-terol (mg)
Total	627.1	107.5	28.0	7.0	2.0	257.0
Per Serving	104.5	17.9	4.7	1.2	0.3	42.8

Cornmeal Pancakes

½ cup flour
1½ tsp. baking powder
½ tsp. salt

1 cup skim milk
2 eggs, slightly
  beaten
½ cup yellow cornmeal

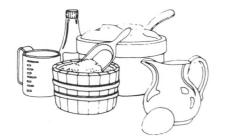

Sift the flour and remeasure to ½ cup. Sift again with the baking powder and salt. Combine the milk with the beaten eggs in a bowl; then add the dry ingredients including cornmeal. Blend the mixture only until the larger lumps disappear. Spray a nonstick skillet with vegetable coating for no-fat frying. Preheat the skillet over medium heat for 1 to 2 minutes. With a tablespoon, drop the batter into the pan to make 4-inch pancakes. Cook until the bubbles break and the edges are cooked. Then turn the pancakes to brown the other side. Serve immediately.

Makes 16 pancakes (8 servings)

	Calories	Carbo-hydrate (gm)	Protein (gm)	Total Fat (gm)	Saturated Fat (gm)	Choles-terol (mg)
Total	699.2	105.5	33.0	15.0	4.5	509.0
Per Serving	87.4	13.2	4.1	1.9	0.6	63.6

Tender Blueberry Pancakes

1⅓ cups unsifted flour
½ tsp. baking soda
1 tsp. salt
¼ tsp. nutmeg
1 egg, beaten

8-oz. container plain
  low-fat yogurt
1 cup skim milk
1 cup blueberries,
  fresh or frozen,
  unsweetened

Stir the dry ingredients together thoroughly. Beat the egg, yogurt and milk smooth. Then add to the dry ingredients. Stir just enough to combine. Fold in the blueberries. Drop ¼ cup for each pancake onto nonstick griddle that has been sprayed with vegetable coating. Cook until the surface is covered with bubbles, turn, and cook until the other side is well browned. Serve with Hot Blueberry Syrup.

Makes 18 pancakes, about 3 inches in diameter (9 servings)

	Calories	Carbo-hydrate (gm)	Protein (gm)	Total Fat (gm)	Saturated Fat (gm)	Choles-terol (mg)
Total	985.2	172.4	4.3	12.3	4.0	277.0
Per Serving	109.4	19.2	0.5	1.4	0.4	30.8

Hot Blueberry Syrup

1 cup blueberries, fresh
  or frozen,
  unsweetened

½ cup unsweetened
  grape juice

Combine the ingredients in saucepan and bring to a boil. Crush the berries with the back of a spoon. Simmer 2 to 3 minutes. Serve hot. Store in the refrigerator. Reheat to serve again.

Makes about 1 cup (8 servings)

	Calories	Carbo-hydrate (gm)	Protein (gm)	Total Fat (gm)	Saturated Fat (gm)	Choles-terol (mg)
Total	169.0	41.9	1.4	1.0	0.0	0.0
Per Serving	21.2	5.2	0.2	0.2	0.0	0.0

gm = grams; mg = milligrams. Nutritional figures are approximate. Figures are based on findings of U.S. Department of Agriculture.

Spiced Apple Syrup

6 -oz. can frozen
    unsweetened apple
    juice concentrate,
    defrosted, undiluted
1 tbsp. arrowroot or
    cornstarch

1 cup cold water
Pinch salt
1/4 tsp. mixed apple
    pie spice or
    cinnamon

Combine all the ingredients in a saucepan. Cook and stir over moderate heat until the mixture simmers and thickens. Serve warm over pancakes or French toast. Store in the refrigerator. Reheat to serve again.

Makes 1¾ cups (12 servings)

	Calories	Carbo-hydrate (gm)	Protein (gm)	Total Fat (gm)	Saturated Fat (gm)	Choles-terol (mg)
Total	385.1	94.3	0.0	0.0	0.0	0.6
Per Serving	32.1	7.9	0.0	0.0	0.0	0.1

Pineapple Pancake Sauce

16-oz. can unsweetened
    crushed pineapple,
    undrained

1 tsp. arrowroot or
    cornstarch
1/4 cup cold water

Combine all the ingredients in blender and blend smooth. Pour into a saucepan. Cook and stir over moderate heat until the mixture simmers. Store in the refrigerator and reheat to serve.

Makes 2¼ cups (18 servings)

	Calories	Carbo-hydrate (gm)	Protein (gm)	Total Fat (gm)	Saturated Fat (gm)	Choles-terol (mg)
Total	310.4	79.1	0.0	0.0	0.0	0.0
Per Serving	17.2	4.4	0.0	0.0	0.0	0.0

Honey-Maple Syrup

1 tbsp. arrowroot or
    cornstarch
5 tbsp. honey

Pinch salt
1 cup water
2 tsp. maple extract

Combine all the ingredients except the maple flavoring in a saucepan. Cook and stir the mixture over moderate heat until it boils. Then lower the heat and simmer for 1 minute. Remove the pan from the heat and stir in the maple flavoring. Store the syrup in the refrigerator.

Makes 1 cup (8 servings)

	Calories	Carbo-hydrate (gm)	Protein (gm)	Total Fat (gm)	Saturated Fat (gm)	Choles-terol (mg)
Total	366.3	95.2	0.0	0.0	0.0	0.0
Per Serving	45.8	11.9	0.0	0.0	0.0	0.0

Pineapple Cheese Danish Squares

1 cup unsweetened
    crushed pineapple
8 to 9 graham crackers,
    plain or cinnamon
1 cup evaporated skim
    milk
4 eggs

1/4 tsp. salt
2 tsp. vanilla
7 tbsp. honey
2 tbsp. cornstarch
2 cups 99% fat-free
    cottage cheese
Dash cinnamon

Drain pineapple, reserving juice. Break up graham crackers and arrange in the bottom of a nonstick 8-inch square cake pan. Cover the crackers with the well-drained pineapple. Combine juice with remaining ingredients, except cinnamon, in a blender and beat until smooth. Pour over pineapple and sprinkle with cinnamon. Bake in a preheated 250° oven for 1 hour, then turn off the heat and let cool in oven. Refrigerate.

Makes 8 squares

	Calories	Carbo-hydrate (gm)	Protein (gm)	Total Fat (gm)	Saturated Fat (gm)	Choles-terol (mg)
Total	1902.7	248.6	107.00	54.0	21.4	1124.8
Per Serving	238.9	31.1	13.4	6.8	2.7	140.6

Savory Sausage

4 lb. lean pork
    shoulder, trimmed
    of all fat and
    ground twice
1 tbsp. onion salt
1 finely chopped garlic
    clove
1 tbsp. sage

1 tsp. ground cloves
1 tsp. mace
2 tsp. pepper
1 tbsp. minced
    parsley
1/4 tsp. ground
    allspice

Combine the ground pork with the other ingredients and mix well. Shape the meat into 3-oz. patties. (This will make 20 patties.) The patties may be broiled 3 to 4 inches from heat source or pan-fried in a nonstick skillet. Cook until they are no longer pink inside.

Makes 20 servings

Note: The raw patties may be frozen for later cooking.

	Calories	Carbo-hydrate (gm)	Protein (gm)	Total Fat (gm)	Saturated Fat (gm)	Choles-terol (mg)
Total	4666.5	0.0	533.2	266.6	80.0	1599.6
Per Serving	233.3	0.0	26.7	13.3	4.0	80.0

Country Sausage

2 tbsp. sage
1 tbsp. salt
1 tsp. pepper
1 tsp. ground cloves

1/2 tsp. ground
    nutmeg
4 lb. lean fresh pork,
    trimmed of all fat
    and ground

Add the seasonings to the meat and mix until well blended. Shape the meat into 3-oz. patties. Broil 3 to 4 inches from the heat source or pan-fry in a nonstick skillet until they are no longer pink inside.

Makes 20 servings

Note: The raw patties may be frozen for later cooking.

	Calories	Carbo-hydrate (gm)	Protein (gm)	Total Fat (gm)	Saturated Fat (gm)	Choles-terol (mg)
Total	4666.5	0.0	533.2	266.6	80.0	1599.6
Per Serving	233.3	0.0	26.7	13.3	4.0	80.0

gm = grams; mg = milligrams. Nutritional figures are approximate. Figures are based on findings of U.S. Department of Agriculture.

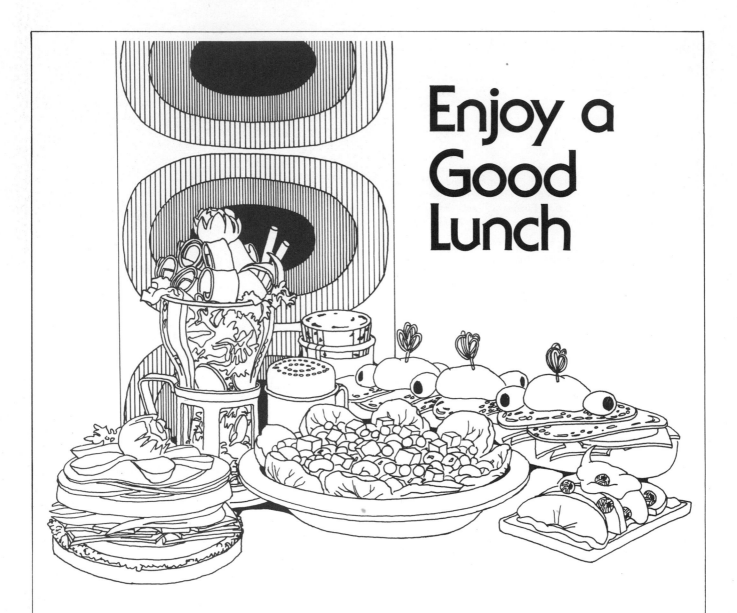

Enjoy a Good Lunch

Whether you brown-bag it to an office or lunch alone at home, munch on a quick hamburger or an expense-account steak, unthought-out lunches can pile on lots of extra calories. Worst of all, they often are not satisfying, and thus take an even higher toll when late-day hunger and fatigue bring on a nibble fit. So plan ahead. Don't take lunch for granted.

There are times when a sandwich is the most practical luncheon choice — if you carry your lunch, for example. Slimming down a sandwich without shortcutting protein takes some careful bargain-hunting among the possible ingredients.

Slimming Sandwiches on the Outside

The fewer calories you spend on bread, the more you'll have for the inside of the sandwich. Here is a rundown on the bread options.

• Ordinary white bread is around 65 calories per slice.

• Slim-sliced breads range from 43 to 53 calories per slice. Their smaller size is what makes the calories lower.

• Diet and protein breads range from 35 to 50 calories per slice, sometimes more, so be a label reader to get the best calorie buy for your money. (If the label won't say, why buy?) Protein-enriched breads are usually made from part soy flour, so they offer a nutrition boost and are more filling than ordinary breads. Gluten breads made from high-protein flour are among the least fattening, about 35 calories per slice. Do not be turned off by the name; they do not taste chewy-gluey.

• Bran breads, depending on the brand, can contain as much as six times the fiber of white bread, but because of added fats, sugars and syrups, the calories can average 85 or 90 per slice.

• Special fiber breads, depending on the brand, contain about five times the fiber of regular whole wheat bread, but only 50 calories per slice. These calorie bargains are the same size as ordinary white or wheat bread, but are formulated with refined cellulose bulking agents. Special fiber breads can be toasted, French-toasted, grilled or used in recipes as replacements for regular breads. Because of the high fiber content, both special fiber breads and bran breads are very filling.

• Rye and pumpernickel breads are generally lower in calories than white bread, but the slices are larger, so they average around 65 calories a slice. Buy it unsliced and cut it superthin for a calorie bargain.

• French and Italian breads will be low in calories if no fat is used in the dough. Check the label.

• Whole wheat and cracked wheat breads are lower than many breads, about 55 to 60 calories per slice.

• Quality and premium-priced breads are usually richer and more fattening but the slices are thinner than white bread, so the calorie count is about the same, 65 per slice.

• Hard rolls average around 150 calories each. So do soft hamburger rolls. You can decalorize a roll to around 100 calories by pulling out the doughy center.

• Toast is no lower in calories than the same bread untoasted.

• Bakery or specialty breads are anybody's guess.

Slimming Sandwiches on the Inside

• Sliced meats from homemade roasts can make the tastiest sandwiches. They can also be the most economical in cost and calories. But choose with care. Dark meat turkey is 176 calories for a three-ounce serving but white meat turkey or roast veal adds up to only 150 calories. Roast beef, ham, or lamb, if really lean and fat-trimmed, can be under 160 calories; but hidden or untrimmed fat can double the count. For example, lean roast round of beef is low, but three ounces of fatty rib roast can go as high as 375 calories. Leg of lamb is low, but fatty shoulder roast may be 250 calories or more. Lean smoked ham is relatively low, but a fatty pork roast or greasy glazed ham adds up to more than 300 calories. And don't forget: a calorie-conscious, nongreasy, homemade meat loaf of lean chopped beef makes a delicious sandwich, too.

• Cold cuts can be a calorie bargain or a fatty disaster. Here are some of the popular choices found at the deli counter, given in three-ounce portions because the calories per slice depend on the slice. These are averages only, based on government, industry, or processors' data; individual brands may vary.

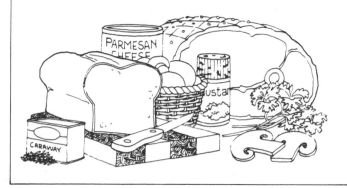

COLD CUT COMPARISONS

Meat	Calories per 3-Ounce Serving
Corned beef	204
Beef bologna	237
Turkey bologna	193
Braunschweiger	270
Smoked chicken	135
Cooked (boiled) ham	120
Beef-pork loaf	297
Ham and cheese loaf	228
Head cheese	206
Liverwurst	261
Olive loaf	156
Pickle-pimiento loaf	234
Pastrami	171
Dry salami	384
Cooked salami	264
Turkey salami	176
Thuringer	254
Turkey loaf	100
Smoked turkey	136

What's turkey bologna? Or turkey salami? These calorie-shy newcomers may not yet be available in your area. A boon to cholesterol counters, too, they are processed from low-calorie turkey, but they have the same spices, the same color, taste, and texture as their more fattening namesakes.

• Cheeses can make or break a low-cal sandwich. Are natural cheeses slimmer than the processed types? What about cheese foods, cheese spreads, and skim milk or diet cheeses? Here are some guidelines:

CHEESE COMPARISONS

Cheese	Calories per Ounce
Most natural hard cheeses: cheddar, American, Swiss, Romano and other grating cheeses	110 or more
Most processed cheeses and soft cheeses: Limburger, bleu, Roquefort, cream cheese	100 to 110
Most processed cheese foods	90 to 100
Most cheese spreads and some part-skim cheeses: mozzarella, pizza cheese, Scamorze, sapsago, Neufchatel	75 to 90
Farmer cheese, cottage cheese. Low calorie or diet cheese such as imitation cream cheese or imitation processed American cheese slices. The word imitation is used on the label because the products don't meet the federal standard of fat content (fortunately!), although they generally contain more protein than the real thing.	under 40

Recipes

Hot Tuna Sandwiches

1 tbsp. diet margarine
1½ tsp. minced green
   pepper
1 tsp. minced onion
4 eggs, slightly beaten
¼ cup skim milk
½ tsp. salt

7-oz. can water-
   packed tuna
   (lobster or
   crabmeat may
   be used)
4 slices toasted
   high-fiber or
   protein bread

Preheat a nonstick saucepan over low heat for 2 minutes. Melt the margarine. Add the green pepper and onion and sauté about 5 minutes. Remove the pan from the heat and add the eggs, milk, salt, and tuna. Cook the mixture over low heat for about 10 minutes, stirring constantly, until it is thick and creamy. Serve over the toast. *Makes 4 servings*

	Calories	Carbo-hydrate (gm)	Protein (gm)	Total Fat (gm)	Saturated Fat (gm)	Choles-terol (mg)
Total	868.7	46.8	92.0	34.8	9.6	1138.9
Per Serving	217.2	11.7	23.0	8.7	2.4	284.7

Cottage Cheese Egg Salad

3 hard-cooked eggs,
   chopped
½ cup 99% fat-free
   cottage cheese
1 tbsp. yogurt
2 tsp. prepared mustard

1½ tsp. chopped
   chives
¼ tsp. salt
⅛ tsp. Worcester-
   shire sauce
¼ tsp. dill

Combine all the ingredients in a small bowl. Cover and chill to blend the flavors. Serve on toast, crackers, or lettuce leaves if desired. *Makes 2 servings*

	Calories	Carbo-hydrate (gm)	Protein (gm)	Total Fat (gm)	Saturated Fat (gm)	Choles-terol (mg)
Total	415.8	23.6	33.5	19.2	6.7	766.9
Per Serving	207.9	11.8	16.8	9.6	3.4	383.5

Crabmeat Louis

1 small head of lettuce
1½ cups cooked or
   canned lump crab-
   meat, chilled

1 large tomato cut
   into wedges
2 hard-cooked eggs,
   sliced
6 pimiento-stuffed
   olives, sliced

Arrange the lettuce in 4 salad serving bowls. Mound the crabmeat on top and garnish with the tomato wedges, egg slices and olives. Serve with Louis Dressing listed next. *Makes 4 servings*

	Calories	Carbo-Hydrate (gm)	Protein (gm)	Total Fat (gm)	Saturated Fat (gm)	Choles-terol (mg)
Total	607.5	30.0	71.5	23.0	4.0	805.0
Per Serving	151.9	7.5	17.9	5.8	1.0	201.3

Louis Dressing

1 cup diet mayonnaise
½ cup tomato purée
¼ tsp. Tabasco sauce
1½ tsp. grated onion
2 tsp. horseradish

¼ tsp. pepper
1 tsp. fresh lemon
   juice
¼ tsp. tarragon
½ tsp. salt

Combine all the ingredients and chill. Serve on chilled lobster, crabmeat, or shrimp.
Makes 1½ cups (12 servings)

	Calories	Carbo-hydrate (gm)	Protein (gm)	Total Fat (gm)	Saturated Fat (gm)	Choles-terol (mg)
Total	372.4	27.9	2.1	32.0	0.0	128.0
Per Serving	31.0	2.3	0.2	2.7	0.0	10.7

Curried Crab Salad

1 cup cooked or canned
   crabmeat, drained
2 unpeeled red apples,
   diced
1 green pepper cut in
   narrow strips
6 pimiento-stuffed
   olives, sliced

2 tbsp. diet
   mayonnaise
2 tbsp. low-fat
   yogurt
1 tbsp. fresh lemon
   juice
½ tbsp. curry powder
Lettuce leaves

Combine the crabmeat, apples, green pepper, and olives. Stir in the mayonnaise, yogurt, lemon juice, and curry. Chill the salad before serving it on the lettuce. *Makes 4 servings*

	Calories	Carbo-hydrate (gm)	Protein (gm)	Total Fat (gm)	Saturated Fat (gm)	Choles-terol (mg)
Total	594.8	45.1	37.1	30.2	4.3	222.9
Per Serving	148.7	11.3	9.3	7.6	1.0	55.7

French Steak and Onion Luncheon Soup

10½-oz. can onion soup
1 soup can of water

7 oz. sliced leftover
   broiled steak,
   lean only (about
   1 cup)
2 tbsp. grated
   Parmesan
   cheese

Heat the onion soup and water until simmering. Add the thinly sliced steak and reheat to boiling. Pour into two flameproof serving bowls and sprinkle with cheese. Slip under the broiler for a minute or so, until the cheese is melted. *Makes 2 servings*

	Calories	Carbo-hydrate (gm)	Protein (gm)	Total Fat (gm)	Saturated Fat (gm)	Choles-terol (mg)
Total	728.8	14.3	90.5	30.0	26.1	273.8
Per Serving	364.4	7.2	45.3	15.0	13.0	136.9

gm = grams; mg = milligrams. Nutritional figures are approximate. Figures are based on findings of U.S. Department of Agriculture.

Fruited Curry Luncheon Salad

½ cup (2 oz.) cooked white meat of turkey or chicken (lean leftover pork or lamb may be substituted)
1 tbsp. soy sauce
1 unpeeled red apple, cored and diced
1 eating orange, peeled, seeded and diced
2 tbsp. raisins

2 stalks celery, diagonally sliced
Shake of apple or pumpkin pie spice
Shake of curry powder (to taste)
Dash of Tabasco (to taste)
2 tbsp. low-calorie mayonnaise
2 tbsp. plain low-fat yogurt
Lettuce leaves

Combine the meat with the soy sauce and set aside to marinate, 15 minutes or longer. Meanwhile, combine the remaining ingredients and mound onto lettuce leaves. Top with the cold, marinated meat.

Makes 2 servings

	Calories	Carbo-hydrate (gm)	Protein (gm)	Total Fat (gm)	Saturated Fat (gm)	Choles-terol (mg)
Total	364.1	57.2	21.8	6.8	0.9	61.9
Per Serving	182.1	28.6	10.9	3.4	0.5	30.9

Chinese Chicken-Cashew-Apple Salad

1 cup cooked chicken (or turkey), white meat only
3 tbsp. soy sauce
1 tbsp. sherry
Shake of monosodium glutamate (optional)
1 red unpeeled apple, cored and diced

3 stalks celery, diagonally sliced
2 tbsp. dry-roasted cashews, broken
2 tbsp. low-calorie mayonnaise
2 tbsp. plain low-fat yogurt

Combine the cooked poultry with the soy sauce, sherry and monosodium glutamate. Set aside 15 minutes to marinate. Combine with the remaining ingredients and serve immediately.

Makes 2 servings

	Calories	Carbo-hydrate (gm)	Protein (gm)	Total Fat (gm)	Saturated Fat (gm)	Choles-terol (mg)
Total	711.9	36.3	87.9	22.3	4.2	207.2
Per Serving	356.0	18.2	44.0	11.2	2.1	103.6

Melon Boats with Seafood

1 lb. cooked shrimp, crabmeat, and/or lobster
½ cup diet salad dressing
¼ tsp. dill
2 cups 99% fat-free cottage cheese
½ tsp. seasoned salt

½ tsp. fresh grated lime peel
1 tsp. fresh lime juice
2 medium cantaloupes
4 leaves romaine or leaf lettuce
4 lime wedges

Place the seafood in a bowl. Pour the dressing over it; sprinkle it with dill and chill it for several hours. Meanwhile, in another bowl, blend together the cottage cheese, seasoned salt, lime peel and lime juice. Cover this mixture and chill it. Cut the cantaloupes in half; remove the seeds and chill. To serve, divide the cottage cheese mixture into fourths and spoon a fourth into each melon half. Drain the seafood from the marinade and arrange it on lettuce next to the melon. Garnish each with a lime wedge. *Makes 4 servings*

	Calories	Carbo-hydrate (gm)	Protein (gm)	Total Fat (gm)	Saturated Fat (gm)	Choles-terol (mg)
Total	1019.7	73.7	144.0	9.3	2.4	721.0
Per Serving	254.5	18.4	36.0	2.3	0.6	180.3

Turkey Salad Veronique

1 cup diced cooked turkey (white meat only)
2 cups diced crisp celery
2 tbsp. plain low-fat yogurt
2 tbsp. low-calorie mayonnaise

2 tbsp. dry sherry
Nutmeg, salt (or onion salt) and pepper to taste
Lettuce leaves
½ cup seedless green grapes, halved

Combine the turkey, celery, yogurt, mayonnaise and wine. Season to taste with nutmeg, salt and pepper. Place the lettuce leaves in 2 large individual salad bowls and add the turkey mixture. Arrange the grapes on top of the salads. *Makes 2 servings*

	Calories	Carbo-hydrate (gm)	Protein (gm)	Total Fat (gm)	Saturated Fat (gm)	Choles-terol (mg)
Total	588.1	29.2	82.4	14.3	2.8	191.4
Per Serving	294.1	14.6	41.2	7.2	1.4	95.7

Steak and Mushroom Luncheon Salad

3½ oz. sliced leftover broiled steak, lean only (about ½ cup)
½ cup sliced raw mushrooms
½ small red onion, thinly sliced

2 cups shredded romaine lettuce
2 tbsp. diet French dressing
¼ tsp. salt or garlic salt
Freshly ground pepper to taste

Toss the ingredients and serve in an oversized salad bowl.

Makes 1 serving

	Calories	Carbo-hydrate (gm)	Protein (gm)	Total Fat (gm)	Saturated Fat (gm)	Choles-terol (mg)
Total	341.7	23.1	38.9	13.5	3.5	89.3
Per Serving	341.7	23.1	38.9	13.5	3.5	89.3

gm = grams; mg = milligrams. Nutritional figures are approximate. Figures are based on findings of U.S. Department of Agriculture.

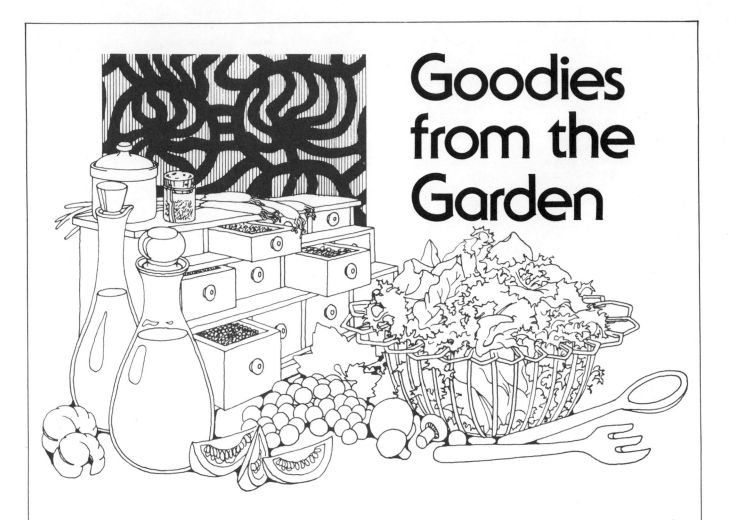

Goodies from the Garden

Salads, as everybody knows, are slimming. Or are they? Although the business end of a salad is slim, the toppings and trimmings are often a weight-inflating wipeout. A whole bowlful of shredded lettuce weighs in at less than 100 calories, but 2 tablespoons of bottled French dressing add 120 calories or more. Mayonnaise is almost as fattening as butter, close to 1600 calories a cupful.

Luckily for waistline-watchers, salad dressing makers have come to the rescue with a variety of slimmed-down toppings with only a fraction of the usual fat and calories. Low-cal versions of nearly every favorite are available: French, Italian, Russian, bleu cheese, Caesar, coleslaw, mayonnaise. Name it and you'll find it somewhere.

The savings are not to be sneered at. Consider, for example, the caloric comparison of a tuna salad made with a 7-ounce can of water-packed tuna and 5 tablespoons diet mayonnaise: total, 320 calories. The same tuna salad made with oil-packed tuna and regular mayonnaise would add up to a whopping 1077 calories.

Because salads are chock full of vitamins and appetite-appeasing fiber, they should be a daily part of every dieter's slim-down plan. Here's a variety of salad ideas, proof that salads can be delicious and exciting. For do-it-yourself dressing makers, we also have included a number of decalorized variations of fattening favorites — all designed to take salad dressings off the forbidden list.

Recipes

Waldorf Salad

3 red apples, cored and diced	5 tbsp. plain low-fat yogurt
1/8 tsp. salt	2 cups diced celery
5 tbsp. diet mayonnaise	4 tbsp. raisins

Combine all of the ingredients except the raisins and chill before serving. When you are ready to serve the salad, garnish it with the raisins.   *Makes 6 servings*

	Calories	Carbo-hydrate (gm)	Protein (gm)	Total Fat (gm)	Saturated Fat (gm)	Choles-terol (mg)
Total	485.2	102.5	2.5	11.2	0.6	46.2
Per Serving	80.9	17.1	0.4	1.9	0.1	7.7

gm = grams; mg = milligrams. Nutritional figures are approximate. Figures are based on findings of U.S. Department of Agriculture.

Polynesian Waldorf Salad

4 small or 2 large tart
    apples, peeled and
    chopped
2 cups juice-packed
    unsweetened
    pineapple chunks,
    drained

2 cups chopped
    celery
4 tbsp. chopped
    walnuts
½ cup diet
    mayonnaise

Combine all the ingredients and chill before serving.
Makes 10 servings

	Calories	Carbo-hydrate (gm)	Protein (gm)	Total Fat (gm)	Saturated Fat (gm)	Choles-terol (mg)
Total	823.7	136.8	6.5	34.8	1.0	64.0
Per Serving	82.4	13.7	0.7	3.5	0.1	6.4

Bleu Pear Salad

1 fresh pear, cored and
    diced
1 cup diced celery

½ cup low-calorie
    bleu cheese
    dressing

Combine all of the ingredients and serve on lettuce.
Makes 4 servings

	Calories	Carbo-hydrate (gm)	Protein (gm)	Total Fat (gm)	Saturated Fat (gm)	Choles-terol (mg)
Total	203.0	35.8	4.2	7.4	0.0	0.0
Per Serving	50.8	9.0	1.1	1.9	0.0	0.0

Tangy Apple Coleslaw

¼ tsp. celery seeds
1 tsp. salt
¼ cup evaporated
    skim milk
¼ cup diet
    mayonnaise
2 tbsp. cider vinegar

1 tsp. dry mustard
1 large red apple, diced
6 lightly packed cups
    shredded green
    cabbage (about a
    2¼ lb. head)

Whisk together all of the ingredients, except the apple and cabbage, in a medium mixing bowl. Then mix in the apple and cabbage. Cover the coleslaw and chill it until ready to serve.
Makes 6 servings

	Calories	Carbo-hydrate (gm)	Protein (gm)	Total Fat (gm)	Saturated Fat (gm)	Choles-terol (mg)
Total	358.2	60.0	10.5	13.0	2.7	51.5
Per Serving	59.7	10.0	1.8	2.2	0.5	8.6

Colorful Coleslaw

5 cups finely shredded
    green cabbage
1 cup shredded raw
    carrot
1 red apple, peeled,
    cored, and diced

¼ cup chopped green
    pepper
½ cup evaporated
    skim milk
¼ tsp. salt
⅛ tsp. pepper
¼ cup cider vinegar

Combine the cabbage, carrot, apple, and green pepper. Blend evaporated skim milk, salt, and pepper to-

gether in a small bowl. Gradually stir in the vinegar. Pour the dressing over the vegetables, and toss lightly to blend. Cover the coleslaw and chill it until you are ready to serve.
Makes 6 servings

	Calories	Carbo-hydrate (gm)	Protein (gm)	Total Fat (gm)	Saturated Fat (gm)	Choles-terol (mg)
Total	390.3	70.0	16.3	10.0	5.5	39.0
Per Serving	65.1	11.7	2.7	1.7	0.9	6.5

Coleslaw

4 cups shredded
    cabbage
½ small onion, minced

4 tbsp. diet
    mayonnaise
4 tbsp. plain low-fat
    yogurt

Combine all ingredients and chill before serving.
Makes 4 servings

	Calories	Carbo-hydrate (gm)	Protein (gm)	Total Fat (gm)	Saturated Fat (gm)	Choles-terol (mg)
Total	211.3	32.3	7.0	9.0	0.5	37.0
Per Serving	52.8	8.1	1.8	2.3	0.1	9.3

Walnut Celery Slaw

4 cups thinly sliced
    celery
⅓ cup coarsely
    shredded carrots
3 tbsp. raisins
3 tbsp. coarsely
    chopped walnuts

1 tbsp. cider vinegar
2 tsp. salt
½ tsp. ground white
    pepper
⅔ cup plain low-fat
    yogurt

Combine the celery, carrots, raisins, and walnuts in a large bowl. Set this mixture aside. Blend the vinegar, salt, and pepper together in a bowl. Stir in the yogurt. Pour the dressing over the celery mixture and toss lightly.
Makes 8 servings

	Calories	Carbo-hydrate (gm)	Protein (gm)	Total Fat (gm)	Saturated Fat (gm)	Choles-terol (mg)
Total	546.8	106.5	10.9	16.9	2.1	13.2
Per Serving	68.4	13.3	1.4	2.1	0.3	1.7

Orange Raisin Carrot Slaw

4 cups shredded raw
    carrot
8 tbsp. raisins
3 tbsp. unsweetened
    orange juice
    concentrate,
    defrosted but not
    diluted

5 tbsp. low-calorie
    mayonnaise
5 tbsp. plain low-fat
    yogurt
½ tsp. salt
⅛ tsp. pepper

Combine all the ingredients well and chill before serving.
Makes 8 servings

	Calories	Carbo-hydrate (gm)	Protein (gm)	Total Fat (gm)	Saturated Fat (gm)	Choles-terol (mg)
Total	625.9	131.7	8.6	11.3	0.6	40.0
Per Serving	78.2	16.5	1.1	1.4	0.1	5.0

gm = grams; mg = milligrams. Nutritional figures are approximate. Figures are based on findings of U.S. Department of Agriculture.

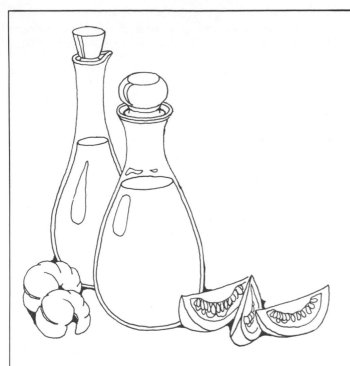

Combine the oil, vinegar, cumin, wine, salt, pepper, and parsley in a bowl. Then add the onion, green pepper, and tomato cubes. Toss the mixture well, and refrigerate it until it is thoroughly chilled. When serving, sprinkle more chopped parsley over the top as garnish. *Makes 6 servings*

	Calories	Carbo- hydrate (gm)	Protein (gm)	Total Fat (gm)	Saturated Fat (gm)	Choles- terol (mg)
Total	335.6	44.7	9.0	14.0	2.0	0.0
Per Serving	55.9	7.5	1.5	2.3	0.3	0.0

Shrimp Cocktail Mold

1 lb. shrimp, cooked, shelled, and deveined
¾ cup water
2 tbsp. (2 envelopes) unflavored gelatin
2 cups 99% fat-free cottage cheese
1 cup plain low-fat yogurt
1 cup tomato purée
¼ tsp. Tabasco sauce
¼ cup finely chopped celery
Salad greens

Split a few of the shrimp lengthwise and then cut up the rest. Place the water in a small saucepan. Sprinkle the gelatin over it and let it stand for a few minutes until it softens. Then heat the water slowly, stirring constantly, until the gelatin has dissolved. Allow it to cool slightly. In a large bowl, combine the cottage cheese, yogurt, tomato purée, Tabasco sauce, celery, cut-up shrimp and gelatin; blend thoroughly. Arrange the split shrimp in a mold; fill the mold with the cottage cheese mixture. Chill the mold until it is firm. Unmold it onto salad greens to serve. *Makes 8 servings*

	Calories	Carbo- hydrate (gm)	Protein (gm)	Total Fat (gm)	Saturated Fat (gm)	Choles- terol (mg)
Total	1043.2	52.9	164.0	13.3	4.4	741.1
Per Serving	130.4	6.6	20.5	1.7	0.6	92.6

Salade Vinaigrette

3 tbsp. vinegar
1 tbsp. corn or safflower oil
½ tsp. salt
¼ tsp. ground black pepper
¼ tsp. basil
1 tsp. instant minced onion
1 medium cucumber, peeled and sliced
3 large tomatoes, sliced and chilled

Combine the vinegar, oil, salt, pepper, basil, and onion in a jar or shaker. Shake the mixture well and pour it over the cucumber slices. Cover this mixture and chill it for 1 hour. Before serving, pour the cucumber mixture over the sliced tomatoes and mix gently. *Makes 8 servings*

	Calories	Carbo- hydrate (gm)	Protein (gm)	Total Fat (gm)	Saturated Fat (gm)	Choles- terol (mg)
Total	401.2	64.7	13.1	14.0	1.0	0.0
Per Serving	50.2	8.1	1.6	1.8	0.1	0.0

Moroccan Salad

1 tbsp. olive oil
3 tbsp. wine vinegar
2 tsp. ground cumin
3 tbsp. dry wine
1 tsp. salt
1 tsp. pepper
1 tbsp. chopped parsley
1 small onion, thinly sliced
2 large green peppers, cut up
3 medium tomatoes, peeled and cubed

Garden Salad

1½ cups 99% fat-free cottage cheese
5 tbsp. diet mayonnaise
1½ tsp. salt
1 cup shredded carrot
2 cups thinly sliced celery
1 cup diced cucumber, unpeeled
½ cup chopped green or red pepper
¼ cup sliced radishes
¼ cup chopped onion

Combine the ingredients and chill before serving. *Makes 8 servings*

	Calories	Carbo- hydrate (gm)	Protein (gm)	Total Fat (gm)	Saturated Fat (gm)	Choles- terol (mg)
Total	482.3	46.1	48.7	13.0	1.8	69.1
Per Serving	60.3	5.8	6.1	1.6	0.2	8.6

gm = grams; mg = milligrams. Nutritional figures are approximate. Figures are based on findings of U.S. Department of Agriculture.

Instant Salade Nicoise

16-oz. can sliced white potatoes, drained
10-oz. pkg. frozen kitchen-cut green beans, defrosted
1 red onion, thinly sliced
7-oz. can water-packed white-meat tuna, flaked
4 pitted black olives, thinly sliced
3 tbsp. olive liquid from the can
1 tbsp. olive oil

3 tbsp. red wine vinegar
Dash Worcestershire sauce
1/4 tsp. instant garlic (or 2 cloves garlic, minced)
1/2 tsp. oregano
1/2 tsp. dried parsley flakes
4 ripe plum tomatoes, thinly sliced
2 hard-cooked eggs, sliced

Combine all the ingredients except the tomatoes and eggs. Mix well and divide into 3 large individual salad bowls. Garnish with the tomato and egg.

Makes 3 servings

	Calories	Carbo-hydrate (gm)	Protein (gm)	Total Fat (gm)	Saturated Fat (gm)	Choles-terol (mg)
Total	1076.8	114.1	87.2	32.0	6.0	630.0
Per Serving	358.9	38.0	29.1	10.7	2.0	210.0

Lean Bean Salad

16-oz. can sliced green beans, drained
16-oz. can French-style sliced yellow beans, drained
1/4 cup onion flakes
1 cup diced celery

1/2 envelope French salad dressing mix
1 cup buttermilk
2 tbsp. finely chopped pimiento
1/2 tsp. oregano
Dash of salt

Mix the beans, onion flakes, and celery in bowl. In another bowl, combine the salad dressing mix with the buttermilk. Add the rest of the ingredients. Pour this mixture over the beans and toss lightly. Chill the bean salad for several hours before serving.

Makes 8 servings

	Calories	Carbo-hydrate (gm)	Protein (gm)	Total Fat (gm)	Saturated Fat (gm)	Choles-terol (mg)
Total	313.3	63.8	21.1	0.3	0.0	5.0
Per Serving	39.2	8.0	2.6	0.0	0.0	0.6

Fresh Mushroom Medley

1 lb. fresh mushrooms, sliced
1 cup diced celery
1 cup diced green pepper
2 tbsp. finely chopped onion

1 tbsp. olive oil
1 tbsp. wine vinegar
2 tsp. salt
1/8 tsp. ground black pepper
2 tbsp. lemon juice

Place the sliced mushrooms, celery, green pepper, and onion in a salad bowl. Mix the remaining ingredients in another bowl. Then pour this mixture over the vegetables and toss gently.

Makes 6 servings

	Calories	Carbo-hydrate (gm)	Protein (gm)	Total Fat (gm)	Saturated Fat (gm)	Choles-terol (mg)
Total	509.0	69.9	36.4	19.0	2.0	0.0
Per Serving	84.8	11.7	6.1	3.2	0.3	0.0

Almond Asparagus Mold

1 1/2 cups 99% fat-free cottage cheese
1 tbsp. unflavored gelatin (1 envelope)
1/4 cup water
14 1/2-oz. can cut asparagus, drained reserving liquid

2 tbsp. lemon juice
1/2 tsp. prepared mustard
1/2 tsp. salt
1/4 cup chopped blanched almonds
Salad greens

Force the cottage cheese through a sieve to remove the lumps, or beat it in a blender. Sprinkle the gelatin over the 1/4 cup water to soften it. In a 1-quart saucepan bring to a boil the asparagus liquid combined with enough water to equal 1 cup. Stir in the softened gelatin until it is dissolved and let the mixture cool slightly. Combine the cottage cheese, lemon juice, mustard, salt, almonds, and asparagus in a bowl. Add this mixture to the saucepan. Turn the contents of the saucepan into a mold and chill it until it is firm. Unmold it onto salad greens.

Makes 8 servings

	Calories	Carbo-hydrate (gm)	Protein (gm)	Total Fat (gm)	Saturated Fat (gm)	Choles-terol (mg)
Total	608.6	34.8	65.9	24.0	3.3	29.1
Per Serving	76.1	4.4	8.2	3.0	0.4	3.6

Chinese Celery and Tomato Salad

2 cups finely chopped Chinese celery cabbage
1/2 tsp. garlic salt
2 medium tomatoes, chopped

1/2 tsp. dry mustard
1 tbsp. water
1 tbsp. soy sauce
1 tbsp. corn oil

Combine all ingredients and chill before serving.

Makes 6 servings

	Calories	Carbo-hydrate (gm)	Protein (gm)	Total Fat (gm)	Saturated Fat (gm)	Choles-terol (mg)
Total	235.0	23.0	7.0	14.0	1.0	0.0
Per Serving	39.2	3.8	1.2	2.3	0.2	0.0

gm = grams; mg = milligrams. Nutritional figures are approximate. Figures are based on findings of U.S. Department of Agriculture.

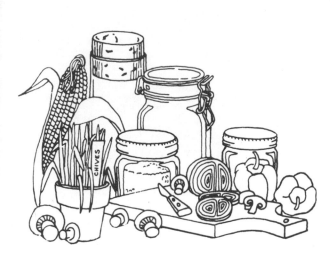

celery salt, and lemon peel. Blend in the milk. Cover the dressing and chill until serving.

Makes 20 tablespoons (10 servings)

	Calories	Carbo- hydrate (gm)	Protein (gm)	Total Fat (gm)	Saturated Fat (gm)	Choles- terol (mg)
Total	210.7	12.8	31.3	2.0	1.2	20.1
Per Serving	21.1	1.3	3.1	0.2	0.1	2.0

French-Cheese Salad Dressing

1½ cups 99% fat-free   ¼ cup crumbled bleu
   cottage cheese   cheese
½ cup diet French   1 tbsp. prepared
   dressing   horseradish

Beat the cottage cheese with an electric mixer on the highest speed until it is fairly smooth. Slowly beat in the French dressing, bleu cheese, and horseradish. Cover the dressing and chill it before serving.

Makes 32 tablespoons (16 servings)

	Calories	Carbo- hydrate (gm)	Protein (gm)	Total Fat (gm)	Saturated Fat (gm)	Choles- terol (mg)
Total	549.7	12.5	60.2	25.8	14.5	89.8
Per Serving	34.4	0.8	3.8	1.6	0.9	5.6

Thousand Island Dressing

1 cup diet mayonnaise   1 tbsp. finely
½ cup tomato purée   chopped
¼ tsp. Tabasco sauce   pimiento
3 tbsp. chopped green   2 tbsp. chopped
   pepper   onion

Combine all of the ingredients and blend thoroughly. Chill before serving. If the dressing becomes too thick, stir in 1 or 2 tablespoons skim milk (there are about 6 calories in 1 tablespoon skim milk).

Makes 24 tablespoons (12 servings)

	Calories	Carbo- hydrate (gm)	Protein (gm)	Total Fat (gm)	Saturated Fat (gm)	Choles- terol (mg)
Total	356.5	24.5	1.7	32.2	0.0	128.0
Per Serving	29.7	2.0	0.1	2.7	0.0	10.7

Salad Dressing Parisienne

1 tbsp. chopped onion   ½ tsp. dry mustard
¼ cup white wine   ¼ tsp. salt
1½ tbsp. corn oil   Pinch of pepper
1 tbsp. chopped parsley

Buzz everything together in a blender and use immediately. *Makes 8 tablespoons (4 servings)*

	Calories	Carbo- hydrate (gm)	Protein (gm)	Total Fat (gm)	Saturated Fat (gm)	Choles- terol (mg)
Total	286.2	10.9	0.2	2.0	1.5	0.0
Per Serving	71.6	2.7	0.1	0.5	0.4	0.0

gm = grams; mg = milligrams. Nutritional figures are approximate. Figures are based on findings of U.S. Department of Agriculture.

Cheese-Stuffed Tomatoes

6 medium tomatoes   ¼ cup chopped
2 cups 99% fat-free   pecans
   cottage cheese   2 tbsp. chopped
¼ cup chopped   onion
   pimiento-stuffed 6 large lettuce
   olives   leaves
¼ cup shredded carrot

Turn the tomatoes stem end down and cut each one into 6 sections, cutting only ⅔ of the way down. Gently spread the sections apart. Chill the tomatoes before filling them.

Combine the cottage cheese, olives, carrot, pecans, and onion in a bowl. Toss the mixture lightly. Just before serving, place the tomatoes on the lettuce and fill them with the cottage cheese mixture.

Makes 6 servings

	Calories	Carbo- hydrate (gm)	Protein (gm)	Total Fat (gm)	Saturated Fat (gm)	Choles- terol (mg)
Total	845.2	73.8	75.3	29.3	3.7	38.8
Per Serving	140.9	12.3	12.6	4.9	0.6	6.5

Creamy Dill Dressing

1 cup 99% fat-free   ⅛ tsp. grated lemon
   cottage cheese   peel
1 tbsp. lemon juice   2 tbsp. skim milk
1 tsp. dill weed
½ tsp. celery salt

Beat the cottage cheese in a small mixing bowl at the highest speed of the electric mixer until it is fairly smooth. Then slowly beat in the lemon juice, dill weed,

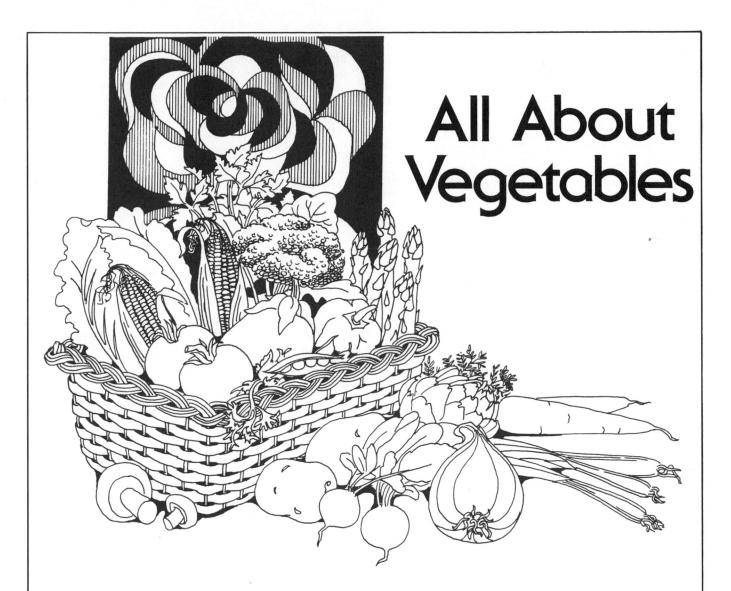

All About Vegetables

Vegetables, unfortunately, are victims of their own virtue. Anything that is good for you is bound to be a bore — or so it must seem if you grew up in a home where clean plates were equated with godliness.

Many an adult aversion to vegetables got its start when Mama began negotiating deals over parsnips, and pudding: "Finish your spinach or you don't get any pie." Right then and there Junior decided that dessert must be more valuable than vegetables and that when he grew up to be an insurance salesman, nobody was going to dictate how much broccoli he had to eat before starting on the seven-layer cake. As a result, many an otherwise intelligent and mature adult still operates on a two-year-old level where vegetables are concerned, insisting that he dislikes varieties he may never have even tried or tasted.

Maybe Mother's vegetables tasted awful because she didn't know how to cook them. Most people and most restaurants don't. If you have never tried a certain vegetable or have tried it only once, or only one way, you haven't given it a fair chance. You may be depriving yourself of a food friend that can stand you in good stead for the rest of your slim days.

Become a Vegetable Adventurer

• Try a new variety every week. When you shop, look for a vegetable you have never tried before and give it a go.

• Combine vegetables. Put together a blend of old favorites with a vegetable you've never tasted or one you decided you disliked back when you were 10 years old.

• Try a vegetable raw if it is usually served cooked. Or cook a vegetable that is normally served in salad — braised celery or raw mushrooms for example.

• Try vegetables in season, preferably from a local farm. The deteriorated taste and texture of stored or processed produce may be what turns you off.

• Stir-fry vegetables the Oriental way. One tablespoon of diet margarine (50 calories) is all you need to stir up a skilletful of crisp onions and green beans laced with soy sauce.

• Simmer vegetables in soup or stock from which you have skimmed the fat.

• Try cooking vegetables in dry wine. The alcohol calories evaporate.

- Add perennial favorites like chopped onions or sliced green pepper for a fresh taste, especially when cooking canned or frozen vegetables.
- Cook vegetables in canned unsweetened fruit juice. Apple, orange, and pineapple are some you might try.
- Turn the cooking water into a low-cal sauce. Stir a little flour into skim milk and stir it into the saucepan after the vegetables are cooked. A cream sauce without the cream — or cream calories.
- Spice and season your vegetables by adding a small amount of bottled diet dressing to the cooking water. The water evaporates as the vegetables simmer and leaves behind a tangy sauce — no butter needed.

FRESH VEGETABLE COOKING GUIDE

Vegetable	Maximum Cooking Time	Buy for 8 Servings
Asparagus		
Whole spears	10 to 20 min.	2½ lb.
Cuts and tips	5 to 15 min.	1¾ lb.
Beans, Lima	25 to 30 min.	2¾ lb. in pods
Beans, Snap (green or wax in 1-in. pieces)	12 to 16 min.	1 lb.
Beets		
Young, whole	30 to 45 min.	2½ lb. with tops
Older, whole	45 to 90 min.	or 1½ lb. without
Sliced or diced	15 to 25 min.	tops
Broccoli (heavy stalk, split)	10 to 15 min.	2 lb.
Brussels Sprouts	15 to 20 min.	1½ lb.
Cabbage		
Shredded	3 to 10 min.	1¼ lb.
Wedges	10 to 15 min.	1½ lb.
Carrots		
Young, whole	15 to 20 min.	1½ lb. without tops
Older, whole	20 to 30 min.	1½ lb. without tops
Sliced or diced	10 to 20 min.	1½ lb. without tops
Cauliflower		
Separated	8 to 15 min.	2 lb.
Whole	15 to 25 min.	2 lb.
Celery (cut up)	15 to 18 min.	1½ lb. untrimmed
Corn (on cob)	3 to 5 min.	3 lb. in husks
Kale	10 to 15 min.	1¼ lb. untrimmed
Okra	10 to 14 min.	1¼ lb.
Onions (mature)	15 to 30 min.	1¾ lb.
Parsnips		
Whole	20 to 40 min.	1½ lb.
Quartered	8 to 15 min.	1½ lb.
Peas	12 to 16 min.	3 lb. in pods
Potatoes		
Whole, medium	25 to 40 min.	1½ lb.
Quartered	20 to 25 min.	1½ lb.
Diced	10 to 15 min.	1¼ lb.
Spinach	3 to 10 min.	1½ lb. trimmed
Squash		
Summer, sliced	8 to 15 min.	1½ lb.
Winter, cut up	15 to 20 min.	2½ lb.
Tomatoes (cut up)	7 to 15 min.	1¼ lb.
Turnips		
Whole	20 to 30 min.	1¾ lb. without tops
Cut up	10 to 20 min.	1¾ lb. without tops

Vegetables Do's and Don'ts

• Do use a sharp knife when preparing vegetables for fewer bruises and less loss of nutrients.

• Don't pare, peel, slice, or cut up fresh vegetables until just before cooking to preserve nutrients.

• Do use as little water as possible to retain both flavor and nutrients. If possible, cook vegetables in so little water that no draining is needed and no vitamins are lost. But watch the pot carefully so they don't stick.

• Don't overcook vegetables. Almost every vegetable is better undercooked and still crunchy.

• Do use a pot with a tight-fitting lid to steam green vegetables.

• Do keep the heat low when steaming vegetables. Otherwise, the steam will escape.

• Do steam white, yellow, and red vegetables. Place them on a rack over boiling water, and cover the pot with a tight lid. This method takes longer than boiling the vegetables, but is well worth it in the savings of nutrients.

• Do add ½ to 1 teaspoon salt to the pot for each six servings of vegetables. Try seasoned salts like butter, onion, garlic, or celery. A little butter-flavored salt added to the cooking water gives vegetables a buttery flavor without the butter or the butter calories.

• Don't use baking soda for preserving color while cooking vegetables. It makes them mushy and flavorless. You can preserve color by undercooking.

• Do cook strong-flavored vegetables like cabbage, broccoli, cauliflower, brussels sprouts, and turnips in an uncovered pan. Add water if needed to prevent burning.

• Do add butter-flavored salt and freshly ground pepper to vegetables just before serving. Herbs and spices as seasonings go a long way, and the calorie contribution is fractional.

Recipes

Spring Artichoke Hearts

9-oz. pkg. frozen artichoke hearts	½ tsp. salt
3 cups thinly sliced celery	10-oz. pkg. frozen peas
½ cup boiling water	2 tsp. lemon juice
	¼ tsp. butter salt

Cook the artichokes and celery in a covered saucepan for 3 minutes in boiling water to which the salt has been added. Add the peas and return to boiling. Cover the pot and cook the vegetables for 5 minutes more. Drain them well. Add the lemon juice and butter salt before serving.

Makes 8 servings

	Calories	Carbo-hydrate (gm)	Protein (gm)	Total Fat (gm)	Saturated Fat (gm)	Choles-terol (mg)
Total	305.0	77.8	21.7	0.0	0.0	0.0
Per Serving	38.1	9.7	2.7	0.0	0.0	0.0

Asparagus Stir-Fry

½ cup chicken broth	½ cup chopped onion
1 tbsp. cornstarch	1 lb. fresh asparagus, sliced diagonally
2 tbsp. soy sauce	
1 tbsp. diet margarine	

Skim the fat from the broth by chilling it until the fat rises to the top and can be whisked away. Mix the broth, cornstarch, and soy sauce together in a bowl. Set the bowl aside. Melt the margarine in a nonstick skillet and sauté the onion until it is golden brown. Add the asparagus and stir-fry it for 3 minutes. Add the broth mixture. Cook and stir until the sauce is clear.

Makes 4 servings

	Calories	Carbo-hydrate (gm)	Protein (gm)	Total Fat (gm)	Saturated Fat (gm)	Choles-terol (mg)
Total	218.8	30.7	14.4	6.0	1.0	18.3
Per Serving	54.7	7.7	3.6	1.5	0.3	4.6

Dilly Green Beans

¼ cup diet Italian salad dressing	½ cup diced celery
2 pkg. (9-oz.) frozen cut green beans, partially thawed	1 large onion, sliced and separated into rings
	2 tsp. dill

Combine the salad dressing, green beans, and celery in a nonstick skillet. Cover and cook just until the beans are fully thawed, separating them with a fork as they cook. Add the onion and dill; continue cooking for about 3 minutes, stirring occasionally, just until the vegetables are tender but still crisp.

Makes 6 servings

	Calories	Carbo-hydrate (gm)	Protein (gm)	Total Fat (gm)	Saturated Fat (gm)	Choles-terol (mg)
Total	220.7	46.4	11.1	4.0	0.0	0.0
Per Serving	36.8	7.7	1.9	0.7	0.0	0.0

Italian Green Beans

½ cup chicken broth	½ tsp. oregano
2 lb. fresh green beans	1 medium garlic clove, minced
1 tomato, peeled and chopped	

Skim the fat from the broth by chilling it until the fat rises to the top and can be whisked away. Combine all of the ingredients in a saucepan. Cook the mixture over low heat for about 20 minutes until the vegetables are tender.

Makes 8 servings

	Calories	Carbo-hydrate (gm)	Protein (gm)	Total Fat (gm)	Saturated Fat (gm)	Choles-terol (mg)
Total	265.7	60.2	17.8	0.0	0.0	7.0
Per Serving	33.2	7.5	2.2	0.0	0.0	0.9

gm = grams; mg = milligrams. Nutritional figures are approximate. Figures are based on findings of U.S. Department of Agriculture.

Canadian Green Beans

1 lb. fresh green beans, French-cut, or 9-oz. pkg. frozen beans	1 clove garlic, minced
¼ cup boiling water	½ tsp. salt
1 tbsp. diet margarine	¼ tsp. pepper
½ cup finely diced Canadian bacon	1 tomato, cut in wedges

Cook the fresh or frozen green beans in the water until they are tender. Then drain them. Melt the margarine in a nonstick skillet and sauté the bacon and garlic until they are brown. Add the beans, salt, and pepper to the skillet, and top with the tomato wedges. Cover the pan and heat the contents through. *Makes 4 servings*

Hint: The calorie-conscious cook can save 50 calories (about 12 per serving) by omitting the diet margarine. Spray a nonstick skillet with spray-on vegetable coating, so you can brown the bacon and garlic without calories.

	Calories	Carbo-hydrate (gm)	Protein (gm)	Total Fat (gm)	Saturated Fat (gm)	Choles-terol (mg)
Total	351.1	25.0	25.1	18.5	4.3	58.9
Per Serving	87.8	6.3	6.3	4.6	1.1	14.7

Granada Green Beans

3 cups canned French-style green beans, drained	1 tsp. chili powder
	Pinch cayenne
2 tbsp. minced onion	1 tsp. salt
2 tbsp. minced green pepper	⅛ tsp. pepper
2½ cups canned tomato pieces, drained	6 tbsp. grated Parmesan cheese

Place the beans in a 1½-quart casserole. Combine the onion, green pepper, tomatoes, and seasonings in a bowl. Pour this mixture over the beans. Sprinkle the cheese over all. Cover the casserole and bake it in a preheated 350° oven for about 20 minutes. *Makes 6 servings*

	Calories	Carbo-hydrate (gm)	Protein (gm)	Total Fat (gm)	Saturated Fat (gm)	Choles-terol (mg)
Total	689.6	51.3	54.5	34.9	18.0	97.2
Per Serving	114.9	8.6	9.1	5.8	3.0	16.2

Green Beans Parmesan

½ tsp. salt	2 tbsp. diet Italian salad dressing
1 lb. fresh green beans, sliced	3 tbsp. grated Parmesan cheese
1 cup boiling water	

Add the salt and beans to the boiling water, cover the pan, and cook until the beans are just tender — 8 or 9 minutes. Drain the beans and stir in the salad dressing and cheese. *Makes 6 servings*

	Calories	Carbo-hydrate (gm)	Protein (gm)	Total Fat (gm)	Saturated Fat (gm)	Choles-terol (mg)
Total	357.7	26.9	28.8	18.2	9.0	48.6
Per Serving	59.6	4.5	4.8	3.0	1.5	8.1

Beets with Orange Sauce

¾ tsp. salt	3 cups canned sliced beets, drained
2 tbsp. cornstarch	
¾ cup unsweetened orange juice	

Mix salt, cornstarch, and orange juice in a saucepan. Cook the mixture, stirring constantly, until it has thickened. Add the beets to the sauce and stir carefully. Heat the mixture through and serve. *Makes 6 servings*

	Calories	Carbo-hydrate (gm)	Protein (gm)	Total Fat (gm)	Saturated Fat (gm)	Choles-terol (mg)
Total	345.4	79.2	6.4	0.8	0.0	0.0
Per Serving	57.6	13.2	1.1	0.1	0.0	0.0

Quick Pickled Beets

1-lb. can sliced beets, drained reserving liquid	¼ cup unsweetened apple juice
	1 tsp. whole mixed pickling spice
¼ cup cider vinegar	

Combine the liquid from the beets with the vinegar, apple juice, and pickling spice in a small saucepan. Boil gently for 5 minutes. Remove the pot from the heat and add the beets. Cover the pot and let it stand for several hours. At serving time, reheat the beets, then drain off the liquid. *Makes 4 servings*

	Calories	Carbo-hydrate (gm)	Protein (gm)	Total Fat (gm)	Saturated Fat (gm)	Choles-terol (mg)
Total	188.6	45.9	3.6	0.0	0.0	0.0
Per Serving	47.2	11.5	0.9	0.0	0.0	0.0

Russian Beets

4 tbsp. low-fat nondairy sour cream substitute	½ tsp. salt
	Dash cayenne
2 tsp. vinegar	3 cups halved cooked beets, drained

Combine all the ingredients, except the beets, in a bowl. Mix the sauce well and add it to the beets. Heat the beets with the sauce slowly, stirring to coat. *Makes 6 servings*

	Calories	Carbo-hydrate (gm)	Protein (gm)	Total Fat (gm)	Saturated Fat (gm)	Choles-terol (mg)
Total	370.0	62.8	8.1	9.7	8.8	0.0
Per Serving	61.7	10.5	1.4	1.6	1.5	0.0

gm = grams; mg = milligrams. Nutritional figures are approximate. Figures are based on findings of U.S. Department of Agriculture.

Lemon Buttered Broccoli

1 tbsp. margarine	¾ cup cold water
1 tsp. arrowroot or cornstarch	5 or 6 drops yellow food coloring
2 tbsp. fresh lemon juice	2 pkg. (10-oz.) frozen broccoli, cooked

Melt the margarine in a small saucepan and stir in the arrowroot or cornstarch. Add the lemon juice and water and cook the mixture over moderate heat until it simmers. Stir in the food coloring a drop at a time until the sauce is buttery yellow. Serve the sauce over the hot broccoli. *Makes 6 servings*

	Calories	Carbo-hydrate (gm)	Protein (gm)	Total Fat (gm)	Saturated Fat (gm)	Choles-terol (mg)
Total	252.2	29.2	18.9	11.0	2.0	0.0
Per Serving	42.0	4.9	3.2	1.8	0.3	0.0

Creamed Broccoli

1 bunch fresh broccoli (2 pkg. frozen)	⅓ cup plain low-fat yogurt
¼ cup boiling salted water	1 tsp. onion flakes
⅓ cup diet mayonnaise	Dash cayenne
	¾ tsp. salt

Cook the broccoli, covered, in the boiling salted water until it is barely tender. In a bowl, combine the mayonnaise, yogurt, onion flakes, cayenne, and salt. Serve the sauce over the hot broccoli. *Makes 4 servings*

	Calories	Carbo-hydrate (gm)	Protein (gm)	Total Fat (gm)	Saturated Fat (gm)	Choles-terol (mg)
Total	362.5	47.9	30.8	16.7	0.7	49.2
Per Serving	90.6	12.0	7.7	4.2	0.2	12.3

Broccoli Capri

1 bunch fresh broccoli	3 tbsp. water
1 tbsp. olive oil	¾ tsp. salt
1 garlic clove, minced	Pinch cayenne
3 tbsp. minced onion	½ tsp. oregano

Split broccoli stems lengthwise into quarters and then cut the strips into 1-inch pieces. Cut the flowerets into coarse pieces. Heat the oil in a large nonstick skillet. Sauté the garlic and onion slowly until tender. Then add the broccoli, water, salt, cayenne, and oregano. Cover the pan tightly and cook the broccoli slowly for about 15 minutes until it is tender. *Makes 6 servings*

Diet hint: The heart-conscious cook should substitute corn or safflower oil for the olive oil to save 1 gram of saturated fat. Also, if fresh broccoli isn't available, you may use 2 10-oz. packages of frozen broccoli spears for this recipe.

	Calories	Carbo-hydrate (gm)	Protein (gm)	Total Fat (gm)	Saturated Fat (gm)	Choles-terol (mg)
Total	343.2	39.3	28.5	18.7	2.0	0.0
Per Serving	57.2	6.6	4.8	3.1	0.3	0.0

Chinese Broccoli with Mushrooms

2 pkg. (10-oz.) frozen broccoli, partially thawed	1 tsp. beef bouillon or 1 bouillon cube
1 tsp. arrowroot or cornstarch	1 tbsp. soy sauce
½ cup cold water	1 small onion, sliced
	8-oz. can mushroom stems and pieces

If broccoli spears are used, slice them into 1-inch diagonal pieces. Combine the arrowroot (or cornstarch) in a saucepan with the water, bouillon, and soy sauce. Bring the mixture to a boil and then add the rest of the ingredients. Cook and stir the vegetables over moderate heat, uncovered, for about 2 minutes until the sauce thickens and simmers and the vegetables are just crunchy. Serve immediately. *Makes 6 servings*

	Calories	Carbo-hydrate (gm)	Protein (gm)	Total Fat (gm)	Saturated Fat (gm)	Choles-terol (mg)
Total	265.6	47.1	29.8	4.2	0.0	3.0
Per Serving	44.3	7.9	5.0	0.7	0.0	0.5

Zesty Brussels Sprouts

3 pkg. (10-oz.) frozen brussels sprouts	1 cup plain low-fat yogurt
½ cup chopped onion	1 tsp. parsley flakes or 1 tbsp. chopped fresh parsley
1 tbsp. flour	
1 tsp. salt	
2 tsp. prepared mustard	

Simmer the brussels sprouts in 1 or 2 tablespoons water just until they are tender. Combine the rest of the ingredients in a separate saucepan, stirring until blended. Cook and stir the sauce over moderate heat until it thickens and bubbles. Serve the sauce over the brussels sprouts. *Makes 8 servings*

	Calories	Carbo-hydrate (gm)	Protein (gm)	Total Fat (gm)	Saturated Fat (gm)	Choles-terol (mg)
Total	549.7	97.3	48.0	9.6	2.0	20.0
Per Serving	68.7	12.2	6.0	1.2	0.3	2.5

Bombay Brussels Sprouts

3 tbsp. diet mayonnaise	Pinch curry
1 tbsp. grated Parmesan cheese	10-oz. pkg. frozen brussels sprouts, cooked and drained
Pinch celery seed	

Blend together the mayonnaise, cheese, celery seed, and curry. Pour over hot sprouts. *Makes 3 servings*

	Calories	Carbo-hydrate (gm)	Protein (gm)	Total Fat (gm)	Saturated Fat (gm)	Choles-terol (mg)
Total	248.0	23.6	21.2	13.4	3.0	40.2
Per Serving	82.7	7.9	7.1	4.5	1.0	13.4

gm = grams; mg = milligrams. Nutritional figures are approximate. Figures are based on findings of U.S. Department of Agriculture.

Cabbage New Orleans

1 head green cabbage,
   quartered
1/4 cup chopped onion
1/4 cup chopped green
   pepper

8-oz. can tomatoes,
   undrained
1/2 tsp. salt
1 cup water
Dash pepper

Combine all of the ingredients in a saucepan. Cover the pan and simmer for 10 minutes. *Makes 4 servings*

	Calories	Carbo-hydrate (gm)	Protein (gm)	Total Fat (gm)	Saturated Fat (gm)	Choles-terol (mg)
Total	179.0	36.3	48.9	1.0	0.0	0.0
Per Serving	44.8	9.1	12.2	0.3	0.0	0.0

German-Style Red Cabbage

1-lb. head red cabbage,
   shredded
1/2 cup sliced onion
2 cups unsweetened
   applesauce

1 tsp. salt
Pinch coarsely
   ground pepper
1 tbsp. caraway
   seeds

Combine all of the ingredients in a saucepan. Cover and simmer over very low heat for 30 to 40 minutes, stirring occasionally. *Makes 6 servings*

	Calories	Carbo-hydrate (gm)	Protein (gm)	Total Fat (gm)	Saturated Fat (gm)	Choles-terol (mg)
Total	348.0	89.0	9.4	0.0	0.0	0.0
Per Serving	58.0	14.8	1.6	0.0	0.0	0.0

Stir-Fried Cabbage

1 tbsp. corn or safflower
   oil
5 cups shredded
   cabbage (about 1
   lb.)

1/2 cup unsweetened
   apple juice
1 tsp. salt
Pinch black
   pepper
1 tbsp. vinegar

Heat the oil in a nonstick skillet. Stir-fry the cabbage for 3 minutes. Add the apple juice, salt, pepper and vinegar. Cook, stirring constantly, until cabbage is tender but crisp, about 3 minutes. *Makes 4 servings*

	Calories	Carbo-hydrate (gm)	Protein (gm)	Total Fat (gm)	Saturated Fat (gm)	Choles-terol (mg)
Total	284.8	40.6	5.0	14.1	1.0	0.0
Per Serving	71.2	10.2	1.2	3.5	0.3	0.0

Pineapple Carrots

3 cups sliced carrots,
   fresh or frozen
6-oz. can unsweetened
   pineapple juice
1/2 tsp. arrowroot or
   cornstarch

1/2 cup water
1/4 tsp. cinnamon
1/4 tsp. salt
Dash pepper

Combine all the ingredients in a saucepan. Cover the pan tightly and simmer until the carrots are nearly tender. Then uncover the pan and continue to simmer, stirring occasionally, until nearly all of the liquid has evaporated. *Makes 4 servings*

	Calories	Carbo-hydrate (gm)	Protein (gm)	Total Fat (gm)	Saturated Fat (gm)	Choles-terol (mg)
Total	224.9	56.4	6.8	0.0	0.0	0.0
Per Serving	56.2	14.1	1.7	0.0	0.0	0.0

California Carrots with Orange Glaze

4 cups sliced carrots
   (fresh or frozen)
1 tsp. butter-flavored
   salt
3/4 cup water
4 tbsp. defrosted
   unsweetened
   orange juice
   concentrate,
   undiluted

1 tbsp. arrowroot
1/4 tsp. salt
1/8 tsp. pepper
Cinnamon to taste

Cook carrots in salted water about 10 to 15 minutes, just until tender. Drain the cooking water into a measuring cup. Add the juice concentrate and water to the measuring cup to make a total of 1 1/4 cups liquid. Stir the arrowroot into this liquid until well blended. Pour the liquid over the carrots in the saucepan. Cook and stir over low heat until sauce simmers and thickens. Season with salt, pepper and cinnamon.

Makes 8 servings

	Calories	Carbo-hydrate (gm)	Protein (gm)	Total Fat (gm)	Saturated Fat (gm)	Choles-terol (mg)
Total	305.9	75.3	9.6	0.0	0.0	0.0
Per Serving	38.1	9.4	1.2	0.0	0.0	0.0

Gourmet Cauliflower

2 pkg. (10-oz.) frozen
   cauliflower, cooked
1/4 tsp. salt
Dash pepper
Dash paprika

1/2 cup nondairy low-
   fat sour cream
   substitute
4 tbsp. bread crumbs

Place the cauliflower in a nonstick baking dish and season it with salt, pepper, and paprika. Cover it with the imitation sour cream and bread crumbs and bake in a preheated 350° oven just until brown.

Makes 6 servings

	Calories	Carbo-hydrate (gm)	Protein (gm)	Total Fat (gm)	Saturated Fat (gm)	Choles-terol (mg)
Total	434.3	50.2	21.8	20.3	17.8	1.3
Per Serving	72.4	8.4	3.6	3.4	3.0	0.2

gm = grams; mg = milligrams. Nutritional figures are approximate. Figures are based on findings of U.S. Department of Agriculture.

Easy Cheesy Cauliflower

10¾-oz. can condensed cheddar cheese soup
¼ cup skim milk
Generous dash nutmeg
2 pkg. (10-oz.) frozen cauliflower, cooked and drained

Blend the soup, milk, and nutmeg in a saucepan. Cook and stir the sauce until it is bubbling. Pour over the hot cauliflower and serve. *Makes 6 servings*

	Calories	Carbo-hydrate (gm)	Protein (gm)	Total Fat (gm)	Saturated Fat (gm)	Choles-terol (mg)
Total	525.8	52.1	29.2	25.8	12.9	65.8
Per Serving	87.6	8.7	5.0	4.3	2.2	11.0

Celery Braised in Broth

2 cans (10½-oz.) chicken broth
1 onion, sliced
2 carrots, sliced
4 bunches of celery, trimmed and sliced

Skim the fat from the broth by chilling it until the fat rises to the top and can be whisked away. Place the onion and carrot slices in a large skillet and arrange the celery on top. Add the broth and just enough water to cover the vegetables. Cover the skillet and bring the mixture to a boil. Then lower the heat and simmer about 45 minutes until the vegetables are tender. *Makes 8 servings*

	Calories	Carbo-hydrate (gm)	Protein (gm)	Total Fat (gm)	Saturated Fat (gm)	Choles-terol (mg)
Total	375.3	102.5	19.7	0.0	0.0	73.4
Per Serving	46.9	12.8	2.5	0.0	0.0	9.2

Italian Celery

4 cups celery cut into 2-in. chunks
½ cup minced onion
1 clove of garlic, minced
15-oz. can tomato sauce
1¼ tsp. salt
1¼ tsp. basil

Combine all the ingredients in a medium saucepan and bring the mixture to the boiling point. Then lower the heat, cover the pot, and simmer the celery for about 10 minutes until it is tender-crisp. *Makes 6 servings*

	Calories	Carbo-hydrate (gm)	Protein (gm)	Total Fat (gm)	Saturated Fat (gm)	Choles-terol (mg)
Total	215.9	60.0	6.9	0.7	0.0	0.0
Per Serving	36.0	10.0	1.2	0.1	0.0	0.0

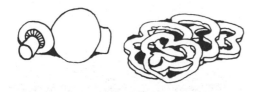

Creamed Celery

2 cups thinly sliced celery
1 cup boiling water
2 tbsp. flour
¼ tsp. paprika
1 cup skim milk
¼ tsp. salt
Dash white pepper

Boil the celery in the water just until it is tender-crisp. Then drain it. Combine the flour, paprika, milk, salt, and pepper and add this to the celery. Heat the entire mixture slowly until it is creamy. *Makes 4 servings*

	Calories	Carbo-hydrate (gm)	Protein (gm)	Total Fat (gm)	Saturated Fat (gm)	Choles-terol (mg)
Total	174.6	35.4	10.6	0.1	0.0	5.0
Per Serving	43.7	8.9	2.7	0.0	0.0	1.3

Corn-Plus-Protein Casserole

2 cups skim milk
1 onion, chopped
2 red or green peppers
1½ cups canned or cooked frozen corn, drained
2 eggs, beaten
2 tsp. butter-flavored salt
Pinch pepper

Scald the milk. Stir in the rest of the ingredients and turn the whole mixture into a casserole. Bake the casserole in a preheated 325° oven for about 1¼ hours until a knife inserted in the center comes out clean. *Makes 8 servings*

	Calories	Carbo-hydrate (gm)	Protein (gm)	Total Fat (gm)	Saturated Fat (gm)	Choles-terol (mg)
Total	713.0	112.0	46.0	13.5	4.0	514.0
Per Serving	89.1	14.0	5.8	1.7	0.5	64.3

Easy Eggplant Parmesan

3 tbsp. Italian-seasoned bread crumbs
1½ tbsp. grated Parmesan cheese
½ tsp. garlic salt
Pinch cayenne
1 eggplant, peeled and cubed
8-oz. can tomato sauce
3 thin slices part-skim mozzarella cheese (3 oz.)

Mix the bread crumbs, Parmesan cheese, garlic salt, and cayenne together in a bowl. Arrange the eggplant in the bottom of a baking dish. Spread the bread crumb mixture over this and then pour on the tomato sauce. Top with the slices of mozzarella cheese. Bake in a preheated 350° oven for 25 minutes.

Makes 6 servings

	Calories	Carbo-hydrate (gm)	Protein (gm)	Total Fat (gm)	Saturated Fat (gm)	Choles-terol (mg)
Total	556.6	43.6	65.2	25.4	8.2	82.0
Per Serving	92.8	7.3	10.9	4.2	1.4	13.7

gm = grams; mg = milligrams. Nutritional figures are approximate. Figures are based on findings of U.S. Department of Agriculture.

Peppers Neopolitan

5 Italian frying peppers, sliced	2 tsp. olive oil
1 medium onion, sliced	½ tsp. Italian seasoning
2 cloves garlic, minced	¼ tsp. salt
2 tbsp. water	Dash pepper

Combine all of the ingredients in a nonstick skillet. Cover and cook over moderate heat for 2 minutes. Then remove the cover and continue cooking until the moisture has evaporated and the vegetables begin to brown slightly. *Makes 4 servings*

	Calories	Carbo-hydrate (gm)	Protein (gm)	Total Fat (gm)	Saturated Fat (gm)	Choles-terol (mg)
Total	197.5	25.0	7.0	9.2	1.3	0.0
Per Serving	49.4	6.3	1.8	2.3	0.3	0.0

Springtime Minted Peas

1 tbsp. diet margarine	1 tbsp. finely chopped fresh mint leaves
½ cup chopped green onion	
2 cups fresh-shelled peas	1 tsp. lemon juice
2 tbsp. water	¼ tsp. salt

Melt the margarine in a nonstick skillet and sauté the onions until they are tender. Then add the rest of the ingredients. Cover and simmer 7 or 8 minutes. Add a little more water, if necessary, to keep the peas from burning. *Makes 4 servings*

	Calories	Carbo-hydrate (gm)	Protein (gm)	Total Fat (gm)	Saturated Fat (gm)	Choles-terol (mg)
Total	301.2	43.4	19.0	8.0	1.0	0.0
Per Serving	75.3	10.9	4.8	2.0	0.3	0.0

Baked Rutabagas

| 2 lb. rutabagas, pared and diced | 1½ tsp. butter-flavored salt |
| | ⅓ cup water |

Spray a casserole with vegetable coating. Spread the rutabagas in the casserole and sprinkle with salt and water. Cover the casserole and bake in a preheated 350° oven about 1 hour until rutabagas are tender. *Makes 6 servings*

	Calories	Carbo-hydrate (gm)	Protein (gm)	Total Fat (gm)	Saturated Fat (gm)	Choles-terol (mg)
Total	319.9	73.1	9.1	0.0	0.0	0.0
Per Serving	53.3	12.2	1.5	0.0	0.0	0.0

Spinach Stir-Fry

1 tsp. lemon juice	6-oz. can sliced mushrooms, drained
1½ tbsp. soy sauce	
1 tbsp. corn oil	
1½ cups diagonally sliced celery	½ cup thinly sliced onion
	6 cups fresh spinach leaves

Combine the lemon juice, and soy sauce in a cup and set it aside. Heat the oil in a nonstick skillet. Add the celery, mushrooms and onion, and stir-fry for 1 minute. Then add the spinach and lemon juice mixture. Stir-fry the vegetables for about 2 minutes longer until the celery and onion are tender-crisp and the spinach is just limp. Do not overcook! *Makes 4 servings*

Hint: The careful calorie-counter can save an extra 75 calories by using diet margarine instead of corn oil. That's almost 19 calories per serving!

	Calories	Carbo-hydrate (gm)	Protein (gm)	Total Fat (gm)	Saturated Fat (gm)	Choles-terol (mg)
Total	481.6	60.6	39.8	20.0	1.0	0.0
Per Serving	120.4	15.2	10.0	5.0	0.2	0.0

Spinach with Sesame

| 2 tbsp. sesame seeds | 1½ lb. fresh spinach |
| | ½ tsp. butter-flavored salt |

Toast sesame seeds by sprinkling them on a cookie sheet and baking them in a preheated 350° oven until they are brown. Watch them carefully so they do not burn. Cut the tough stems off the spinach and wash the spinach carefully. Place the spinach in a saucepan with just the water that clings to the leaves. Add the salt. Cook the spinach over moderate heat, uncovered, just until it is tender. Sprinkle the sesame seeds over the cooked spinach. *Makes 4 servings*

	Calories	Carbo-hydrate (gm)	Protein (gm)	Total Fat (gm)	Saturated Fat (gm)	Choles-terol (mg)
Total	256.1	27.2	22.8	12.7	1.3	0.0
Per Serving	64.0	6.8	5.7	3.2	0.3	0.0

Baked Acorn Squash

3 small acorn squash, halved	¾ cup unsweetened apple juice
1 tsp. salt	6 tsp. diet margarine
Dash pepper	Cinnamon to taste

Sprinkle the cut surfaces of the squash with salt and pepper and place them cut side down in a baking dish. Bake in a preheated oven at 400° for 25 minutes. Turn the squash cut side up and spoon 2 tablespoons of apple juice and 1 teaspoon of margarine into each cavity. Bake them for about 30 minutes longer until they are tender. *Makes 6 servings*

	Calories	Carbo-hydrate (gm)	Protein (gm)	Total Fat (gm)	Saturated Fat (gm)	Choles-terol (mg)
Total	775.2	166.0	18.0	16.5	2.0	0.0
Per Serving	129.2	27.7	3.0	2.8	0.3	0.0

gm = grams; mg = milligrams. Nutritional figures are approximate. Figures are based on findings of U.S. Department of Agriculture.

The I-Love-To-Eat Gallery of Photos

These photographs will make you hungry. But, for once, there is no need to feel guilty when you see cheese blintzes, waffles, sausage, spaghetti and meatballs. All of these attractive dishes have been cleverly decalorized to make dieting a pleasure instead of a punishment. Below, spicy Moroccan Salad (recipe on page 24) could be part of a Mediterranean feast.

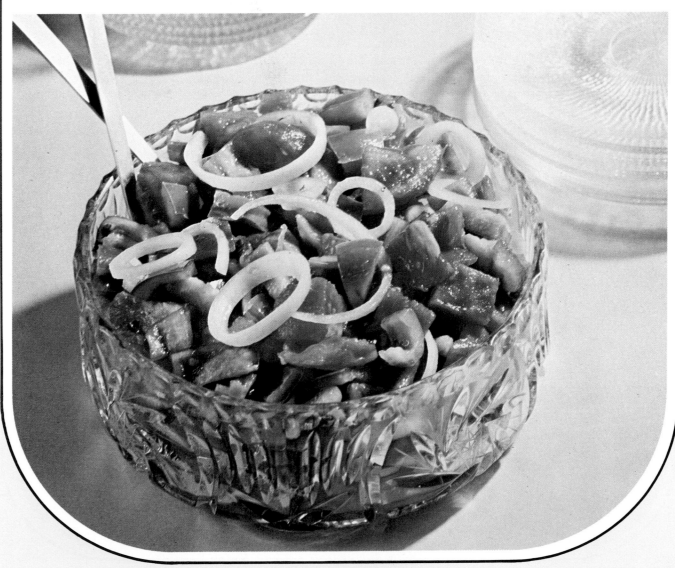

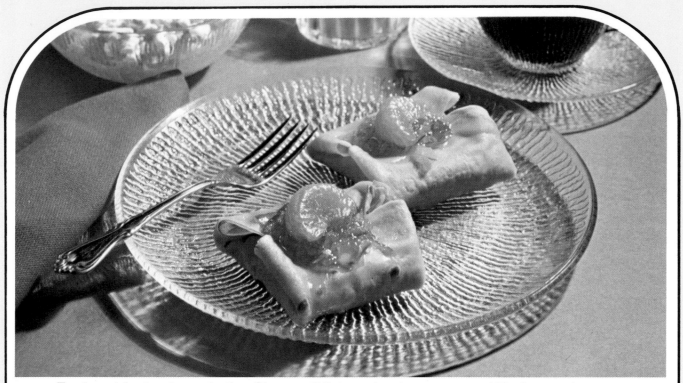

For breakfast or brunch, the Cheese Blintzes (recipe on page 15) shown above are a surprise treat. They can be topped with fresh fruit or one of the low-calorie preserves found in the "Unforbidden Sweets" chapter. Shown below, Shell Salad (recipe on page 42) makes a tasty side dish for lunch or a picnic.

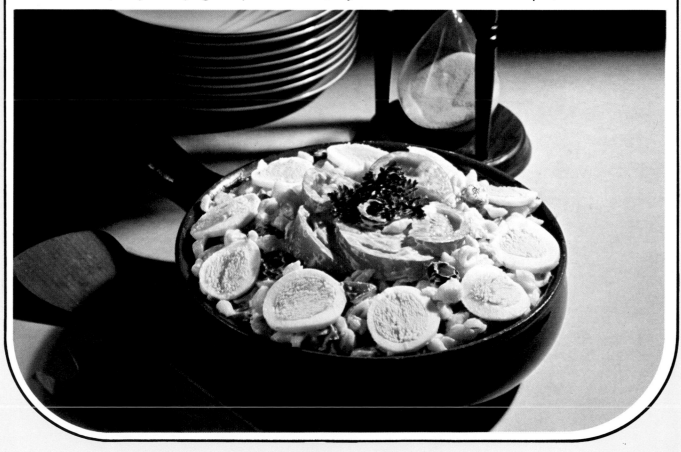

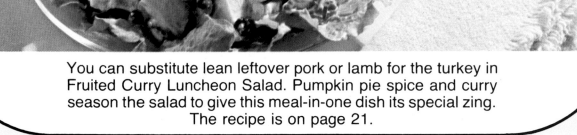

You can substitute lean leftover pork or lamb for the turkey in Fruited Curry Luncheon Salad. Pumpkin pie spice and curry season the salad to give this meal-in-one dish its special zing. The recipe is on page 21.

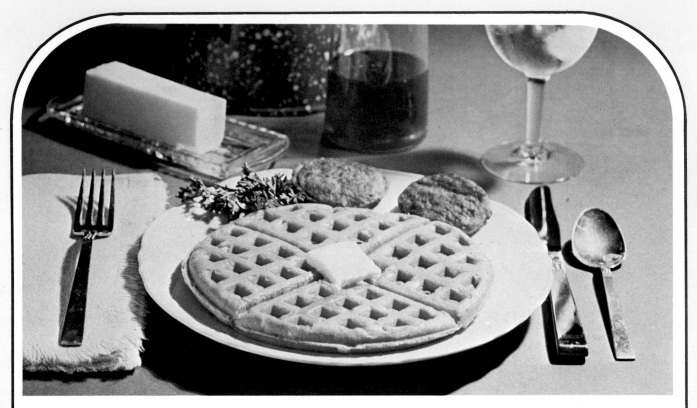

You can resist coffee-and-junk at midmorning if you enjoy a hearty breakfast like High Protein Waffles and Savory Sausage (recipes on pages 16 and 17), shown above. Below, easy Eggplant Parmesan (recipe on page 33) tastes so rich you'll think you shouldn't be eating it.

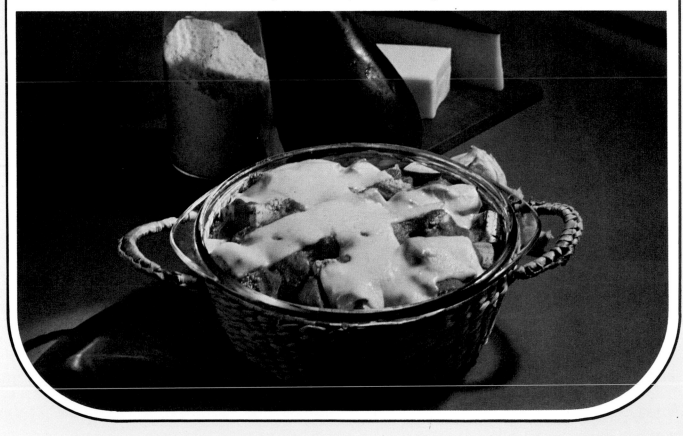

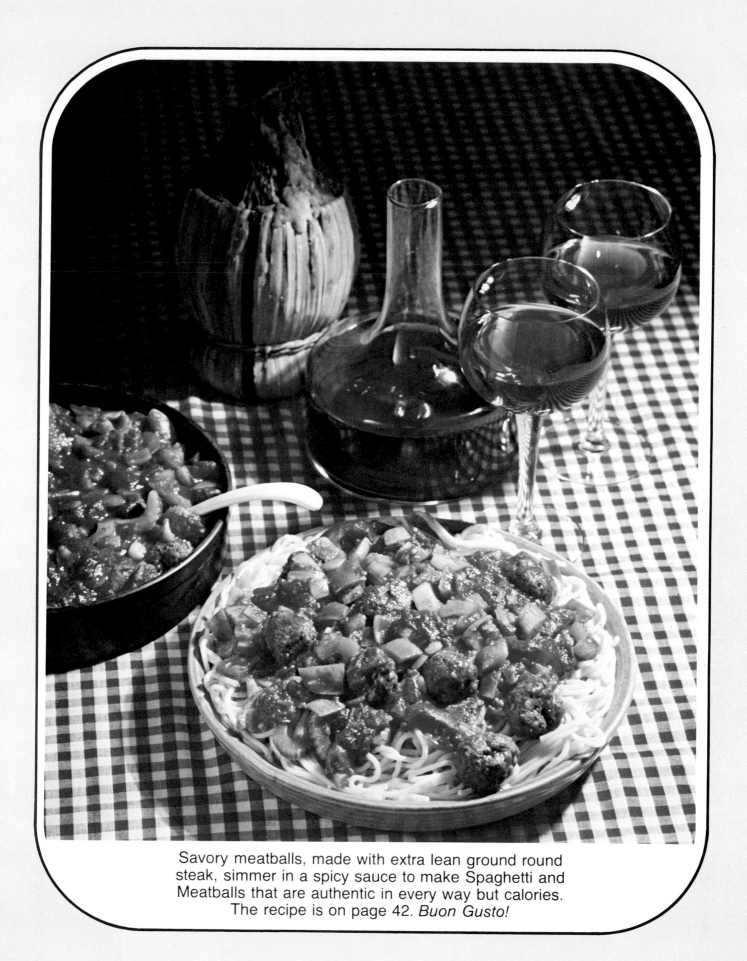

Savory meatballs, made with extra lean ground round
steak, simmer in a spicy sauce to make Spaghetti and
Meatballs that are authentic in every way but calories.
The recipe is on page 42. *Buon Gusto!*

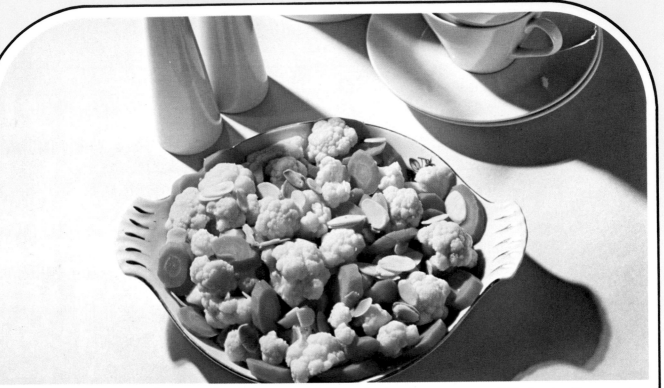

Above, Almond Crusted Cauliflower and Carrots (recipe on page 36), looks like a dinner-party side dish. Below, Steak and Mushroom Salad (recipe on page 21) tastes like it comes from a fancy restaurant—but really it's leftovers.

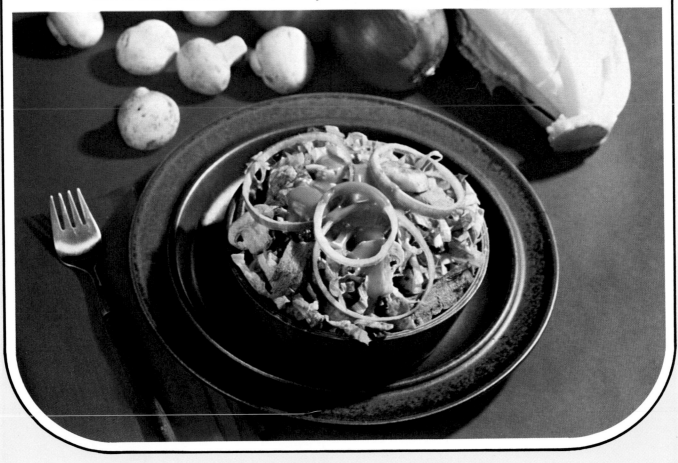

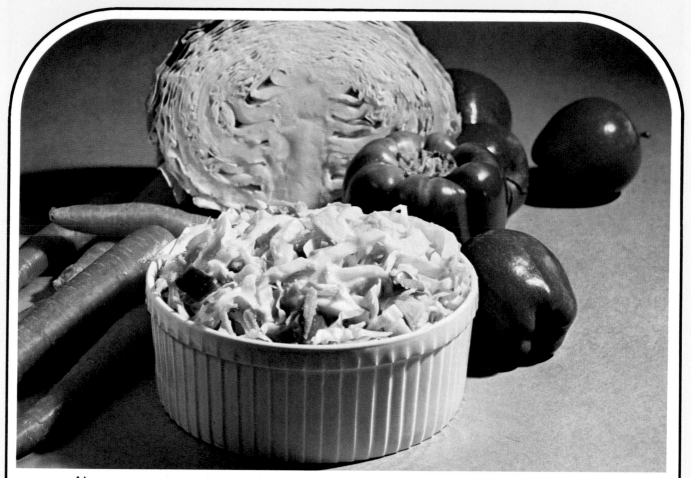

Above, carrot, apple and green pepper combine with cabbage for a crunchy, sweet-tart Colorful Coleslaw (recipe on page 23). Below, creamy-smooth Stuffed Potatoes (recipe on page 39) tempt you. Each half has only 85 calories, so enjoy! Prepared correctly, potatoes and pasta, too, can be eaten by diet watchers.

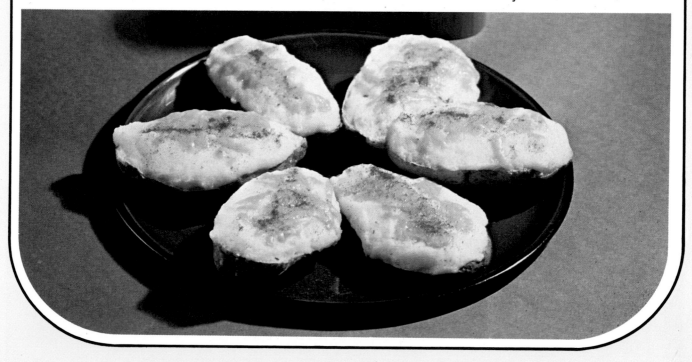

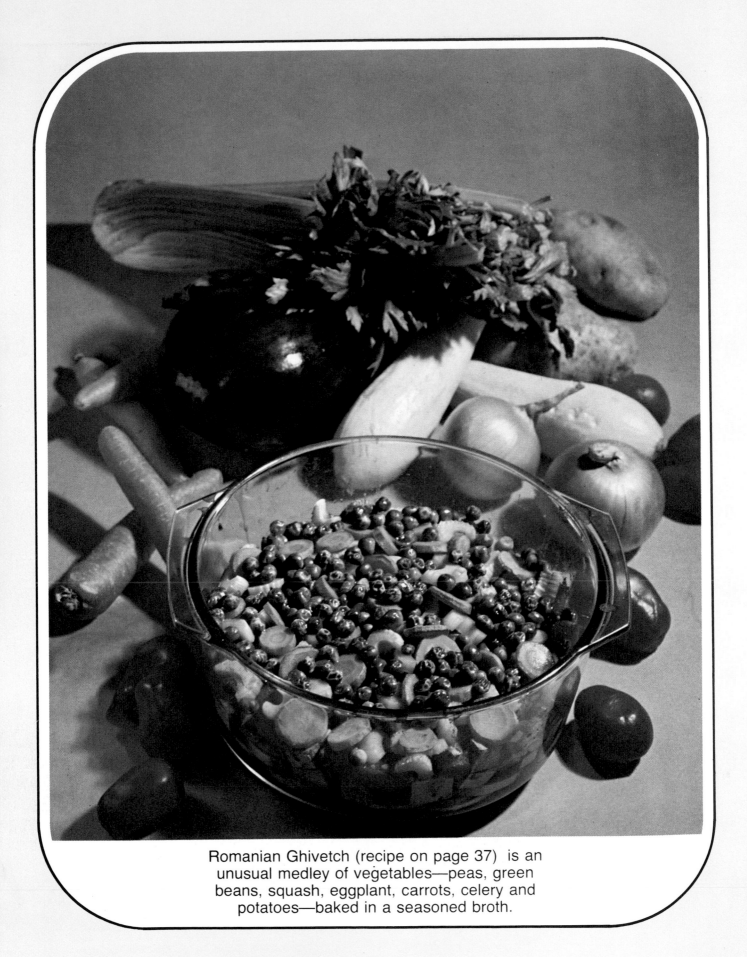

Romanian Ghivetch (recipe on page 37) is an unusual medley of vegetables—peas, green beans, squash, eggplant, carrots, celery and potatoes—baked in a seasoned broth.

Spicy Mashed Acorn Squash

2 medium acorn
    squash, halved
1 tbsp. skim milk
1/2 tsp. cinnamon

1/2 tsp. allspice
1/2 tsp. butter-flavored
    salt

Place the squash halves cut side down in a baking pan. Bake them for about 30 minutes in a preheated 400° oven until they are tender. Scoop the squash from the shells, and place it in a bowl. Mash the squash, stirring in the remaining ingredients. *Makes 8 servings*

	Calories	Carbo-hydrate (gm)	Protein (gm)	Total Fat (gm)	Saturated Fat (gm)	Choles-terol (mg)
Total	503.3	123.3	15.8	3.8	0.0	0.3
Per Serving	62.9	15.4	2.0	0.5	0.0	0.0

Summer Squash Bake

2 lb. yellow summer
    squash, sliced in 1/2-
    in. pieces
1/4 cup water
3 tbsp. chopped onion
3 eggs, beaten

1/2 tsp. hot pepper
    sauce
2 tsp. parsley flakes
1 tsp. salt
1/4 tsp. pepper
5 tbsp. cracker
    crumbs

Boil the squash about 3 minutes in the water until it is tender. Drain the squash and add all the remaining ingredients except the cracker crumbs and mix well. Pour the mixture into a 1-quart casserole that has been sprayed with vegetable coating. Sprinkle the cracker crumbs over the top. Bake the casserole uncovered in a preheated 350° oven for 35 to 40 minutes until the squash is brown. *Makes 6 servings*

	Calories	Carbo-hydrate (gm)	Protein (gm)	Total Fat (gm)	Saturated Fat (gm)	Choles-terol (mg)
Total	438.2	41.8	28.2	19.3	6.0	756.0
Per Serving	73.0	7.0	4.7	3.2	1.0	126.0

Sunshine Squash

3/4 lb. yellow summer
    squash, sliced
6-oz. can unsweetened
    orange juice
1/2 tsp. arrowroot or
    cornstarch

2 green onions,
    sliced
1/4 tsp. salt
Dash pepper

Combine all of the ingredients in a shallow saucepan. Leaving the pan uncovered, simmer the contents, stirring occasionally, until most of the liquid has evaporated. *Makes 4 servings*

	Calories	Carbo-hydrate (gm)	Protein (gm)	Total Fat (gm)	Saturated Fat (gm)	Choles-terol (mg)
Total	148.2	34.8	5.0	0.0	0.0	0.0
Per Serving	37.1	8.7	1.3	0.0	0.0	0.0

Baked Tomatoes

2 large ripe tomatoes,
    halved
2 green onions, minced

1 tsp. minced fresh
    parsley
1/4 tsp. salt
Dash pepper

Place each tomato half cut side up on a large square of double-thick foil. Sprinkle the surface of the tomato halves with green onion, parsley, salt, and pepper. Bring the foil up and around the tomato half. Seal the sides of the foil, but leave a space at the top for steam to escape. Bake the tomatoes in a preheated 350° oven for 20 minutes. *Makes 4 servings*

	Calories	Carbo-hydrate (gm)	Protein (gm)	Total Fat (gm)	Saturated Fat (gm)	Choles-terol (mg)
Total	82.2	18.3	4.1	0.0	0.0	0.0
Per Serving	20.6	4.6	1.0	0.0	0.0	0.0

Swiss-Broiled Tomatoes

1/4 cup diet mayonnaise
2 oz. Swiss cheese,
    grated

1/2 tsp. paprika
6 medium tomatoes,
    halved

Mix the mayonnaise, cheese and paprika together, and spread this mixture over the cut surface of the tomatoes. Broil the tomatoes about 5 minutes until the tops are brown. *Makes 6 servings*

	Calories	Carbo-hydrate (gm)	Protein (gm)	Total Fat (gm)	Saturated Fat (gm)	Choles-terol (mg)
Total	527.9	58.0	27.4	23.4	7.7	88.7
Per Serving	88.0	9.7	4.6	3.9	1.3	14.8

Savory Tomato Stew

2 lb. tomatoes, peeled
    and cut in wedges
4 green onions,
    chopped

1 1/2 tsp. garlic salt
1/4 tsp. seasoned
    pepper

Combine all of the ingredients and cook over moderate heat for 10 minutes, stirring occasionally. *Makes 6 servings*

Hint: Fresh tomatoes are easier to peel if they are first plunged into boiling water.

	Calories	Carbo-hydrate (gm)	Protein (gm)	Total Fat (gm)	Saturated Fat (gm)	Choles-terol (mg)
Total	192.4	43.6	9.7	0.0	0.0	0.0
Per Serving	32.1	7.3	1.6	0.0	0.0	0.0

gm = grams; mg = milligrams. Nutritional figures are approximate. Figures are based on findings of U.S. Department of Agriculture.

Apple-Glazed Zucchini

2 zucchini squash (¾ lb.), sliced
6-oz. can unsweetened apple juice
½ tsp. arrowroot or cornstarch
1 tsp. instant dried onion
½ tsp. dried parsley flakes
¼ tsp. salt
Dash pepper

Combine all of the ingredients in a shallow saucepan. Simmer the mixture, uncovered, over moderate heat, stirring occasionally, until most of the liquid has evaporated, leaving a thick sauce. *Makes 4 servings*

	Calories	Carbo-hydrate (gm)	Protein (gm)	Total Fat (gm)	Saturated Fat (gm)	Choles-terol (mg)
Total	145.1	35.4	3.3	0.0	0.0	0.0
Per Serving	36.3	8.9	0.8	0.0	0.0	0.0

Skillet Zucchini Parmesan

2 tbsp. diet margarine
6 medium zucchini, sliced
¼ tsp. butter-flavored salt
½ tsp. oregano
½ cup grated Parmesan cheese

Melt the margarine in a heavy nonstick skillet. Add the zucchini and season it with salt and oregano. Cover the pan tightly and cook over low heat about 5 minutes, just long enough to heat the slices through. Sprinkle the zucchini with the cheese and serve immediately. *Makes 12 servings*

	Calories	Carbo-hydrate (gm)	Protein (gm)	Total Fat (gm)	Saturated Fat (gm)	Choles-terol (mg)
Total	904.0	46.8	69.6	55.2	26.0	129.6
Per Serving	75.3	3.9	5.8	4.6	2.2	10.8

Tomato-Pepper Sauté

1 tbsp. diet margarine
1½ cups sliced sweet onions
2 green peppers, cut in thin strips
3 medium tomatoes, peeled and cut in 8 wedges
1 tsp. salt
¼ tsp. pepper
¼ tsp. oregano

Melt the diet margarine in a nonstick skillet over low heat. Add the onions and saute them until tender. Add the green pepper and tomatoes and the seasonings. Cover and simmer about 10 minutes, just until the peppers are tender-crisp. *Makes 6 servings*

Hint: Fresh tomatoes are easier to peel if they are first plunged into boiling water.

	Calories	Carbo-hydrate (gm)	Protein (gm)	Total Fat (gm)	Saturated Fat (gm)	Choles-terol (mg)
Total	260.0	48.0	11.0	6.0	1.0	0.0
Per Serving	43.3	8.0	1.8	1.0	0.2	0.0

Almond-Crusted Cauliflower and Carrots

1 small head cauliflower, broken into flowerets
2 cups diagonally sliced carrots
4 tbsp. slivered, blanched almonds
2 tsp. lemon juice
Coarsely ground pepper to taste

Cook the cauliflower and carrots in a small amount of boiling, salted water for about 15 minutes until they are just tender. Then drain them. Place the almonds in a nonstick skillet over moderate heat for about 1 minute until they are lightly browned. Remove them from the heat and stir in the lemon juice. Pour the lemon and almonds over the vegetables and sprinkle them generously with the pepper. *Makes 8 servings*

	Calories	Carbo-hydrate (gm)	Protein (gm)	Total Fat (gm)	Saturated Fat (gm)	Choles-terol (mg)
Total	411.4	51.1	24.5	19.3	1.5	0.0
Per Serving	51.4	6.4	3.1	2.4	0.2	0.0

Vegetable Medley

1 tbsp. diet margarine
2 cups diagonally sliced carrots
2 cups snap beans, broken into 1-in. pieces
2 cups sliced summer squash
1 cup thinly sliced onion
½ tsp. salt
Dash ground black pepper

Melt the margarine in a nonstick skillet. Add the vegetables and salt. Cover the pan, and cook the vegetables, stirring occasionally, 10 to 15 minutes until they are crisp-tender. Season with the pepper according to your taste and serve the vegetables hot. *Makes 6 servings*

	Calories	Carbo-hydrate (gm)	Protein (gm)	Total Fat (gm)	Saturated Fat (gm)	Choles-terol (mg)
Total	290.0	58.0	14.0	6.0	1.0	0.0
Per Serving	48.3	9.7	2.3	1.0	0.2	0.0

Ratatouille

3 onions, sliced
4 green peppers, cut in eighths
1 medium eggplant, peeled and cubed
4 small zucchini, sliced
4 tomatoes, sliced
2 garlic cloves, minced
1 tsp. salt
¼ tsp. freshly ground black pepper
1 tbsp. chopped black olives

gm = grams; mg = milligrams. Nutritional figures are approximate. Figures are based on findings of U.S. Department of Agriculture.

Arrange the vegetables in layers in a baking dish. Sprinkle the garlic, salt, pepper, and olives over each layer. Cover the dish and bake in a preheated 275° oven for about 40 minutes until the vegetables are soft. Then remove the cover, raise the heat to 500° and cook another 5 minutes, until the liquid is reduced.

Makes 6 servings

	Calories	Carbo-hydrate (gm)	Protein (gm)	Total Fat (gm)	Saturated Fat (gm)	Choles-terol (mg)
Total	518.3	115.1	28.3	2.0	0.0	0.0
Per Serving	86.4	19.2	4.7	0.3	0.0	0.0

Romanian Ghivetch

10½-oz. can condensed beef bouillon
1 potato, pared and diced
1 carrot, thinly sliced
1 eggplant, pared and diced
2 stalks of celery, sliced
1 yellow squash, thinly sliced
2 medium onions, sliced

17-oz. can Italian plum tomatoes, drained
½ cup green peas
½ cup green beans
1½ tsp. salt
½ tsp. hot pepper sauce
1 garlic clove, minced
1 tsp. dried dill weed

Skim the fat from the bouillon by chilling it until the fat rises to the top and can be whisked away. Arrange the vegetables in layers in a 3- or 4-quart casserole, sprinkling each layer with salt. In a saucepan heat together the hot pepper sauce, bouillon, and garlic. Pour this over the vegetables and sprinkle the dill over the top. Cover the casserole, and bake in a preheated 350° oven for 1 hour or longer until all the vegetables are tender.

Makes 6 servings

	Calories	Carbo-hydrate (gm)	Protein (gm)	Total Fat (gm)	Saturated Fat (gm)	Choles-terol (mg)
Total	516.4	104.5	34.0	2.5	0.0	62.9
Per Serving	86.1	17.4	5.7	0.4	0.0	10.5

Cheesy Tomato-Spinach Bake

4 tbsp. flour
1 tbsp. chopped onion
1-lb. can tomatoes, undrained

1 cup cooked spinach, well drained
1 cup 99% fat-free cottage cheese
2 eggs, beaten
1 tsp. salt

Combine the flour, onion, and tomatoes (with the liquid) in a saucepan. Cook the mixture over moderate heat until it has thickened slightly. Then add the remaining ingredients and mix well. Pour the entire mixture into a 1½-quart casserole that has been sprayed with vegetable coating. Bake the casserole for 20 minutes in a preheated 375° oven. *Makes 6 servings*

	Calories	Carbo-hydrate (gm)	Protein (gm)	Total Fat (gm)	Saturated Fat (gm)	Choles-terol (mg)
Total	594.2	55.0	54.1	17.2	5.2	523.4
Per Serving	99.0	9.2	9.0	2.9	0.9	87.2

Mini-Caloried Marinated Vegetables

1 cup crisp-cooked, unbuttered green beans or other vegetable such as asparagus, broccoli, carrots, or cauliflower
1 tbsp. minced onion (1 tsp. onion flakes)

2 tbsp. low-calorie salad dressing
2 tbsp. olive juice (from jar of olives)
¼ pimiento, diced and drained (optional)
½ fresh red bell pepper, chopped (optional)

Combine all ingredients and chill until serving time.

Makes 2 servings

	Calories	Carbo-hydrate (gm)	Protein (gm)	Total Fat (gm)	Saturated Fat (gm)	Choles-terol (mg)
Total	71.8	10.5	2.3	2.0	0.0	0.0
Per Serving	35.9	5.3	1.2	1.0	0.0	0.0

Rutabaga-Onion Casserole

2 lb. rutabagas (yellow turnips), pared and thinly sliced
3 cups thinly sliced onion

½ tsp. salt
Dash pepper
1 chicken bouillon cube
½ cup boiling water

Arrange alternate layers of rutabaga and onion slices in a 2½-quart casserole. Sprinkle each layer lightly with salt and pepper. Dissolve the bouillon cube in the boiling water and pour the bouillon over the vegetables. Cover and bake in a preheated 350° oven about 1¼ hours until the rutabagas are tender.

Makes 6 servings

	Calories	Carbo-hydrate (gm)	Protein (gm)	Total Fat (gm)	Saturated Fat (gm)	Choles-terol (mg)
Total	446.9	121.6	24.8	7.0	2.0	0.0
Per Serving	74.5	20.3	4.1	1.2	0.3	0.0

Peas and Cauliflower

10-oz. pkg. frozen cauliflower, cooked
10-oz. pkg. frozen peas, cooked

½ tsp. butter-flavored salt
¼ tsp. pepper
2 tbsp. chopped pimiento

Combine hot cooked vegetables with remaining ingredients and serve immediately. *Makes 4 servings*

	Calories	Carbo-hydrate (gm)	Protein (gm)	Total Fat (gm)	Saturated Fat (gm)	Choles-terol (mg)
Total	255.6	46.4	21.3	0.3	0.0	0.0
Per Serving	63.9	11.6	5.3	0.1	0.0	0.0

gm = grams; mg = milligrams. Nutritional figures are approximate. Figures are based on findings of U.S. Department of Agriculture.

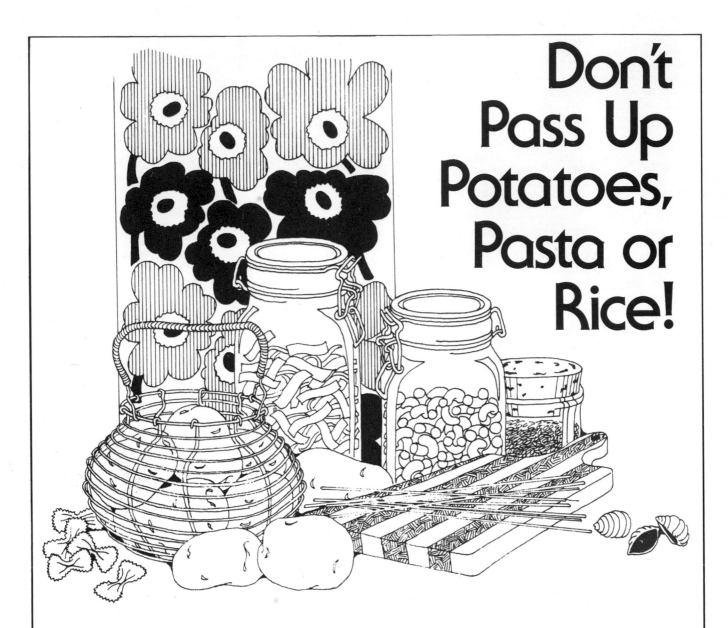

Don't Pass Up Potatoes, Pasta or Rice!

If you pass up potatoes, skip spaghetti, or refuse rice in favor of a second helping of steak, you are probably a victim of the carbohydrate myth. Low-carb dieters seem to think some calories are more fattening than others and that somehow they can achieve slimness on limitless meat, cheese, cream, and other high-fat foods. As a matter of fact, the so-called starchy foods are relatively low in calories. Most cost between 70 and 90 calories a serving, considerably less than the second helping of high-fat foods most low-carb dieters would replace them with. In fact, the only time these appetite-appeasers become fattening is when fat is added to them in the form of butter, cream sauce, gravy, cheese, or other calorie-rich toppings. A half-cup serving of mashed potatoes is only 63 calories, but a level tablespoon of butter adds 100 more. Here is just how low-cal most of these palate-pleasers are before the extra calories are added on.

	Serving	Calories
Baked potato	1 medium, no fat	90
Boiled potato	1 medium, peeled	65
Boiled potato	1 medium, unpeeled	76
Mashed potato	½ cup, milk, no fat	63
Spaghetti	½ cup, cooked firm	108
	½ cup, cooked tender	83
Macaroni	½ cup, cooked firm	104
	½ cup, cooked tender	75
Egg noodles	½ cup, cooked	100
Brown rice	½ cup, cooked	89
White rice	½ cup, cooked	82
Long grain rice	½ cup, cooked	79
Instant rice	½ cup, prepared, no fat	80

A frozen stuffed potato is nearly triple the calories of a plain potato. Heat-and-serve fried rice is 40 percent more fattening than regular rice. And macaroni and cheese made from a convenience mix is double the calories of plain pasta. But who wants plain potatoes or naked noodles? In this chapter, we offer a variety of variations from standard fattening recipes all aimed at keeping calorie counts low.

Recipes

Savory Bacon Potatoes

10¾-oz. can condensed cream of celery soup
4 tbsp. water
4 tbsp. minced onion
Pinch of pepper

3 potatoes (1lb. total) peeled, boiled, cut in chunks
1 tbsp. bacon-flavored bits

In a saucepan, combine the soup, water, onion, and pepper. Cook this mixture over low heat for 5 to 10 minutes, stirring occasionally. Then add the potatoes and continue to heat thoroughly. Serve the potatoes garnished with the bacon-flavored bits.

Makes 8 servings

	Calories	Carbo-hydrate (gm)	Protein (gm)	Total Fat (gm)	Saturated Fat (gm)	Choles-terol (mg)
Total	475.3	80.1	11.7	13.1	0.0	18.3
Per Serving	59.4	10.0	1.5	1.6	0.0	2.3

Stuffed Potatoes

.4 baking potatoes
1 tsp. butter-flavored salt
2 egg whites
Pinch of cream of tartar
Pinch of pepper

1 tsp. freeze-dried chives
½ to ¾ cup skim milk
3 tbsp. grated extra-sharp cheddar cheese
Paprika

Scrub the potatoes, pierce them with a fork and bake them in a preheated 400° oven for about 1 hour until they are soft. Remove the potatoes from the oven and carefully slice them in half, lengthwise. Combine the salt, egg whites, and cream of tartar in a bowl. Using an electric mixer, whip the egg whites until stiff peaks form. Carefully scoop out the pulp of the potatoes and place them in another bowl. Add the pepper and chives and whip them with the electric mixer, adding a little milk at a time until they are fluffy. Fold the egg white mixture into the potatoes and pile the mixture back into the potato skins. Sprinkle the top of each potato with grated cheese and paprika and return the potatoes to the oven. Bake them in a preheated 425° oven until the cheese is melted and the potatoes are hot.

Makes 8 servings

	Calories	Carbo-hydrate (gm)	Protein (gm)	Total Fat (gm)	Saturated Fat (gm)	Choles-terol (mg)
Total	686.6	94.8	40.8	18.0	10.0	59.8
Per Serving	85.8	11.9	5.1	2.3	1.3	7.5

Cheesy Creamed Potatoes

3 potatoes, peeled and boiled
¼ cup skim milk
4 oz. low-calorie cream cheese

1 egg, beaten
1 tbsp. chopped chives
Paprika

Mash the potatoes, adding the skim milk a little at a time, until the potatoes are smooth. Then add the diet cream cheese, and beat the mixture well. Stir in the egg and chives and spoon the mixture into a 1-quart casserole that has been sprayed with vegetable coating. Sprinkle paprika on the top and bake the potato casserole in a preheated 400° oven for 30 minutes.

Makes 8 servings

	Calories	Carbo-hydrate (gm)	Protein (gm)	Total Fat (gm)	Saturated Fat (gm)	Choles-terol (mg)
Total	626.0	61.8	22.6	30.0	18.0	337.3
Per Serving	78.3	7.7	2.8	3.8	2.3	42.2

Parsley Potatoes en Casserole

6 potatoes (2 lb. total), peeled and cubed
4 tbsp. chopped fresh parsley
2 tbsp. minced green onion

4 tbsp. lemon juice
1 tsp. grated lemon peel
1 tsp. butter-flavored salt

Toss all of the ingredients together and turn the mixture into a nonstick baking dish. Cover the dish, and bake the potatoes in a preheated 425° oven for 45 minutes.

Makes 12 servings

	Calories	Carbo-hydrate (gm)	Protein (gm)	Total Fat (gm)	Saturated Fat (gm)	Choles-terol (mg)
Total	505.3	114.6	12.6	0.0	0.0	0.0
Per Serving	42.1	9.6	1.1	0.0	0.0	0.0

Protein-Enriched Potato Pancakes

2 cups shredded raw potatoes
2 eggs, beaten
3 tbsp. grated onion

1 tbsp. flour
½ tsp. salt
2 tbsp. diet margarine

Combine the shredded potatoes with the eggs, onion, flour, and salt. Melt the margarine in a nonstick skillet. Drop the potato mixture from a tablespoon into the hot margarine and fry the patties on both sides until they are crisp.

Makes 10 servings

	Calories	Carbo-hydrate (gm)	Protein (gm)	Total Fat (gm)	Saturated Fat (gm)	Choles-terol (mg)
Total	455.3	43.8	17.2	24.1	6.0	504.0
Per Serving	45.5	4.4	1.7	2.4	0.6	50.4

gm = grams; mg = milligrams. Nutritional figures are approximate. Figures are based on findings of U.S. Department of Agriculture.

Skinny Scalloped Potatoes

2 cups thinly sliced
   potatoes
½ cup sliced
   mushrooms
½ cup sliced onions
4 beef bouillon cubes

1½ cups boiling water
1 tsp. butter-flavored
   salt
Pinch of pepper
Pinch of nutmeg

Mix the potatoes, mushrooms, and onions in a nonstick baking dish. Dissolve the bouillon cubes in the water; blend in the salt, pepper and nutmeg, and pour this mixture over the vegetables. Cover and bake for 45 minutes in a preheated 350° oven. Then uncover and bake 20 minutes longer. *Makes 6 servings*

	Calories	Carbo-hydrate (gm)	Protein (gm)	Total Fat (gm)	Saturated Fat (gm)	Choles-terol (mg)
Total	254.0	52.5	14.5	0.5	0.0	12.0
Per Serving	42.3	8.8	2.4	0.1	0.0	2.0

Omelette Pommes de Terre

1 tbsp. diet margarine
1 potato, peeled and
   diced
⅓ cup minced onion
2 tbsp. chopped
   green pepper

½ tsp. salt
Pinch of pepper
4 tsp. tomato paste
4 eggs, slightly
   beaten

Melt the margarine in a large nonstick skillet. Add the potato, onion, and green pepper to the skillet and season them with the salt and pepper. Sauté them for about 20 minutes, stirring occasionally, until they are tender and lightly browned. Stir in tomato paste and cook and stir for 2 to 3 minutes longer. Add the beaten eggs. Tilt the pan until the eggs flow evenly through and around the potato mixture. Cook just until the eggs are set. Fold the omelet in half and slide it out of the pan onto a serving dish. *Makes 4 servings*

	Calories	Carbo-hydrate (gm)	Protein (gm)	Total Fat (gm)	Saturated Fat (gm)	Choles-terol (mg)
Total	480.6	24.4	27.3	30.0	9.0	1008.0
Per Serving	120.2	6.1	6.8	7.5	2.3	252.0

Oven French Fries au Naturel

2 medium potatoes,
   unpeeled
1 tbsp. corn or safflower
   oil

Dash salt
Dash pepper

Scrub unpeeled potatoes well, then cut in half lengthwise. Slice each half into lengthwise wedges, so that each wedge has some peel. Soak the potato strips in a bowl of cold water and ice cubes 20 minutes. Preheat oven at highest setting. Meanwhile, spray a nonstick cookie sheet with vegetable coating for no-fat cooking. Drain and dry the potatoes and spread on the cookie sheet. Sprinkle with oil; stir the potatoes to coat evenly. Use an oven thermometer to check temper-ature. When oven temperature reaches 450°, put the tray in the oven. Bake, uncovered, for about 20 minutes, or until potatoes are golden and crisp. Stir occasionally while baking. Salt and pepper to taste. *Makes 4 servings*

	Calories	Carbo-hydrate (gm)	Protein (gm)	Total Fat (gm)	Saturated Fat (gm)	Choles-terol (mg)
Total	305.0	42.0	6.0	14.0	1.0	0.0
Per Serving	76.2	10.5	1.5	3.5	0.3	0.0

Dieter's Dumplings for Stew

2 large potatoes,
   peeled, cooked,
   and drained
¼ cup skim milk
1 egg
4 tbsp. flour

1 tbsp. minced onion
1 tbsp. chopped
   parsley
½ tsp. salt
Dash paprika

Mash the potatoes, adding the skim milk a little at a time, until they are smooth. Then add all the rest of the ingredients, except the paprika. Scoop up rounded spoonfuls of the potato mixture and place them on top of the stew. Sprinkle them with paprika. Cover the pot and simmer the stew with the potatoes for 20 minutes. *Makes 12 dumplings (6 servings)*

	Calories	Carbo-hydrate (gm)	Protein (gm)	Total Fat (gm)	Saturated Fat (gm)	Choles-terol (mg)
Total	469.7	77.4	19.7	8.3	2.0	261.3
Per Serving	78.3	12.9	3.3	1.4	0.3	43.6

Twice-Baked Spuds

4 well-shaped baking
   potatoes
½ cup plain low-fat
   yogurt
1 cup 99% fat-free
   cottage cheese
1 tbsp. onion flakes

½ tsp. butter-flavored
   salt
Pinch pepper
Pinch paprika
½ tsp. dried parsley
   flakes

Pierce well-scrubbed potatoes with a fork. Bake in a preheated 400° oven 1 hour until they are soft. Remove them from the oven; carefully slice the potatoes in half. Scoop out the potato pulp and place it in a bowl. Mash together the potato pulp, yogurt, cottage cheese, onion flakes, salt, and pepper; or whip the mixture on the high speed of your electric mixer. Pile the potato mixture back into the baked potato skins and sprinkle the top with paprika and parsley. Turn the oven heat up to 425° and bake the potatoes until they are lightly browned. *Makes 8 servings*

	Calories	Carbo-hydrate (gm)	Protein (gm)	Total Fat (gm)	Saturated Fat (gm)	Choles-terol (mg)
Total	613.0	99.0	46.3	4.0	2.2	29.4
Per Serving	76.6	12.4	5.8	0.5	0.3	3.7

gm = grams; mg = milligrams. Nutritional figures are approximate. Figures are based on findings of U.S. Department of Agriculture.

Potatoes au Gratin

3 potatoes, peeled, boiled, and sliced
½ cup celery chunks
10¾-oz. can cheddar cheese soup
1 tbsp. prepared mustard

Arrange the potato slices and the celery chunks in a nonstick baking dish. Mix the cheese soup and the mustard together in a bowl, and pour this mixture over the potatoes. Bake in a preheated 375° oven for 30 minutes. *Makes 8 servings*

	Calories	Carbo-hydrate (gm)	Protein (gm)	Total Fat (gm)	Saturated Fat (gm)	Choles-terol (mg)
Total	750.5	111.8	18.9	0.0	12.9	64.5
Per Serving	93.8	14.0	2.4	0.0	1.6	8.1

Tangy Potato Salad

1 tbsp. vinegar
2 tbsp. corn or safflower oil
1½ tsp. garlic salt
1 tsp. dill weed
¼ tsp. pepper
8 cups boiled potatoes, pared and diced
¼ cup chopped pimiento-stuffed olives
1½ cups sliced celery
⅓ cup sliced green onion
8 oz. plain low-fat yogurt
1 tsp. prepared mustard

Mix the vinegar, oil, salt, dill weed, and pepper together. Pour this mixture over the potatoes and mix them gently. Chill the potato mixture for several hours. At serving time, add the olives, celery, and onion. Mix together the yogurt, and mustard, and fold this mixture into the potatoes gently but thoroughly. *Makes 16 servings*

	Calories	Carbo-hydrate (gm)	Protein (gm)	Total Fat (gm)	Saturated Fat (gm)	Choles-terol (mg)
Total	1142.4	183.6	24.1	37.7	3.9	18.6
Per Serving	71.4	11.5	1.5	2.4	0.2	1.2

Decalorized Potato Salad

7 cups boiled potatoes, pared and diced
1½ cups diced celery
3 tbsp. finely chopped parsley
1 onion, chopped
1 cup diet mayonnaise
3 tbsp. vinegar
1 tsp. salt
Dash paprika
Dash pepper

Combine all ingredients thoroughly. Cover and chill before serving. *Makes 16 servings*

	Calories	Carbo-hydrate (gm)	Protein (gm)	Total Fat (gm)	Saturated Fat (gm)	Choles-terol (mg)
Total	948.5	164.0	16.0	32.0	0.0	128.0
Per Serving	59.3	10.3	1.0	2.0	0.0	8.0

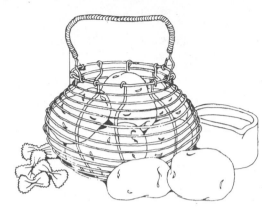

Cottage Potato Salad

¼ cup plain low-fat yogurt
2 tbsp. diet Italian salad dressing
2 cups peeled, diced cooked potatoes
2 hard-cooked eggs, chopped
2 cups 99% fat-free cottage cheese
½ cup sliced celery
⅓ cup chopped ripe olives
⅓ cup sliced radishes
⅓ cup chopped green onions
½ tsp. salt

Blend the yogurt and salad dressing together in a bowl. Add the potatoes and eggs and allow them to marinate at room temperature while you slice and chop the rest of the ingredients. Then combine all of the ingredients well and refrigerate for several hours before serving. *Makes 8 servings*

	Calories	Carbo-hydrate (gm)	Protein (gm)	Total Fat (gm)	Saturated Fat (gm)	Choles-terol (mg)
Total	834.4	59.0	78.7	29.7	6.9	547.8
Per Serving	104.3	7.4	9.8	3.7	0.9	68.5

Simple Macaroni Salad

8 oz. protein-enriched elbow macaroni
½ cup diet mayonnaise
1 cup chopped celery
½ cup plain low-fat yogurt
2 tbsp. chopped onion
1½ tsp. salt
¼ tsp. pepper
Dash paprika

Cook the macaroni according to the directions on the package; drain it, and rinse it with cold water. Add the rest of the ingredients to the macaroni, mixing thoroughly. Chill several hours. *Makes 8 servings*

	Calories	Carbo-hydrate (gm)	Protein (gm)	Total Fat (gm)	Saturated Fat (gm)	Choles-terol (mg)
Total	490.8	73.0	12.2	19.6	1.0	74.0
Per Serving	61.4	9.1	1.5	2.5	0.1	9.3

gm = grams; mg = milligrams. Nutritional figures are approximate. Figures are based on findings of U.S. Department of Agriculture.

Shell Salad

4½ tsp. dried onion flakes
2 tbsp. vinegar
1 cup diet mayonnaise
1¾ tsp. salt
¼ tsp. pepper
2 tsp. paprika
8 oz. small shell macaroni, cooked and drained

3 medium tomatoes, cut in wedges
½ cup chopped green pepper
2 tbsp. pitted black olives, sliced
3 hard-cooked eggs, sliced
2 tbsp. snipped parsley

Combine the onion and vinegar and let it stand for a few minutes. Then add the mayonnaise, salt, pepper, and paprika and mix well. Mix the macaroni, tomatoes, green pepper, and olives in a large salad bowl; and pour the mayonnaise mixture over all. Toss lightly. Chill the salad for several hours before serving. When serving, garnish with the egg slices and parsley.

Makes 8 servings

	Calories	Carbo-hydrate (gm)	Protein (gm)	Total Fat (gm)	Saturated Fat (gm)	Choles-terol (mg)
Total	985.0	102.3	33.0	55.7	6.0	884.0
Per Serving	164.2	17.1	5.5	9.3	1.0	147.3

Macaroni and Cheese Salad

3 cups cooked elbow macaroni
1½ cups 99% fat-free cottage cheese
1 onion, minced
½ cup minced green pepper

1 carrot, grated
1 tsp. salt
¼ tsp. pepper
Dash chili powder

Toss all ingredients together lightly and chill before serving.

Makes 10 servings

	Calories	Carbo-hydrate (gm)	Protein (gm)	Total Fat (gm)	Saturated Fat (gm)	Choles-terol (mg)
Total	802.5	122.0	63.5	6.0	1.8	29.1
Per Serving	80.3	12.0	6.4	0.6	0.2	2.9

Viva Macaroni and Cheese

1 tbsp. diet margarine
½ cup chopped onion
½ cup chopped celery
1 garlic clove, crushed
3½ cups water
6-oz. can tomato paste
½ lb. large #4 macaroni

2 tsp. salt
1 tsp. oregano
½ cup chopped parsley
2 cups 99% fat-free cottage cheese
5 tbsp. grated extra-sharp Romano

Melt the margarine in a large nonstick skillet. Sauté the onion, celery, and garlic until they are tender. Then stir in the water, tomato paste, macaroni, salt, and oregano. Cover the pan and simmer the mixture, stir-

ring occasionally, until the macaroni is tender. Stir in parsley. Turn half the mixture into a baking dish. Top it with 1 cup of cottage cheese, and sprinkle it with Romano cheese. Repeat the layers, ending with Romano cheese. Bake the macaroni in a preheated 350° oven for about 15 minutes or until it is bubbly.

Makes 6 servings

	Calories	Carbo-hydrate (gm)	Protein (gm)	Total Fat (gm)	Saturated Fat (gm)	Choles-terol (mg)
Total	1530.5	664.7	119.9	40.6	18.4	119.8
Per Serving	255.1	110.8	20.0	6.8	3.1	20.0

Canadian Spaghetti Supper Casserole

1 lb. Canadian bacon, cubed
1 cup chopped onion
1 cup chopped green pepper
16-oz. can tomatoes, undrained
1½ tsp. salt

2 tsp. chili powder
1 tsp. paprika
8-oz. pkg. protein-enriched spaghetti, cooked
1 cup shredded cheddar cheese

Brown the bacon cubes slowly in a nonstick skillet. Do not add any oil to the pan because the meat will release enough of its own fat for frying. Add the onion and green pepper, continuing to cook until they are tender. Then add the tomatoes, salt, chili powder, paprika, and spaghetti. Place the mixture in a baking dish and spread the cheese on top. Bake in a preheated 350° oven for about 45 minutes until the mixture bubbles and the cheese has melted. *Makes 8 servings*

	Calories	Carbo-hydrate (gm)	Protein (gm)	Total Fat (gm)	Saturated Fat (gm)	Choles-terol (mg)
Total	2878.5	93.5	212.3	179.7	74.7	678.2
Per Serving	359.8	11.7	26.5	22.5	9.3	84.8

Spaghetti and Meatballs

¾ lb. extra-lean round steak, ground
½ tsp. oregano
1 tsp. basil
½ tsp. salt
Pepper to taste
1 cup water
1-lb. 3-oz. can Italian tomatoes, undrained
6-oz. can tomato paste
1 cup chopped onion

1 green pepper, chopped
1 tbsp. oregano or mixed herbs
1 garlic clove, minced
½ cup chopped celery
6 cups tender-cooked spaghetti

Combine the meat with the oregano, basil, salt, and pepper. Shape the mixture into 18 small meatballs, and

gm = grams; mg = milligrams. Nutritional figures are approximate. Figures are based on findings of U.S. Department of Agriculture.

brown them under the broiler, turning them once. In a large saucepan bring all of the remaining ingredients (except the spaghetti) to a boil. Add the meatballs; cover the pot and simmer over low heat for 1 hour or longer. Pour sauce over spaghetti. *Makes 6 servings*

	Calories	Carbo-hydrate (gm)	Protein (gm)	Total Fat (gm)	Saturated Fat (gm)	Choles-terol (mg)
Total	1787.6	260.0	148.7	21.5	4.4	315.2
Per Serving	297.9	43.4	24.8	3.6	0.7	52.5

Italian Pasta Soup

2 cans chicken broth	1 cup chopped
½ cup chopped onion	canned
½ tsp. oregano	tomatoes,
	undrained
	1 tbsp. chopped
	parsley
	¼ cup uncooked
	elbow macaroni

Skim the fat from the broth by using a bulb-type baster. In a large saucepan combine all of the ingredients except the macaroni. Bring the mixture to a boil. Then add the macaroni. Cook over low heat until the macaroni is tender, stirring ccasionally.

Makes 6 servings

	Calories	Carbo-hydrate (gm)	Protein (gm)	Total Fat (gm)	Saturated Fat (gm)	Choles-terol (mg)
Total	273.5	43.4	21.6	1.6	0.0	73.6
Per Serving	45.6	7.2	3.6	0.3	0.0	12.3

Curried Mushroom Rice

2 cups chicken broth	4-oz. can sliced
1 tbsp. diet margarine	mushrooms,
1 cup chopped onions	drained
1 garlic clove, minced	1 tsp. curry
1 cup uncooked rice	1 tsp. salt
	¼ tsp. pepper
	1 tbsp. lemon juice

Skim the fat from the broth with a bulb-type baster; or chill until the fat rises and can be whisked away. Melt the margarine in a nonstick skillet. Sauté the onions and garlic until the onions are tender. Then add the rice, broth, mushrooms, seasonings, and lemon juice. Heat the mixture to boiling; then cover the pan, lower the heat, and simmer about 15 minutes until the rice is tender. Before serving, fluff the rice lightly with a fork. *Makes 6 servings*

Hint: If you don't have chicken broth you may use 2 chicken bouillon cubes mixed with 2 cups of water.

	Calories	Carbo-hydrate (gm)	Protein (gm)	Total Fat (gm)	Saturated Fat (gm)	Choles-terol (mg)
Total	796.4	163.6	19.0	7.0	1.0	6.0
Per Serving	132.7	27.3	3.2	1.2	0.2	1.0

Wild Rice and Mushrooms

10½-oz. can condensed	2 medium onions,
beef or chicken	chopped
broth	½ cup wild rice
4-oz. can sliced	1 cup long-grain rice
mushrooms,	2 tbsp. parsley
drained reserving	
liquid	

Skim the broth with a bulb-type baster; or chill until the fat rises and can be whisked away. Combine the broth with enough water to equal 2 cups. Bring the broth, mushroom liquid, and onions to a boil in a saucepan. Add the wild rice, reduce the heat, and simmer about 20 minutes. Then add the long-grain rice and mushrooms. Return the mixture to boiling. Again, reduce heat and simmer about 20 minutes until the rice is tender. Serve garnished with parsley. *Makes 10 servings*

	Calories	Carbo-hydrate (gm)	Protein (gm)	Total Fat (gm)	Saturated Fat (gm)	Choles-terol (mg)
Total	1179.1	249.2	44.9	1.5	0.0	55.7
Per Serving	117.9	24.9	4.5	0.2	0.0	5.6

gm = grams; mg = milligrams. Nutritional figures are approximate. Figures are based on findings of U.S. Department of Agriculture.

Celery-Rice Casserole

2½ cups boiling chicken broth
1 cup uncooked rice
3 cups celery, sliced ½-in. thick
½ cup finely chopped onion
½ tsp. marjoram
⅛ tsp. salt
⅛ tsp. pepper
Celery leaves, chopped for garnish

Skim the fat from the broth, using a bulb-type baster. Combine all the ingredients in a 2-quart casserole. Cover the casserole and bake it in a preheated 400° oven for about 30 minutes until the rice and celery are tender. Garnish with chopped celery leaves.

Makes 6 servings

	Calories	Carbo-hydrate (gm)	Protein (gm)	Total Fat (gm)	Saturated Fat (gm)	Choles-terol (mg)
Total	790.0	177.0	20.5	1.0	0.0	35.0
Per Serving	131.7	29.5	3.4	0.2	0.0	5.8

Skinny Spanish Rice

1 tbsp. diet margarine
1½ cups chopped onion
1 cup uncooked converted white rice
1 cup chopped green pepper
1 cup chopped celery
1 tsp. chili powder
8-oz. can whole tomatoes, undrained
1 tsp. salt
2 cups water
3 tbsp. bacon bits

Melt the margarine in a heavy skillet, and sauté the onion. Stir in the rice, green pepper, celery, chili powder, canned tomatoes, and salt. Add the water. Bring the mixture to a boil. Reduce the heat and simmer, covered, for about 20 minutes until the liquid is absorbed and the rice is cooked. Garnish with the bacon bits to serve.

Makes 8 servings

	Calories	Carbo-hydrate (gm)	Protein (gm)	Total Fat (gm)	Saturated Fat (gm)	Choles-terol (mg)
Total	928.5	186.8	24.2	11.5	1.0	0.0
Per Serving	116.1	23.4	3.0	1.4	0.1	0.0

Cheese and Rice Bake

3 cups hot cooked rice
½ cup chopped parsley
¼ cup minced onion
¼ cup finely chopped green pepper
1 tsp. garlic salt
½ cup grated sharp cheese
1 cup skim milk
2 tbsp. grated Parmesan cheese

Combine all of the ingredients except the Parmesan. Turn the mixture into a 1½-quart casserole that has been sprayed with vegetable coating. Sprinkle the top of the rice mixture with the Parmesan cheese. Bake for 20 minutes in a preheated 350° oven. *Makes 6 servings*

	Calories	Carbo-hydrate (gm)	Protein (gm)	Total Fat (gm)	Saturated Fat (gm)	Choles-terol (mg)
Total	1555.8	171.8	73.5	58.8	32.7	186.6
Per Serving	259.3	28.6	12.3	9.8	5.5	31.1

Kaleidoscope Rice

10½-oz. can chicken broth
1 cup chopped celery
½ cup chopped onion
½ cup shredded carrot
¼ cup chopped green pepper
1 cup uncooked rice
Dash pepper

Skim the fat from the broth by using a bulb-type baster, or by chilling the broth until the fat rises to the top and can be whisked away. Combine all of the ingredients in a saucepan and bring them to a boil. Cover the pan, and continue cooking over low heat, stirring occasionally, about 20 minutes until the liquid is absorbed.

Makes 8 servings

	Calories	Carbo-hydrate (gm)	Protein (gm)	Total Fat (gm)	Saturated Fat (gm)	Choles-terol (mg)
Total	786.4	171.0	22.2	1.0	0.0	36.7
Per Serving	98.3	21.4	2.8	0.1	0.0	4.6

Slender Rice

1 cup finely minced celery
¼ cup finely minced onion
1 cup water
1 cup quick or instant rice
½ tsp. salt or butter-flavored salt
⅛ tsp. pepper

The celery and onion should be chopped as fine as the grains of rice. Combine all of the ingredients in a covered saucepan and simmer for 2 minutes. Remove the pan from the heat, and set it aside for 5 minutes or more, until serving time. *Makes 6 servings*

	Calories	Carbo-hydrate (gm)	Protein (gm)	Total Fat (gm)	Saturated Fat (gm)	Choles-terol (mg)
Total	205.0	48.5	4.5	0.0	0.0	0.0
Per Serving	34.2	8.1	0.8	0.0	0.0	0.0

Clam Rice

1 tbsp. diet margarine
1 cup sliced green onions
1 cup uncooked rice
7½-oz. bottle clam juice
1 cup water
1 tsp. salt
Dash pepper

Melt the margarine in a nonstick skillet. Using low heat, cook the onions and rice in the diet margarine until the rice is golden. Add the remaining ingredients. Heat the mixture to boiling. Stir once, cover the pan, reduce the heat and simmer 15 minutes. Toss the mixture lightly before serving. *Makes 6 servings*

	Calories	Carbo-hydrate (gm)	Protein (gm)	Total Fat (gm)	Saturated Fat (gm)	Choles-terol (mg)
Total	800.7	163.3	18.3	7.0	1.0	19.3
Per Serving	133.5	27.2	3.1	1.2	0.2	3.2

gm = grams; mg = milligrams. Nutritional figures are approximate. Figures are based on findings of U.S. Department of Agriculture.

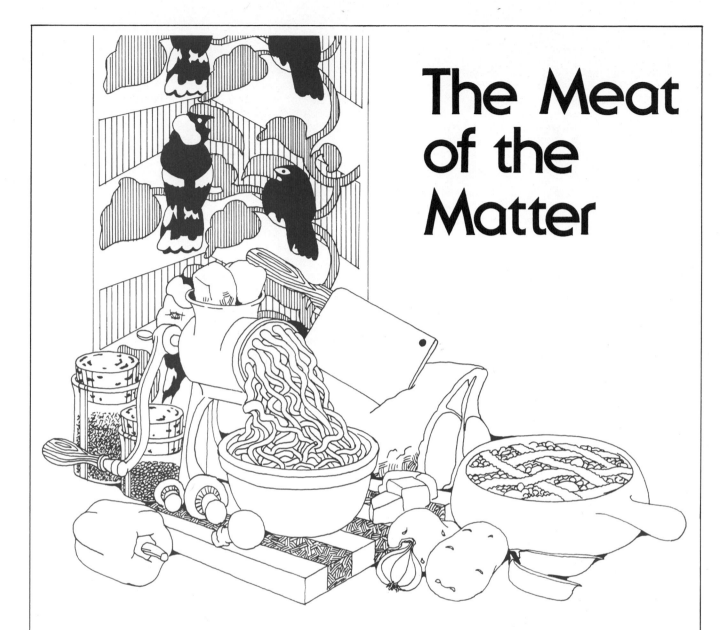

The Meat of the Matter

Meat! What red-blooded American doesn't love it? If you're like most homemakers, meat is the most expensive item in your food budget. It may also be the most costly category in your calorie budget. Many well-intentioned but misinformed dieters are wasting their money and calories on meat — too much and the wrong kind — in the mistaken notion that a high-meat diet is necessary to achieve slimness. Meat is good, yes. But too much of a good thing is not only fattening, it's boring!

How many of these fallacies about meat do you believe?

Fallacy: Meat is all protein, and the more you eat, the thinner you'll be.

Fact: Meat is only part protein. The rest is fat, and fat is the most fattening basic food there is. Some of the most popular cuts of meat have nearly five times as many fat calories as protein calories. And the more

calories you eat, the fatter you'll be.

Fallacy: You need meat every day.

Fact: Other animal foods are an equal or better source of complete protein. Eggs, skim milk, cottage cheese and yogurt are low-fat, low-calorie foods that are extra-rich in protein. Eight ounces of 99 percent fat-free cottage cheese alone is enough to satisfy most people's daily protein needs. Remember, meat is also balanced by the smaller amounts of less complete protein found in vegetable foods. Nuts and beans are especially rich in vegetable protein. And soy products such as soy flours, protein-enriched mixes and meat extenders are particularly important sources of inexpensive, low-calorie protein.

Fallacy: You can never eat too much meat.

Fact: Some steak-lovers may feel that way, but a superabundance of protein, especially meat protein, can be harmful. Meat contains cholesterol and saturated fat that have been implicated in heart disease. Too much protein in the diet is especially bad for anyone with latent kidney trouble. Recent studies have demonstrated that high-protein diets can upset calcium balance and accelerate osteoporosis, loss of bone tissue.

Fallacy: Simple steaks and roasts are better for calorie counters than combination dishes like stews or casseroles.

Fact: The cuts of meat most amenable to simple broiling or roasting are generally the most expensive, in calories as well as cost, while the leanest and least costly cuts are ideally suited to imaginative combinations and gourmet creations. And, since most of the other ingredients in casseroles are less fattening than meat, combination dishes allow dieters to satisfy their appetites with fewer calories. Of course, it's necessary to prepare these dishes in a way that eliminates excess fat.

Fallacy: Rare meat is less fattening than meat that is well done.

Fact: The longer meat is cooked, the more fat is melted out and eliminated, presuming that the fat is drained away or skimmed off. This does not mean that you should overcook an expensive porterhouse, but rather that you should concentrate on the less expensive, less fattening cuts, the kinds that are usually slow-simmered to a well-done tenderness.

Fallacy: Fat meat is juicy; lean meat is dry.

Fact: Fat meat is greasy, and because of its greasiness, fatty meat is better able to withstand the mishandling of too-high temperatures. Too-quick cooking at too-high temperatures robs lean meat of its juiciness.

Fallacy: Beef is less fattening than most other meats.

Fact: Many cuts of lamb, pork, and ham are lower in fat and calories than the most popular cuts of beef. Veal, poultry, and seafood are much more slimming.

How to Cook Meat

Broiling is the dry-heat method for quick cooking. When broiling, the heat source is above the meat.

1. Set your oven regulator for broiling, the highest heat.

2. Place the meat on a rack in your broiler pan 3 to 6 inches away from the heat. Thick cuts of meat should be placed further away from the heat.

3. Broil the meat until the top side is brown.

4. Sprinkle the browned surface with salt, pepper, and any other seasonings you desire.

5. Turn the meat and brown the other side. Make a small cut in the center of the meat to see if the desired doneness has been reached.

Barbecuing is another form of dry-heat cookery, usually done outdoors over glowing charcoal. Electric and gas barbecues are also available; some are built right into the kitchen. In barbecuing, the source of heat is beneath the meat. For best results, the meat should not be closer than 3 inches from the heat. When the meat is brown on one side, turn it with tongs and brown the other side.

Pan-broiling is yet another dry-heat method of cooking.

1. Place the meat in an uncovered nonstick skillet or griddle.

2. The pan may be sprinkled with a thin layer of salt or sprayed with vegetable coating for nonstick cooking. Do not add fat or water. Do not cover the pan.

3. Cook slowly over low heat, turning the meat occasionally.

4. Pour off or remove all fat as it accumulates.

5. Brown the meat on both sides, being careful not to overcook it.

6. Season the meat and serve it at once.

Oven-roasting is the slow method of dry cooking.

1. To achieve tenderness with lean cuts, treat the meat with meat tenderizer according to package directions; or for a more interesting flavor, marinate the meat for several hours. Check the index for a variety of marinade recipes.

2. Place the meat on a rack in an open shallow roasting pan.

3. Insert a meat thermometer so that the bulb or tip of the thermometer is in the center of the meat.

4. Do not add water and do not cover the pan.

5. Roast the meat in a slow oven, approximately 325°, to the desired degree of doneness. If you like your beef rare, roast it until the thermometer reads 140°; if medium is your taste, the thermometer should read 160°. Never allow the thermometer to reach more than 170°. Lamb is rare at 165° to 170°; medium at 174°; and well done at 180°. Pork should be roasted to an internal temperature of 170°.

6. Let the roast stand about 10 minutes before carving.

Braising or pot-roasting is the preferred method of moist-heat cooking. It is particularly suitable for less tender cuts of beef.

1. Brown the meat slowly on all sides in a heavy nonstick utensil without added fat. One low-cal method of browning is to add a tablespoon of water to the meat, cover the utensil, and heat it slowly over moderate heat. The water will evaporate, and the steam will cause the meat to release its own inner fat. Then, uncover the pot and let the meat brown in its own fat. The meat may also be browned under the broiler.

2. If you like, season the meat with salt, pepper, herbs, and spices.

3. Add a small amount of liquid such as water, wine, tomato juice, or fruit juice to the meat.

4. Cover the pot tightly, and cook the meat at a low temperature until it is tender.

5. You can make a sauce or gravy from the liquid in the pot if you like, but first skim the fat from the pan juices.

6. Pot roast is best made a day ahead, then refrigerated until about half-hour before serving time. The refrigeration will cause the fat that rises to the top to harden so it can be lifted off and discarded before the meat is reheated.

Simmering is another method of moist-heat cooking. This method requires more liquid than others and is used with cuts of meat that need longer cooking and more moisture to make them fork-tender.

1. If desired, brown the meat on all sides in a nonstick utensil without added fat. (See step 1 under Braising).

HOW DIFFERENT MEATS COMPARE IN CALORIES

Compare the typical calories in similar cuts from different animals. All calorie counts are for one pound of boneless meat, uncooked, and are derived from U.S. Department of Agriculture data* for "choice" or "medium-fat" grades of meat, the kind most frequently found in supermarkets. Individual cuts will vary.

	BEEF	VEAL	LAMB	PORK AND HAM
From the shoulder	Chuck	Shoulder	Shoulder	Boston Butt
Meat and fat	1,597	785	1,275	1,302
Lean only	853	629	671	816
From the rib	Rib Steak	Rib Chop	Rib Chop	Rib or Loin Chop
Meat and fat	1,819	939	1,252	1,352
Lean only	875	709	612	857
From the leg				
Meat and fat	894	744	1,007	1,397
Lean only	612	592	590	694

*All data approximate, adapted from U.S. Department of Agriculture information.

2. Cover the meat with water or other liquid like wine or juice.

3. Season with salt, pepper, herbs, and spices if you like.

4. Cover the pot and simmer the meat until it is tender. Do not boil.

5. For best results, cook the meat the day before serving and chill it overnight in the stock in which it was cooked. The fat will float to the top and harden, so it can be easily removed before reheating and serving the meat.

6. When vegetables are to be cooked with the meat, add them whole or in pieces after the fat has been removed, and cook them just until they are tender.

What's Your Beef?

Beef is America's favorite food. From filet mignon to hamburger to stew, beef proves its great versatility. You can boil it, broil it, braise it, fry it, and even eat it raw. And it is available in a wide range of prices. Fortunately for the weight-conscious millions, it is the less expensive cuts of beef that are the calorie bargains. Part of what makes prime beef "prime" is the marbling of fat throughout the meat — great for flavor, lousy for waistlines.

Recipes

Pot Roast Olé

2 tsp. diet margarine	1 tsp. chili powder
4-lb. lean boneless	1 tbsp. paprika
bottom round,	2 tsp. onion salt
trimmed of fat and	1/8 tsp. ground clove
rolled for pot roast	1/2 tsp. cinnamon
1/2 cup water	2 tbsp. flour

Melt margarine over low heat in a heavy, nonstick Dutch oven. Brown the meat slowly on all sides in the melted margarine. Add the water and seasonings to the pot. Cover and simmer the meat slowly about 2½ to 3 hours until tender. Remove the meat to a platter, and keep it warm.

Pour the pan drippings into a large measuring cup. Add water and ice cubes to bring it to 2 cups. When the ice cubes have melted and the fat has risen to the surface, skim off all the fat. Stir the flour into the cold drippings, and return it to the pot. Over low heat, cook and stir the liquid, scraping the pan well, until it simmers and thickens. *Makes 12 servings*

	Calories	Carbo-hydrate (gm)	Protein (gm)	Total Fat (gm)	Saturated Fat (gm)	Choles-terol (mg)
Total	3121.7	12.4	570.5	83.2	25.7	1682.7
Per Serving	260.1	1.0	47.5	6.9	2.1	140.2

gm = grams; mg = milligrams. Nutritional figures are approximate. Figures are based on findings of U.S. Department of Agriculture.

Cider-Spicy Pot Roast

3-lb. boneless top round roast, bottom or eye, trimmed of fat
1/4 cup cider vinegar
1 cup unsweetened cider
2 tbsp. mixed pickling spices
2 tsp. salt
1/8 tsp. pepper

Place the meat in a bowl. Combine all the other ingredients and pour over the meat. Cover the bowl and refrigerate for 24 hours. Transfer the meat and liquid into a heavy pot or Dutch oven. Simmer it over low heat, covered, for about 2 1/2 hours until the meat is tender; or roast it, covered, in a 350° oven for about 2 1/2 hours. Remove the meat to a serving platter. Using a bulb-type baster, skim all of the fat from the pan drippings. Simmer the remaining liquid, uncovered, until it is reduced to just enough to pour over the meat. Strain the reduced liquid, pour over the meat and serve.

Makes 10 servings

	Calories	Carbo-hydrate (gm)	Protein (gm)	Total Fat (gm)	Saturated Fat (gm)	Choles-terol (mg)
Total	2344.5	32.2	426.9	53.3	17.8	1262.4
Per Serving	234.5	3.2	42.7	5.3	1.8	126.2

Slim-but-Saucy Pot Roast

3-lb. beef arm pot roast, trimmed of fat
2 tsp. salt
1/8 tsp. pepper
2 medium onions, sliced
1/2 can (10 3/4-oz.) condensed cheddar cheese soup
8-oz. can tomato sauce
4-oz. can mushroom stems and pieces, undrained
1/4 tsp. oregano
1/4 tsp. basil

Place the pot roast in a nonstick roasting pan and roast it, uncovered, in a preheated 475° oven just until the meat is browned. Pour off the pan drippings that have accumulated and lower the oven temperature to 325°. Season the meat with the salt and pepper, and add the onions, cheese soup, tomato sauce, mushrooms, oregano, and basil to the pan. Cover the pan tightly, and roast the meat slowly for about 2 1/2 hours until it is tender. To serve, slice the meat thinly.

Makes 10 servings

	Calories	Carbo-hydrate (gm)	Protein (gm)	Total Fat (gm)	Saturated Fat (gm)	Choles-terol (mg)
Total	2574.9	51.5	442.4	65.7	23.8	1292.4
Per Serving	257.5	5.2	44.2	6.6	2.4	129.2

All Day Chuck Roast

3 tbsp. prepared mustard
3-lb. boneless chuck shoulder, trimmed of all fat
2 tbsp. Worcestershire sauce
2 tsp. salt (or onion salt or garlic salt)
1/8 tsp. coarse freshly ground pepper

Spread the mustard liberally over the surfaces of the meat. Sprinkle the Worcestershire sauce, salt, and pepper all over. Place the meat on a rack in a roasting pan. Slow-roast it, uncovered, at 225° for 5 hours or more — until the meat is tender. If you want a browner roast, you can place it under the broiler briefly just before serving — or you can raise the oven temperature to 450° for the last 20 minutes of roasting.

Makes 9 servings

	Calories	Carbo-hydrate (gm)	Protein (gm)	Total Fat (gm)	Saturated Fat (gm)	Choles-terol (mg)
Total	2570.5	87.0	426.7	53.3	17.8	1262.4
Per Serving	285.6	9.7	47.4	5.9	2.0	140.3

Burgundy Pot Roast

5-lb. boneless bottom round or rolled rump roast, trimmed of fat
2 cups sliced onion
2 garlic cloves, crushed
1 bay leaf
1/2 tsp. thyme
1 tsp. peppercorns
1 tsp. salt
2 cups Burgundy or any other dry red wine
10 1/2-oz. can beef broth
3 tbsp. flour

Put the meat in a stainless steel or glass bowl just large enough to hold the meat and onions. In a separate bowl combine the onions, garlic, herbs, peppercorns, salt, and wine. Pour this mixture over the meat. Cover the meat and refrigerate for 10 to 12 hours, turning occasionally. Skim fat from broth using a bulb-type baster.

Remove the meat from the marinade and pat it dry. Separate the onions from the marinade. Place the meat on a rack in a shallow roasting pan. Insert a meat thermometer so that the bulb is in the center of the roast. Roast the meat for 30 minutes in a preheated 475° oven, basting once or twice with the reserved marinade. Reduce the heat to 400°. Add the reserved onions to the pan and continue to roast the meat for 40 to 45 minutes, basting occasionally with the marinade. When the thermometer reaches 140° to 150°, remove the meat to a warm platter. Let it stand for about 15 minutes before carving.

Pour the pan drippings from the roasting pan into a container. Put the container in the freezer to cool it quickly, bringing the fat to the surface. Skim off the fat. On the top of the range, heat the pan drippings to boiling and boil 1 minute. In a separate bowl, combine the broth and flour, and add this mixture to the hot drippings. Continue to cook, stirring constantly, until the sauce is thick. Serve this over the sliced beef.

Makes 15 servings

	Calories	Carbo-hydrate (gm)	Protein (gm)	Total Fat (gm)	Saturated Fat (gm)	Choles-terol (mg)
Total	4300.3	60.3	724.1	89.1	29.6	2134.9
Per Serving	286.7	4.0	48.3	5.9	2.0	142.3

gm = grams; mg = milligrams. Nutritional figures are approximate. Figures are based on findings of U.S. Department of Agriculture.

Sauerbraten Get-Slim

1 cup cider vinegar	1½ tsp. pepper
1 cup red port wine	3-lb. boned top
1 cup sliced onion	round pot roast,
1 carrot, thinly sliced	trimmed of fat
1 stalk celery, sliced	2 tbsp. diet
3 whole allspice	margarine
6 whole cloves	2 tbsp. unsifted all-
¼ tsp. ground ginger	purpose flour
1 tbsp. salt	⅓ cup cold water

In a large bowl, combine the vinegar, wine, vegetables, spices, and seasonings. Add the meat to the marinade and refrigerate it, covered, for 3 days, turning the meat occasionally.

Remove the meat from the marinade and pat it dry with paper towels. Melt the margarine in a nonstick Dutch oven. Quickly brown the meat on all sides in the melted margarine. Add the marinade to the meat and simmer, covered, for 2½ hours or until the meat is tender.

Remove the meat from the pot. Press the liquid and vegetables through a coarse sieve, or whir them in a blender. Skim off the fat by using a bulb-type baster. Measure 3½ cups of liquid (add water, if necessary) and return this to the Dutch oven. In a separate bowl make a paste of the flour and water. Stir this into the liquid in the Dutch oven and heat to boiling. Return the meat to the Dutch oven and simmer, uncovered, for 15 minutes. Serve the meat, sliced thin, with the gravy.

Makes 10 servings

	Calories	Carbo-hydrate (gm)	Protein (gm)	Total Fat (gm)	Saturated Fat (gm)	Choles-terol (mg)
Total	2816.6	75.3	431.4	65.4	19.8	1262.4
Per Serving	281.7	7.5	43.1	6.5	2.0	126.2

Rare Roast Beef with Teriyaki Sauce

3-lb. lean boneless arm	1 cup unsweetened
roast, trimmed of fat	cider
Meat tenderizer	4 tbsp. soy sauce
Monosodium	1 tbsp. cornstarch
glutamate	¼ cup cold water

Sprinkle the meat with tenderizer and monosodium glutamate. Puncture well with a fork. Put the roast in a plastic bag and set it in a shallow dish. Combine the cider and soy sauce and pour into the bag. Secure the bag with a twist-tie and cover all surfaces of the meat with marinade. Refrigerate 8 hours or longer, up to two days.

Empty the meat and marinade into a small ovenproof baking dish. Insert a meat thermometer into the meat. Bake uncovered at 275° until thermometer indicates 140° for rare, or 150° to 160° for medium, about 2 hours. Don't overcook! Drain the liquid from the pan into a tall glass. Spoon off all fat that rises to the surface. Pour the liquid into a saucepan and heat to boiling. Combine the cornstarch and cold water and stir into the hot liquid. Cook and stir until thickened. Brown the surface of the meat briefly under the broiler. Slice the meat thinly against the grain and serve with sauce.

Makes 10 servings

	Calories	Carbo-hydrate (gm)	Protein (gm)	Total Fat (gm)	Saturated Fat (gm)	Choles-terol (mg)
Total	2404.4	39.5	430.7	53.3	17.8	1262.3
Per Serving	240.4	4.0	43.1	5.3	1.8	126.2

Savory Swiss Steak

1 tbsp. diet margarine	1 cup chopped
2-lb. boneless round	onions
steak, trimmed of	3 cups canned
fat	stewed tomatoes
1 tsp. garlic salt	1 cup chopped
⅛ tsp. pepper	celery

Place the margarine in a nonstick skillet and melt over moderate heat. Add the steak to the pan. Season the meat with the garlic salt and pepper. Raise the heat under the pan to high and brown the meat quickly on both sides. Lower the heat, and before going any further, pour off any fat that has accumulated in the pan. Then add the onions, tomatoes, and celery to the meat and cover the skillet tightly. Simmer — do not boil — over very low heat for 1½ hours or more until the meat is tender and the sauce is thick.

Makes 8 servings

	Calories	Carbo-hydrate (gm)	Protein (gm)	Total Fat (gm)	Saturated Fat (gm)	Choles-terol (mg)
Total	1987.9	46.0	287.9	62.3	27.7	826.5
Per Serving	248.5	5.8	36.0	7.8	3.5	103.3

Smothered Baked Steak

3-lb. lean beef round	3 tbsp. Worcester-
steak, cut 2-in. thick	shire sauce
and trimmed of fat	2 tbsp. lemon juice
½ tsp. salt	1 clove garlic,
¼ tsp. pepper	minced
1 cup unsweetened	4-oz. can sliced
pineapple juice	mushrooms
6-oz. can tomato paste	2 large onions,
	sliced

Place the steak on a rack in a shallow roasting pan; brown under the broiler. Drain the fat. Season with salt and pepper. Combine all the other ingredients. Pour over the meat. Roast uncovered in a preheated 325° oven for 1½ to 2 hours. Cut the meat diagonally. Serve with the pan juices.

Makes 12 servings

	Calories	Carbo-hydrate (gm)	Protein (gm)	Total Fat (gm)	Saturated Fat (gm)	Choles-terol (mg)
Total	3022 7	102.0	434.7	80.0	40.0	1240.0
Per serving	251.9	8.5	36.2	6.7	3.3	103.3

gm = grams; mg = milligrams. Nutritional figures are approximate. Figures are based on findings of U.S. Department of Agriculture.

Braciola Romano (Italian Beef Roll)

1-lb. lean beef round, sliced thin for rolling and trimmed of fat
1 cup dry 99% fat-free cottage cheese
2 tbsp. freshly-grated extra-sharp Romano cheese
3 tbsp. finely minced onion

3 tbsp. chopped Italian parsley
1 egg
2 tsp. oregano
1/2 tsp. salt or garlic salt
Pinch of red pepper flakes
1 cup tomato sauce
1/4 cup Chianti or other dry red wine (or water)

Lay the beef out flat. Combine the cottage cheese, Romano, onion, parsley, egg, oregano, salt and pepper in a small bowl. Spread the filling on top of the beef. Roll the beef over the filling. Tuck in the ends. Place the roll seam side down in a shallow baking dish just large enough to hold it. Combine the tomato sauce and wine or water. (You may add additional onion and oregano if you wish.) Pour over beef roll. Place in a preheated 350° oven and bake 1 hour, uncovered, basting occasionally. *Makes 5 servings*

	Calories	Carbo-hydrate (gm)	Protein (gm)	Total Fat (gm)	Saturated Fat (gm)	Choles-terol (mg)
Total	1454.2	34.4	184.4	38.6	18.5	684.5
Per Serving	290.8	6.9	36.9	7.7	3.7	136.9

Minute Steaks alla Parmigiana

4 tbsp. grated Parmesan cheese
1/3 cup bread crumbs
6 minute steaks, 4 oz. each
1 tbsp. olive oil

8-oz. can tomato sauce
Garlic salt to taste (optional)
3 (1-oz.) slices part-skim mozzarella cheese
1 tsp. oregano

Combine the grated Parmesan and the bread crumbs in a paper bag. Put the steaks in the bag, 1 at a time, and shake the bag until the steaks are well coated with the crumb mixture. Heat the oil in a nonstick skillet over high heat. Add the meat and quickly brown it on both sides. Arrange the meat in a baking dish, and pour the tomato sauce over all. Sprinkle the meat with garlic salt according to your own taste. Cut the mozzarella slices in half and place 1 half atop each steak. Sprinkle the oregano all over. Bake the meat in a preheated 375° oven for about 10 minutes — until the cheese is bubbly. *Makes 6 servings*

Hint: Olive oil is the favorite of Italian cooks. But calorie-conscious cooks can save 75 calories (about 12 per serving) by substituting diet margarine for olive oil.

	Calories	Carbo-hydrate (g)	Protein (gm)	Total Fat (gm)	Saturated Fat (gm)	Choles-terol (mg)
Total	2168.4	44.6	291.3	92.7	37.3	740.5
Per Serving	361.4	7.4	48.6	15.5	6.2	123.4

Savory Beef Roll

2-lb. round steak or flank steak, pounded to 1/4-in. thickness
1/4 cup fresh lemon juice
2 tbsp. soy sauce
2 garlic cloves, minced
1/2 tsp. pepper
1/2 lb. cooked smoked ham, sliced in strips

2 hard-cooked eggs, sliced
2 tbsp. raisins
6 green olives, chopped
2 cups water
1 medium onion, sliced
1/4 cup cider vinegar
8-oz. can tomato sauce

Spread the pounded beef out flat. Sprinkle the surface with the lemon juice, soy sauce, minced garlic, and pepper. Spread the ham strips and egg slices evenly over the meat. Sprinkle the raisins and chopped olives over all. Beginning at a narrow end, carefully roll up the beef, tucking in the ends. Tie the roll with string. Place the rolled beef in a deep skillet or pan, and add the water, sliced onions, vinegar, and tomato sauce. Cover the pan tightly, and simmer the meat slowly for about 1 hour, or until it is tender when a fork is inserted into it. To serve, slice the rolled beef crosswise and serve it with the sauce from the pan.

Makes 10 servings

	Calories	Carbo-hydrate (gm)	Protein (gm)	Total Fat (gm)	Saturated Fat (gm)	Choles-terol (mg)
Total	2779.2	52.1	347.3	120.2	49.3	1532.7
Per Serving	277.9	5.2	34.7	12.0	4.9	153.3

Slim-Down Steak Diane

1/2 tsp. dry mustard
1/4 tsp. garlic salt
1/8 tsp. coarse freshly ground pepper
1 1/2-lb. lean boneless sirloin steak, 1/2-in. thick, trimmed of fat
2 tsp. corn or safflower oil

1 tbsp. chopped chives
1 tbsp. lemon juice
2 tsp. Worcestershire sauce
3 tbsp. brandy

Mix the dry mustard, salt, and pepper together. Sprinkle this mixture over 1 side of the steak and rub it in. Pour the oil into a nonstick skillet and heat it over medium heat. Rotate the pan to spread the oil evenly. Add the steak to the skillet and brown about 1 1/2 minutes on each side. Sprinkle the chives, lemon juice and Worcestershire sauce into the skillet. Heat the brandy in a small saucepan over low heat; or it can be heated at the table over a candle warmer. Bring the steak to the table in the skillet. Pour the brandy over the steak and ignite it. When the flame goes out, transfer the steak to a serving platter. *Makes 6 servings*

	Calories	Carbo-hydrate (gm)	Protein (gm)	Total Fat (gm)	Saturated Fat (gm)	Choles-terol (mg)
Total	1619.6	2.0	216.4	57.2	22.0	612.0
Per Serving	269.9	0.3	36.1	9.5	3.7	102.0

gm = grams; mg = milligrams. Nutritional figures are approximate. Figures are based on findings of U.S. Department of Agriculture.

Beef and Asparagus Stir-fry

2 tbsp. soy sauce
1 tbsp. dry white wine
1 garlic clove, minced
1/4 tsp. ground ginger
1-lb. flank steak, sliced
  diagonally across
  the grain in 1-in.
  strips
1 tbsp. diet
  margarine
1 lb. asparagus, cut
  in 2-in. pieces
1 cup beef broth
1 1/2 tbsp. cornstarch

In a ceramic bowl, mix together the soy sauce, wine, garlic, ginger, and beef. Let this mixture sit uncovered at room temperature for 1 hour. Melt the diet margarine in a nonstick skillet over moderate heat. Add the meat (save marinade), and brown it quickly on all sides. Add the asparagus to the skillet, and stir-fry with the meat for 3 minutes. In a bowl, mix together the broth, cornstarch, and reserved marinade; stir this mixture into the skillet. Cook the entire mixture over moderate heat, stirring constantly, until the sauce has thickened. *Makes 4 servings*

	Calories	Carbo-hydrate (gm)	Protein (gm)	Total Fat (gm)	Saturated Fat (gm)	Choles-terol (mg)
Total	1139.7	45.3	154.6	32.4	14.2	433.2
Per Serving	284.9	11.3	38.7	8.1	3.6	108.3

Steak Oriental

1 tbsp. diet margarine
1-lb. boneless round
  steak or roast,
  trimmed of fat and
  cut in thin strips
2 tbsp. finely chopped
  onion
1 garlic clove, chopped
2 large green peppers,
  sliced into strips
1/2 cup celery, diagonally
  sliced
1/2 cup beef
  consommé
1/2 tsp. salt
1/4 tsp. pepper
2 tbsp. chopped
  pimiento
2 tsp. cornstarch
3 tbsp. water
1 tsp. soy sauce

Place the diet margarine in a nonstick skillet and melt it over low heat. Add the strips of beef and brown on both sides. Pour off any drippings that have accumulated in the pan, then add the onion, garlic, green peppers, and celery. Add the consommé and season the whole mixture with salt and pepper. Cover the skillet tightly and simmer the meat for 20 minutes. Do not boil it. Add the pimiento. Blend cornstarch, water, and soy sauce. Stir into skillet to thicken mixture. Simmer, covered, for an additional 5 minutes. *Makes 4 servings*

	Calories	Carbo-hydrate (gm)	Protein (gm)	Total Fat (gm)	Saturated Fat (gm)	Choles-terol (mg)
Total	1001.4	17.9	145.2	32.8	14.3	424.9
Per Serving	250.4	4.5	36.3	8.2	3.6	106.2

Tangy Steak Bake

1 tbsp. diet margarine
1 1/2-lb. lean, 1/2-in. thick
  round steak,
  trimmed of fat and
  cut in 6 pieces
12 small white onions
1 tsp. salt
1/2 tsp. pepper
1/8 tsp. allspice
1 cup unsweetened
  pineapple juice
1/4 cup vinegar
1 cup canned
  tomatoes

Place the diet margarine in a nonstick skillet and melt it over low heat. Add the steak and onions to the skillet and sauté until they are brown. Then transfer the meat and onions to a roasting pan. Combine salt, pepper, allspice, pineapple juice, vinegar and tomatoes in a bowl. Pour over the meat and onions. Place the roasting pan, uncovered, and roast in a preheated 325° oven 1 1/4 hours. *Makes 6 servings*

	Calories	Carbo-hydrate (gm)	Protein (gm)	Total Fat (gm)	Saturated Fat (gm)	Choles-terol (mg)
Total	1777.2	107.5	223.0	47.0	21.0	620.0
Per Serving	296.2	17.9	37.2	7.8	3.5	103.3

gm = grams; mg = milligrams. Nutritional figures are approximate. Figures are based on findings of U.S. Department of Agriculture.

Versatile Veal

Unlike luxury foods, veal is one extravagance the calorie counter can afford — if the budget permits. While the price per pound is high compared with other meats, veal is actually a better bargain than simple price comparisons might indicate. Veal's relative lack of fat (and fat calories) means a corresponding increase in protein content. And protein, after all, is why you feed your family meat in the first place.

Veal, of course, is baby beef. The best veal comes from animals 4 to 14 weeks old, weighing 100 pounds or less. Because of its tender age, veal is naturally tasty and tender without the fatty marbling of mature beef.

Compare the calorie, fat, and protein content of similar cuts of beef and veal, and you'll see why veal is often a better buy for dieters.

BEEF AND VEAL COMPARISONS

	Protein	Fat	Calories*
Veal chuck	19%	10%	173
Beef chuck	16%	31%	352
Veal rib chops	19%	14%	207
Beef rib steak	14%	43%	444
Veal loin chops	19%	11%	181
Beef porterhouse	15%	36%	390
Veal shank	20%	8%	156
Beef shank	18%	23%	289
Veal rump	19%	9%	164
Beef rump	17%	25%	303

*Per 100 grams (approximately 3½ ounces). All data approximate, adapted from U.S. Department of Agriculture information.

Veal's sophisticated flavor is subtly accented by the judicious use of lemon or wine and herbs, or garlic, cheese, and tomato for more robust dishes. Because of its leanness, veal is at its best when gently cooked; scallopini sautéed lightly in a nonstick skillet, for example, or a tender, rolled rump slow-roasted at low temperature. The less tender cuts of veal can be creatively seasoned and slow-simmered in wine or tomato juice. Under no circumstances, however, should veal be carelessly tossed into a hot frying pan, seared in a hot oven, or scorched under the broiler. Only the tiniest, most tender chops can be broiled or barbecued and then only with patience and care.

Recipes

Veal Marlene

2 tbsp. diet margarine	1 chicken bouillon
2 lb. boneless veal,	cube
trimmed of fat and	2 tbsp. instant
cut in 1-in. cubes	onions
2 tbsp. all-purpose flour	2 strips lemon peel
½ tsp. salt	1 cup boiling water
¼ tsp. pepper	½ cup evaporated
	skim milk

Melt the margarine in a large nonstick skillet. Add the veal and brown it slowly. Then sprinkle the flour, salt, and pepper over the veal. Add the bouillon cube, onion, lemon peel, and 1 cup of boiling water. Cover the skillet and simmer the mixture 30 to 45 minutes until the meat is tender. Remove the lemon peel and discard it. Add the evaporated milk, and continue to cook the mixture until the milk is heated through.

Makes 8 servings

	Calories	Carbo-hydrate (gm)	Protein (gm)	Total Fat (gm)	Saturated Fat (gm)	Choles-terol (mg)
Total	1548.6	48.9	202.4	71.9	30.8	679.2
Per Serving	193.6	6.1	25.3	9.0	3.9	84.9

Veal Pago-Pago

10½-oz. can beef broth	½ cup chopped onion
1 tbsp. diet margarine	½ tsp. salt
1½ lb. lean boneless veal	Dash of pepper
(shoulder or leg),	1 cup sliced celery
trimmed of fat and	2 tbsp. cornstarch
cut in 1-in. cubes	3 tbsp. soy sauce
2 cups juice-packed	2 tbsp. vinegar
unsweetened	½ lb. fresh
pineapple tidbits,	mushrooms,
drained reserving	sliced
juice	

Chill the broth until the fat rises to the top, hardens, and can be lifted away; or skim off the fat using a bulb-type baster.

Melt the margarine in a nonstick skillet. Add the veal and brown it on all sides. Add the pineapple juice, onion, salt, and pepper and pour the broth over all. Cover the skillet and simmer the mixture for 50 minutes. Then add the celery and continue to simmer the mixture, covered, for about 10 minutes until the meat is tender. In a separate bowl, mix together the cornstarch, soy sauce, and vinegar. Stir this into the hot mixture, and cook until the sauce becomes thick and bubbly. Then mix the pineapple and mushrooms into the thickened mixture. *Makes 6 servings*

	Calories	Carbo-hydrate (gm)	Protein (gm)	Total Fat (gm)	Saturated Fat (gm)	Choles-terol (mg)
Total	1536.3	129.1	67.7	38.0	17.0	542.8
Per Serving	256.1	21.5	28.0	6.3	2.8	90.5

Mini-Calorie Veal Marengo

1 lb. lean boneless veal	½ cup dry sherry
from leg or	8-oz. can stewed
shoulder, trimmed	tomatoes
of fat and cut in 1½-	1 cup water
in. cubes	1 tbsp. lemon juice
½ tsp. garlic salt	4-oz. can
⅛ tsp. pepper	mushrooms,
10½-oz. can French onion	drained
soup, skimmed of	
fat	

Spray a nonstick skillet with vegetable coating. Season the meat with garlic salt and pepper and brown it in the skillet over moderate heat. Add all the remaining ingredients, except the mushrooms. Cover the skillet and simmer the contents over low heat for 50 to 60 minutes until the meat is tender. Then uncover the pan and add the mushrooms. Raise the heat to moderate and continue to cook the mixture, uncovered, until the liquid has been reduced to a thick sauce.

Makes 4 servings

	Calories	Carbo-hydrate (gm)	Protein (gm)	Total Fat (gm)	Saturated Fat (gm)	Choles-terol (mg)
Total	995.2	36.3	108.4	27.5	10.7	382.6
Per Serving	248.8	9.1	27.1	6.9	2.7	95.7

gm = grams; mg = milligrams. Nutritional figures are approximate. Figures are based on findings of U.S. Department of Agriculture.

Veal Goulash

1 tbsp. diet margarine
2-lb. lean veal shoulder, trimmed of fat and cut in 1-in. cubes
2 onions, sliced
16-oz. can whole peeled Italian tomatoes in purée

1½ tsp. salt
1 tbsp. paprika
¼ tsp. pepper
1 tsp. caraway seeds

Melt the margarine in a large nonstick skillet. Brown the meat slowly in the melted margarine; then add the remaining ingredients. Heat the mixture to boiling. Then lower the heat, cover the pan and simmer for 1¼ hours, or until the meat is tender. *Makes 8 servings*

	Calories	Carbo-hydrate (gm)	Protein (gm)	Total Fat (gm)	Saturated Fat (gm)	Choles-terol (mg)
Total	1414.4	40.0	189.4	50.7	22.3	640.2
Per Serving	176.8	5.0	23.7	6.3	2.8	80.0

Tangy Veal Spareribs

2½-lean breast of veal, trimmed of fat and cut in 8 individual ribs
1½ cups salt-free tomato juice

¼ cup cider vinegar
1 cup unsweetened applesauce
3 tbsp. soy sauce

Place the ribs in a roasting pan in a single layer. Bake them, uncovered, in a preheated 425° oven for 20 to 25 minutes — just to brown them and remove the excess fat. Pour off all the fat that accumulates in the pan. Then combine the remaining ingredients and pour them over the ribs. Lower the oven temperature to 350°, return the meat to the oven and bake it, covered, for about 1½ hours until the veal is tender, basting occasionally.

Makes 8 servings

	Calories	Carbo-hydrate (gm)	Protein (gm)	Total Fat (gm)	Saturated Fat (gm)	Choles-terol (mg)
Total	1681.1	48.0	233.6	53.3	26.7	799.8
Per Serving	210.1	6.0	29.2	6.7	3.3	100.0

Super-Slimming Casserole

1 tbsp. diet margarine
2-lb. lean veal shoulder, trimmed of fat and cut in 1½-in. cubes
4-oz. can sliced mushrooms, drained

10½-oz. can condensed cream of chicken soup

Melt the margarine in a heavy oven-safe pan. Add the veal and mushrooms and brown them slowly. Pour off any fat that has accumulated in the pan before going any further. Then add soup. Cover the pan and bake the veal at 350° for 1 hour or more until the meat is tender. *Makes 8 servings*

	Calories	Carbo-hydrate (gm)	Protein (gm)	Total Fat (gm)	Saturated Fat (gm)	Choles-terol (mg)
Total	1503.4	24.0	191.7	64.5	24.9	666.4
Per Serving	188.0	3.0	24.0	8.1	3.1	83.3

Skinny Schnitzel

2 tbsp. diet margarine
1½-lb. veal round steak, ¾-inch thick, trimmed of fat
1 envelope or 1 cube chicken or beef bouillon

½ cup boiling water
3 tbsp. lemon juice
½ tsp. butter-flavored salt
⅛ tsp. pepper
¼ cup chopped parsley

Melt the margarine over moderate heat in a large nonstick skillet. Add the veal and brown it on both sides. Dissolve the bouillon in ½ cup boiling water and add this to the skillet. At the same time, add the lemon juice, salt, and pepper. Cover the pan and bring the mixture to boiling. Lower the heat and simmer the meat for about 30 minutes until it is tender. Then stir in the parsley. Remove the steak to a serving platter, and pour the pan juices over it. *Makes 6 servings*

	Calories	Carbo-hydrate (gm)	Protein (gm)	Total Fat (gm)	Saturated Fat (gm)	Choles-terol (mg)
Total	1008.4	3.8	137.2	44.0	18.0	483.0
Per Serving	168.0	0.6	22.9	7.3	3.0	80.5

Low-Fat Veal Parmigiana

1½-lb. lean veal round (thinly sliced), trimmed of fat and cut in 6 pieces
¼ cup bread crumbs
1 tbsp. diet margarine
16-oz. can tomato sauce

2 tsp. Italian seasoning or oregano
1½ tsp. garlic salt
⅛ tsp. pepper
3 oz. part-skim mozzarella cheese, sliced

Dip the veal pieces in the bread crumbs until they are lightly coated. Melt the margarine in a large nonstick skillet. Add the coated veal and brown it slowly, turning once. Remove the veal from the skillet, and arrange it in a single layer in a shallow baking dish. Spoon the tomato sauce over the veal. Then season it with Italian seasoning, garlic salt, and pepper. Top the veal with the mozzarella slices. Bake uncovered in a preheated 350° oven for 20 to 25 minutes, until the cheese is melted and bubbly. *Makes 6 servings*

	Calories	Carbo-hydrate (gm)	Protein (gm)	Total Fat (gm)	Saturated Fat (gm)	Choles-terol (mg)
Total	1411.3	52.9	190.7	55.1	20.3	535.3
Per Serving	235.2	8.8	31.8	9.2	3.4	89.2

gm = grams; mg = milligrams. Nutritional figures are approximate. Figures are based on findings of U.S. Department of Agriculture.

Veal Stroganoff Size Nine

1 tbsp. diet margarine
1½-lb. boneless veal
   shoulder, trimmed
   of fat and cut in thin
   strips
1 tsp. salt
¼ tsp. pepper
½ lb. fresh mushrooms,
   sliced

1 medium onion,
   sliced
⅓ cup sauterne
2 potatoes, peeled
   and sliced
1 tbsp. flour
⅔ cup buttermilk

Melt the margarine in a large nonstick skillet. Season veal with salt and pepper, then add to skillet along with mushrooms and onion. Brown them slowly. Then add the sauterne and potatoes. Cover the pan and simmer for 10 to 15 minutes — until the potatoes are tender. In a separate bowl, mix together the flour and buttermilk. Add this to the skillet and continue cooking and stirring until the mixture has thickened. Then simmer for 3 more minutes. *Makes 6 servings*

	Calories	Carbo-hydrate (gm)	Protein (gm)	Total Fat (gm)	Saturated Fat (gm)	Choles-terol (mg)
Total	1459.3	90.1	166.2	40.6	17.0	483.3
Per Serving	243.2	15.0	27.7	6.8	2.8	80.6

Veal Provençal Petite

10½-oz. can chicken
   consommé
8-oz. can boiled whole
   onions
8-oz. can small carrots
8-oz. can potatoes
4-oz. can mushroom
   caps
2 tsp. diet margarine

1 lb. lean boneless
   veal, trimmed of fat
   and cut in 1-in.
   cubes
Salt
Pepper
2 tbsp.
   Worcestershire
   sauce
1 bay leaf
½ cup dry white wine

Chill the consommé until the fat rises to the top, hardens, and can be lifted off; or skim off the fat by using a bulb-type baster. Drain canned vegetables reserving liquid.

Melt the margarine in a large nonstick skillet. Season the veal with salt and pepper and brown it in the melted margarine. Add the consommé, Worcestershire sauce, bay leaf, wine, and the liquid from all the canned vegetables. Cover the skillet and simmer the mixture over very low heat for 1 hour or more until the meat is tender. Then uncover the pan and add the vegetables. Raise the heat to moderate and continue to simmer the mixture, uncovered, until nearly all of the liquid is evaporated. *Makes 4 servings*

	Calories	Carbo-hydrate (gm)	Protein (gm)	Total Fat (gm)	Saturated Fat (gm)	Choles-terol (mg)
Total	1039.1	68.7	108.5	25.3	11.4	356.4
Per Serving	259.8	17.2	27.1	6.3	2.9	89.1

Hungarian Veal Chops

1 cup chicken broth
1 tbsp. diet margarine
6 veal loin chops, ¾
   inch thick, trimmed
   of fat
½ cup sliced onion

1 tbsp. paprika
1½ tsp. butter-flavored
   salt
¼ tsp. pepper
⅔ cup plain low-fat
   yogurt

Chill the chicken broth until the fat has risen to the top, hardens, and can be lifted off; or skim off the fat, using a bulb-type baster.

Melt the margarine in a large nonstick skillet. Add the chops and brown them well on both sides. Add the onion and sauté the meat and onion a few minutes longer. Pour the chicken broth over the chops and sprinkle the paprika, salt, and pepper over all. Cover the skillet and simmer the chops 20 to 30 minutes until they are nearly tender. Uncover the skillet and continue to simmer the veal for about 10 minutes until most of the liquid has evaporated. Then stir in the yogurt. Cook the mixture for 1 to 2 minutes longer until the yogurt is heated, but be careful not to let it boil. *Makes 6 servings*

	Calories	Carbo-hydrate (gm)	Protein (gm)	Total Fat (gm)	Saturated Fat (gm)	Choles-terol (mg)
Total	1238.5	15.6	145.3	64.6	26.3	506.7
Per Serving	206.4	2.6	24.2	10.8	4.4	84.5

Baked Veal Chops Risotto

1 tbsp. diet margarine
6 lean veal loin chops,
   ¾ to 1 inch thick,
   trimmed of fat
6 tbsp. uncooked rice
16-oz. can tomatoes,
   drained
   reserving liquid
1 medium onion cut into
   6 slices

1 medium green
   pepper, sliced
   into 6 strips
¼ tsp. garlic salt
⅛ tsp. pepper
¼ tsp. oregano

Melt the margarine in a large nonstick skillet. Add the chops and brown them slowly on both sides. Remove the chops from the skillet and place them in a large baking dish. On top of each chop put 1 tbsp. of uncooked rice, some of the tomatoes, 1 slice of onion, and 1 piece of green pepper. Sprinkle with garlic salt, pepper, and oregano. Cover the chops with the liquid from the tomatoes. Cover the baking dish and bake the chops in a preheated 350° oven for 1½ hours. *Makes 6 servings*

	Calories	Carbo-hydrate (gm)	Protein (gm)	Total Fat (gm)	Saturated Fat (gm)	Choles-terol (mg)
Total	1878.7	90.6	193.0	83.1	33.0	640.2
Per Serving	313.1	15.1	32.2	13.9	5.5	106.7

gm = grams; mg = milligrams. Nutritional figures are approximate. Figures are based on findings of U.S. Department of Agriculture.

Calorie-Conscious Cordon Bleu

1 lb. veal for scallopini (from leg), trimmed of fat and cut in 8 pieces
3 oz. part-skim pizza cheese, thinly sliced
3 oz. Canadian bacon, thinly sliced
1/4 cup seasoned bread crumbs
1 tsp. corn oil

Pound the veal slices with a meat tenderizer to make them as thin as possible. Top each piece with a slice of cheese and a slice of bacon. Then top each with another slice of veal to make 4 veal "sandwiches." Combine the bread crumbs with the oil, and brush the mixture lightly on both sides of the sandwiches. Place them on a cookie sheet. Bake in a preheated 350° oven for about 25 minutes until the veal is cooked and the cheese melts. *Makes 4 servings*

	Calories	Carbo-hydrate (gm)	Protein (gm)	Total Fat (gm)	Saturated Fat (gm)	Choles-terol (mg)
Total	1196.4	19.9	161.9	57.3	18.3	446.1
Per Serving	299.1	5.0	40.5	14.3	4.6	111.5

Veal Piccata

1 tbsp. diet margarine
1 1/2 lb. lean veal for scallopini, trimmed of fat and cut in 6 pieces
1 envelope or cube chicken bouillon
1/2 cup dry white wine
1/4 cup water
1 lemon, sliced
6 sprigs parsley

Melt the margarine in a large nonstick skillet. Add the veal and brown it quickly on both sides. Remove the veal to a platter. Stir the bouillon, wine, water, and juice of 1 lemon half into the skillet, scraping the pan to loosen the brown bits. Return the veal to the pan and cook it over high heat for about 5 minutes until it is tender. Return the veal to the serving platter and garnish it with slices of the remaining lemon and parsley sprigs. *Makes 6 servings*

	Calories	Carbo-hydrate (gm)	Protein (gm)	Total Fat (gm)	Saturated Fat (gm)	Choles-terol (mg)
Total	1041.9	23.1	145.0	45.0	19.0	480.0
Per Serving	173.7	3.9	24.2	7.5	3.2	80.0

Learning about Lamb

Once upon a time, lamb was seasonal meat available mainly in the spring. Today lamb is here year-round for patio cookout or a fireside supper.

Lamb is a lean and luscious main course for dieters. It wears most of its fat on the outside, where it is easily trimmable by the calorie-wise cook. Because lamb is young and succulent, it doesn't need fatty marbling to provide tenderness.

If you've served lamb well done and have been disappointed in its taste or texture, next time try it European-style. Broil or sauté it so there's still a tinge of inner pinkness, or roast it to an internal temperature of only about 165°. Lamb is rare at 165° to 170°, medium at 174°, and well done at 180°.

Lamb is just as versatile as beef. Large tender cuts like leg, sirloin, loin, rack, crown, and shoulder can be oven roasted. And smaller cuts such as leg or sirloin steaks, chops, and fat-trimmed ground patties can be broiled, barbecued, or sautéed. (Steaks are the lowest in calories.) The less tender, less expensive cuts of lamb can be braised or simmered to scrumptious tenderness. To check on how to use any of these cooking methods, turn to The Meat of the Matter.

Recipes

Herbed Lamb Chops

2 tbsp. flour
1 tsp. dry mustard
1/2 tsp. salt
1/4 tsp. thyme
1/8 tsp. oregano
8 loin lamb chops, 1-in. thick, trimmed of fat

Mix the flour, mustard, salt, thyme, and oregano together in a paper bag. Add the lamb chops, a few at a time and shake the bag until they are coated with the flour mixture. Place the coated chops on a rack on a broiling pan placed 3 to 4 inches from the heat source. Broil about 7 minutes on each side, or until the desired doneness is reached. *Makes 8 servings*

	Calories	Carbo-hydrate (gm)	Protein (gm)	Total Fat (gm)	Saturated Fat (gm)	Choles-terol (mg)
Total	3259.2	12.4	201.7	264.1	144.0	1072.0
Per Serving	407.4	1.6	25.2	33.0	18.0	134.0

gm = grams; mg = milligrams Nutritional figures are approximate. Figures are based on findings of U.S. Department of Agriculture.

Baked Lamb Chops with Rice

8 lamb shoulder chops, 1-in. thick, trimmed of fat
1 cup uncooked rice
2 medium onions, sliced
2 medium green peppers, sliced
16-oz. can tomatoes
10½-oz. can beef bouillon or broth

Place the lamb chops under the broiler until they are just brown. Place the rice in a baking dish. Then cover the rice with chops, onion, green pepper, and tomatoes. Pour the bouillon over all. Cover the baking dish, and bake the meat and vegetables in a preheated 350° oven for 1½ hours. *Makes 8 servings*

	Calories	Carbo-hydrate (gm)	Protein (gm)	Total Fat (gm)	Saturated Fat (gm)	Choles-terol (mg)
Total	4159.2	204.9	235.2	267.0	144.0	1135.4
Per Serving	519.9	25.6	29.4	33.4	18.0	141.9

Colorado Lamb Stew

1 tbsp. diet margarine
1 lb. lean lamb shoulder, trimmed of fat and cut in 2-in. cubes
1 cup sliced onion
2 tsp. salt
¼ tsp. coarse, freshly ground pepper
¾ tsp. ground allspice
¼ tsp. ground ginger
½ cup water
1 tbsp. flour
8-oz. can tomato sauce
1-lb. can carrots, undrained

Melt the margarine in a large nonstick skillet or saucepan. Add the meat and brown it on all sides. Add the onion and brown lightly. Drain off any fat that has accumulated in the pan. Then stir in the salt, pepper, allspice, ginger, and ½ cup water. Cover the pot tightly, and simmer the mixture for about 2 hours. If necessary, add more water during the simmering period. Using a bulb-type baster, skim the fat from the pan juices. Blend 2 tablespoons cold water into the flour and add this mixture to the meat. Also add the tomato sauce and carrots. Continue to cook the stew, uncovered, until it has thickened, about 15 minutes. *Makes 6 servings*

	Calories	Carbo-hydrate (gm)	Protein (gm)	Total Fat (gm)	Saturated Fat (gm)	Choles-terol (mg)
Total	1158.8	64.2	138.6	38.5	20.2	454.4
Per Serving	193.1	10.7	23.1	6.4	3.4	75.7

Lamb Rib Barbecue

3-lb. breast of lamb, trimmed of fat and sliced into ribs
6-oz. can tomato paste
½ cup apple juice
2 tbsp. cider vinegar
1 medium onion, sliced
1 tsp. salt
¼ tsp. pepper
⅛ tsp. hot pepper sauce

Place the lamb riblets on a rack in a shallow roasting pan. Bake in a preheated 325° oven for about 1½ hours. Drain off the fat that has accumulated in the pan before going any further. Then combine the remaining ingredients in a bowl and mix well. Brush some of this sauce over the riblets, and continue baking for 1½ hours more, basting occasionally with the sauce. Turn the riblets twice to coat the underside. *Makes 9 servings*

	Calories	Carbo-hydrate (gm)	Protein (gm)	Total Fat (gm)	Saturated Fat (gm)	Choles-terol (mg)
Total	2249.5	57.3	249.7	108.0	63.0	900.0
Per Serving	249.1	6.4	27.7	12.0	7.0	100.0

Low-Cal Kebabs

1½ lb. lean boneless leg of lamb, trimmed of fat and cut in 1-in. cubes
⅓ cup fresh lemon juice
1½ tsp. garlic salt
1 tbsp. soy sauce
1 green pepper
1 red pepper
4 onions
3 tomatoes

Place the lamb cubes into a glass or ceramic bowl. Add the lemon juice, garlic salt, soy sauce, and enough water to cover the meat. Marinate the meat at room temperature, uncovered, for 2 hours. Meanwhile, cut the peppers and onions into 2-inch chunks and cut the tomatoes into wedges. Drain the meat, reserving the marinade. Thread the meat onto 6 skewers, alternating it with the pieces of peppers, tomato, and onion. Broil the kebabs for about 15 minutes over hot coals or in a broiler, turning frequently and brushing with the reserved marinade. *Makes 6 servings*

	Calories	Carbo-hydrate (gm)	Protein (gm)	Total Fat (gm)	Saturated Fat (gm)	Choles-terol (mg)
Total	1595.8	83.6	209.3	48.0	28.8	681.6
Per Serving	266.0	13.9	34.9	8.0	4.8	113.6

Trimming Lamb Teriyaki

1¾-lb. slice of lean leg of lamb, trimmed of fat and cut in 6 pieces
2 tsp. ground ginger
2 garlic cloves, minced
1 medium onion, finely chopped
½ cup soy sauce
¼ cup unsweetened white grape juice

Place the meat in a large baking dish. In a separate bowl, combine the ginger, garlic, onion, soy sauce, and grape juice. Pour this mixture over the meat and let it stand at room temperature, uncovered, for 2 hours. Drain the meat well. Place it on a rack in the broiler and broil it for 3 to 5 minutes on each side. *Makes 6 servings*

	Calories	Carbo-hydrate (gm)	Protein (gm)	Total Fat (gm)	Saturated Fat (gm)	Choles-terol (mg)
Total	1615.9	28.5	233.9	55.9	33.6	794.0
Per Serving	269.3	4.8	39.0	9.3	5.6	132.3

gm = grams; mg = milligrams. Nutritional figures are approximate. Figures are based on findings of U.S. Department of Agriculture.

Chinese Sweet 'n Sour Lamb

1 lb. boneless lean leg of lamb, trimmed of fat and sliced thinly across the grain
Unseasoned meat tenderizer
2 onions
8½-oz. can water chestnuts
1 green pepper
2 firm, ripe tomatoes
2 tbsp. soy sauce
8-oz. can unsweetened pineapple chunks or tidbits, packed in juice
2 tbsp. catsup (see index)
1 tbsp. wine vinegar
1 tbsp. cornstarch
3 tbsp. cold water

Moisten the meat with water, and sprinkle it with meat tenderizer. Cut the onions into thin wedges; drain and slice the water chestnuts; cut the green pepper into 1½-inch squares; and cut the tomatoes into eighths.

Heat the soy sauce in a nonstick skillet. Add the lamb and brown it over high heat stirring rapidly until the liquid evaporates. Add the onion, water chestnuts, and green pepper, and continue stir-frying for about 3 minutes. Then add the undrained pineapple, catsup, and vinegar. Heat the contents of the skillet to boiling. In a cup, mix the cornstarch with the cold water until it is smooth. Add this mixture to the sauce in the skillet and continue heating, stirring constantly, until the sauce clears and thickens. Stir in tomato chunks.

Makes 6 servings

	Calories	Carbo-hydrate (gm)	Protein (gm)	Total Fat (gm)	Saturated Fat (gm)	Choles-terol (mg)
Total	1287.8	109.3	141.5	32.0	19.2	454.4
Per Serving	214.6	18.2	23.6	5.3	3.2	75.7

Lamb-Stuffed Acorn Squash

3 small acorn squash
1 lb. lean leg of lamb, trimmed of fat and ground
2 tbsp. grated onion
1 garlic clove, minced
1 tsp. salt
¼ tsp. ginger
¼ tsp. allspice
1 egg, slightly beaten
⅔ cup frozen green peas, defrosted
½ cup crushed high-protein cereal, unsweetened

Cut the squash in half. Place the squash cut side down on a baking sheet and bake in a preheated 350° oven for 35 minutes. In the meantime, heat a large nonstick skillet and add the lamb, onion, and garlic. Brown the meat. Do not add any oil to the pan because the meat will release enough of its own fat for frying. Stir in the salt, ginger, and allspice. Allow the mixture to cool slightly; then stir in the beaten egg, peas, and cereal crumbs. Remove the squash from the oven and turn cut sides up. Pack the lamb mixture firmly into the squash cups and cover the filling in each squash with a small piece of aluminum foil. Continue baking the squash for about another 25 minutes until they are tender.

Makes 6 servings

	Calories	Carbo-hydrate (gm)	Protein (gm)	Total Fat (gm)	Saturated Fat (gm)	Choles-terol (mg)
Total	1628.2	168.1	160.4	42.7	21.2	706.4
Per Serving	271.4	28.0	26.7	7.1	3.5	117.7

Lamb and Artichoke en Brochette

2 pkg. (9 oz. each) frozen artichoke hearts
½ cup low-calorie French salad dressing
¼ cup fresh lemon juice
2 tsp. salt
1 tsp. marjoram or oregano leaves
¼ tsp. pepper
1½ lb. lean boneless leg of lamb, trimmed of fat and cut in 1½-in. cubes
2 large tomatoes

Cook the artichokes according to the package directions, drain and allow to cool. In a large bowl mix together the French dressing, lemon juice, and seasonings. Add the lamb and artichokes and mix lightly. Cover the bowl and refrigerate for several hours or overnight.

Place the lamb on skewers. Cut each of the tomatoes into 6 wedges and alternate the artichokes and tomatoes on another set of skewers. Brush the lamb and vegetables with the marinade. Broil the lamb 3 to 5 inches from the heat source for 5 to 7 minutes on each side, or until they have reached the desired doneness. Broil the artichoke kebabs for 3 to 4 minutes on each side.

Makes 6 servings

	Calories	Carbo-hydrate (gm)	Protein (gm)	Total Fat (gm)	Saturated Fat (gm)	Choles-terol (mg)
Total	1484.6	74.4	211.7	48.0	28.8	681.6
Per Serving	247.4	12.4	35.3	8.0	4.8	113.6

Skinny Skewered Lamb

2 green peppers
3 large carrots
4 celery stalks
½ lb. fresh mushrooms
1½ lb. lean boneless leg of lamb, trimmed of fat and cut in ¾-in. cubes
1½ tsp. salt
Dash black pepper
3 cups tomato sauce
¾ tsp. whole cloves
Dash oregano
2 tbsp. Worcestershire sauce

Add water to a large skillet to a ½-inch depth. Cut the green peppers, carrots and celery, into 1-inch chunks; add them to skillet with the mushrooms. Cover and simmer 10 minutes. Drain well. Arrange the meat and vegetables on 6 skewers and place the skewers in a single layer in a roasting pan. Sprinkle the meat and vegetables with salt and pepper. In a separate bowl, combine the tomato sauce, cloves, oregano, and Worcestershire sauce. Pour this mixture over the kebabs. Bake in a preheated 325° oven for 30 to 45 minutes — or until the lamb is tender — basting frequently with the pan liquid.

Makes 6 servings

	Calories	Carbo-hydrate (gm)	Protein (gm)	Total Fat (gm)	Saturated Fat (gm)	Choles-terol (mg)
Total	1762.0	112.3	224.7	51.7	28.8	681.6
Per Serving	293.6	18.7	37.5	8.6	4.8	113.6

gm = grams; mg = milligrams Nutritional figures are approximate Figures are based on findings of U S Department of Agriculture

Lamb Salonika

2 lb. lean boneless leg of lamb, trimmed of fat and cut in 1-in. cubes	⅓ cup water
1 tsp. salt	10½-oz. can condensed cream of celery soup
⅛ tsp. pepper	1 cup sliced mushrooms
1 tbsp. diet margarine	½ cup low-fat yogurt
1 garlic clove, minced	3 tbsp. chopped parsley
½ cup chopped onion	

Season the lamb cubes with salt and pepper. Melt the diet margarine in a large nonstick skillet. Add the lamb, garlic, and onions to the melted margarine. Sauté over low heat until the lamb is browned on all sides. If any fat has accumulated in the skillet, drain it before going any further. Then add the water, celery soup, and mushrooms. Cook the entire mixture over very low heat for 45 minutes, stirring occasionally. Gradually add the yogurt to the hot mixture, being careful not to let the mixture boil. Add the parsley before serving, or sprinkle it over the top as a garnish.

Makes 8 servings

	Calories	Carbo-hydrate (gm)	Protein (gm)	Total Fat (gm)	Saturated Fat (gm)	Choles-terol (mg)
Total	2093.7	46.2	273.3	86.2	40.4	937.2
Per Serving	261.7	5.8	34.2	10.8	5.1	117.2

Stir-Fried Lamb with Bean Sprouts

1 tbsp. diet margarine	1½ tsp. crushed garlic cloves
1½ lb. lean boneless leg of lamb, trimmed of fat and cut in 1 x 2½-in. strips	2 tbsp. flour
	2 tbsp. soy sauce
4 green onions, sliced	1½ lb. fresh bean sprouts, cooked and drained

Melt the diet margarine in a nonstick skillet. Add the lamb strips and brown them lightly. Then mix the onions and garlic with the meat and continue to cook for about 5 minutes, stirring constantly. Sprinkle the flour over this mixture, cooking and stirring until it is well blended with the lamb and onions. Add the soy sauce and continue cooking and stirring until the lamb is tender. Serve the meat mixture on a bed of bean sprouts.

Makes 6 servings

	Calories	Carbo-hydrate (gm)	Protein (gm)	Total Fat (gm)	Saturated Fat (gm)	Choles-terol (mg)
Total	1580.8	55.8	218.2	54.1	29.8	681.6
Per Serving	263.5	9.3	36.4	9.0	5.0	113.6

gm = grams; mg = milligrams. Nutritional figures are approximate. Figures are based on findings of U.S. Department of Agriculture.

All about Pork and Ham

Once upon a time, pork was plenty pudgy, but thanks to modern breeding techniques, today's pork contains only half as much fat as in the olden days and far fewer calories. Although not as trim as veal, pork does beat out many cuts of beef in the calorie sweepstakes. (Check the comparison chart in The Meat of the Matter to see how some cuts of pork and beef compare.) Another point in pork's favor: it's always served well done, which eliminates even more fat. Comparable cuts of beef that have been broiled or roasted are generally served rare.

Which brings us to another point about pork. Many homemakers, aware that pork must be cooked through, habitually overcook it and thereby ruin its delightful taste and texture. Many old cookbooks and meat thermometers suggest an internal temperature of 185°, but research shows that pork is more tender and tasty when served at 170°, which is perfectly safe, since all trichinae are killed at 140°. When cooking pork, a meat thermometer is doubly important to avoid either undercooking or overcooking.

Much of the cured ham available in supermarkets is "fully cooked" or "ready to eat," which means that it needs only sufficient cooking to warm it through and improve its flavor. Such meat should always be properly identified on the can, label, or wrapper. Reheat ready-to-eat whole or half hams to an internal temperature of 130° in a preheated 300° or 325° oven for the best flavor. Ready-to-eat ham slices can be sautéed in a nonstick skillet or barbecued or broiled until heated through.

Cured or smoked pork that is labeled "cook before eating" must, of course, be cooked. Follow the label directions. Or, roast an uncooked ham to an internal temperature of 160° in a preheated 300° or 325° oven. Uncooked picnic roast (shoulder) or boneless butt (cottage roll) should be roasted to 170° or simmered in liquid until tender.

Even though modern breeding techniques result in leaner stock, some cuts of pork are still exceedingly high in fat and calories. These should be avoided by the committed calorie-counter. Included are bacon (69 percent fat and 3,016 calories per pound), sausage (50 percent fat and 2,259 calories per pound), and spareribs (33 percent fat and 1,637 calories per pound). If you crave these diet crashers, try some substitutions. Canadian bacon (only 980 calories per pound) can be sliced and served in place of fatty bacon, and homemade sausage patties can be prepared from lean ground pork. Veal or lamb ribs cut from the breast make an interesting stand-in for fatty pork spareribs.

Recipe

Pork Chop Barbecue

8 pork chops about 1-in. thick, trimmed of fat	2 tsp. Worcester-shire sauce
1/2 tsp. salt	2 tbsp. prepared mustard
1/8 tsp. pepper	1/4 cup frozen unsweetened apple juice concentrate, defrosted
1 cup tomato purée	
1/4 cup vinegar	

Season the chops with salt and pepper to taste, and place in a baking dish. Cover and bake in a preheated 350° oven for 45 minutes. Pour off the fat. Combine the remaining ingredients and mix well. Pour over the chops and cook for an additional 30 minutes.

Makes 8 servings

	Calories	Carbo-hydrate (gm)	Protein (gm)	Total Fat (gm)	Saturated Fat (gm)	Choles-terol (mg)
Total	3419.2	112.3	186.7	239.8	91.4	993.5
Per Serving	427.4	14.0	23.3	30.0	11.4	124.2

Tomato-Rice Pork Chops

6 lean pork chops, 1-in. thick, trimmed of fat	6 onion slices, 1-in. thick
1/2 tsp. salt	6 tbsp. uncooked rice
1/8 tsp. pepper	16-oz. can tomatoes, undrained

Season the chops with salt and pepper and place in a baking dish. Bake in a preheated 450° oven about 20 minutes — just until brown. Drain off all the fat that has accumulated before going any further. Then place 1 slice of onion and 1 tablespoon of uncooked rice on each chop. Pour tomatoes with the juice over all. Season with salt and pepper again. Cover and bake the chops at 350° for 1 hour.

Makes 6 servings

	Calories	Carbo-hydrate (gm)	Protein (gm)	Total Fat (gm)	Saturated Fat (gm)	Choles-terol (mg)
Total	1994.6	96.6	108.6	128.4	48.0	522.0
Per Serving	332.4	16.1	18.1	21.4	8.0	87.0

Pork Chop Surprise

6 lean pork chops, 1-in. thick, trimmed of fat	8 tsp. tomato paste
1/2 tsp. salt	2 tbsp. chopped onion
1/8 tsp. pepper	1 tbsp. lemon juice
16-oz. can unsweetened juice-packed apricot halves, drained reserving 1/2 cup juice	1/2 tsp. dry mustard
1 tbsp. diet margarine	

With a sharp knife, make a slit in the side of each chop as a pocket for stuffing. Season the pockets with a little salt and pepper and put 2 apricot halves in each. Pin the pockets closed with wooden picks. Cut the remaining apricots in 1/2-inch pieces and set them aside. Melt the margarine in a nonstick skillet. Add the stuffed pork chops, and brown slowly, turning once. Then add the chopped apricots, reserved apricot juice, tomato paste, onion, lemon juice, and mustard to the skillet. Bring mixture to a boil, then reduce heat, cover, and simmer 1 hour or more until meat is tender.

Makes 6 servings

	Calories	Carbo-hydrate (gm)	Protein (gm)	Total Fat (gm)	Saturated Fat (gm)	Choles-terol (mg)
Total	1896.8	71.9	102.1	132.0	49.0	522.0
Per Serving	316.1	12.0	17.0	22.0	8.2	87.0

Pork Pepper Steak

1 1/2-lb. lean boneless pork shoulder, trimmed of fat	1 cup water
1 garlic clove, crushed	1 green pepper, cut in strips
1-lb. can tomatoes, undrained	1 cup chopped onion
6 tbsp. soy sauce	1/2 cup diced celery
1 tsp. Worcestershire sauce	1/4 cup water
1/4 tsp. coarse, freshly ground pepper	2 tbsp. cornstarch

Cut meat across the grain into 1/2-inch thick slices, then slice again, lengthwise, into strips. Spray a non-stick skillet with vegetable coating for no-fat frying and brown the pork strips over low heat. Add the garlic, tomatoes (with juice), sauces, ground pepper and 1 cup water to browned meat. Cover and simmer mixture about 45 minutes until the meat is tender. Then add the green pepper strips, onion, and celery. Cover and simmer 15 minutes longer. Combine the cornstarch with 1/4 cup cold water, stirring until smooth. Add this mixture to the skillet, stirring and cooking until contents have slightly thickened.

Makes 6 servings

	Calories	Carbo-hydrate (gm)	Protein (gm)	Total Fat (gm)	Saturated Fat (gm)	Choles-terol (mg)
Total	1593.2	55.3	213.0	50.0	24.0	600.0
Per Serving	265.5	9.2	35.5	8.3	4.	100.0

gm = grams; mg = milligrams. Nutritional figures are approximate. Figures are based on findings of U.S. Department of Agriculture.

Pork 'n' Kraut

1½ lb. boneless lean pork (from leg), trimmed of fat and cut in 6 pieces
1 tbsp. water
3 cups sauerkraut, drained and rinsed
1 cup peeled and chopped apples
1 cup chopped onion
2 tsp. caraway seeds
1½ cups water

Place the meat with 1 tablespoon water in a large non-stick skillet. Cover and heat over a moderate temperature until the water has evaporated and the steam has caused the meat to release its own inner fat. Then uncover the skillet and brown the meat slowly on both sides. Or you may brown the meat by first spraying the pan with vegetable coating. In a separate bowl, mix together the rinsed sauerkraut, apples, onions, caraway seeds, and 1½ cups water. Pour this mixture over the pork. Cover and simmer over low heat until the meat is very tender — about 1½ hours. *Makes 6 servings*

	Calories	Carbo-hydrate (gm)	Protein (gm)	Total Fat (gm)	Saturated Fat (gm)	Choles-terol (mg)
Total	1971.2	48.9	208.0	100.0	30.0	600.0
Per Serving	328.5	8.1	34.7	16.7	5.0	100.0

Chinese Pork

1½-lb. lean boneless pork shoulder, trimmed of fat and cut in 1-in. cubes
2 beef bouillon cubes
1 cup hot water
11-oz. can unsweetened juice-packed mandarin oranges, drained reserving juice
¼ cup soy sauce
1 tbsp. instant minced onion
½ tsp. ground ginger
2 tbsp. cornstarch
¼ cup cold water
4-oz. can water chestnuts, drained and sliced
2 green peppers, in ¼-in. strips
1 cup sliced mushrooms
1 cup sliced celery cabbage (cut diagonally ½- to ¾- in. thick)

Spray a non-stick skillet with vegetable coating for no-fat frying. Add the meat and brown slowly. Dissolve the bouillon cubes in 1 cup hot water. Add this with the liquid from the oranges, the soy sauce, minced onion, and ginger to the pork. Bring the mixture to a boil; then cover, reduce the heat, and simmer about 30 minutes. In a separate bowl, blend cornstarch with ¼ cup cold water. Gradually add the cornstarch mixture to the meat, cooking and stirring constantly until the sauce is thick and clear. Then add the water chestnuts, green pepper, mushrooms, and celery cabbage. Cover and continue to cook over low heat 7 minutes. Fold in the mandarin oranges just before serving. *Makes 8 servings*

	Calories	Carbo-hydrate (gm)	Protein (gm)	Total Fat (gm)	Saturated Fat (gm)	Choles-terol (mg)
Total	1714.1	80.7	219.0	49.3	24.0	606.0
Per Serving	214.3	10.1	27.3	6.2	3.0	75.8

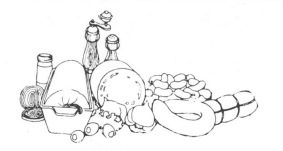

Pork Steak Viennese

1-lb. lean pork leg steak (or fresh ham slice) trimmed of fat
1½ tsp. salt
½ tsp. pepper
1-lb. 11-oz. can sauerkraut, drained
1-lb. can whole tomatoes, undrained
2½ tbsp. instant onion
1 green pepper, cut in 1-in. strips
¼ tsp. thyme

Spray a nonstick skillet with vegetable coating for no-fat frying and brown the meat slowly. Season the browned meat on both sides with the salt and ¼ teaspoon of pepper. In a bowl, combine the other ¼ teaspoon of pepper with the sauerkraut, tomatoes, onion, green pepper, and thyme. Mix well and pour into 7½ x 11¾-inch baking dish. Place the meat on top of the mixture. Cover with aluminum foil and bake 30 minutes in a preheated 325° oven. Then uncover and bake another 30 minutes — or until the pork is tender. *Makes 4 servings*

	Calories	Carbo-hydrate (gm)	Protein (gm)	Total Fat (gm)	Saturated Fat (gm)	Choles-terol (mg)
Total	1556.0	52.0	106.4	103.4	37.3	405.1
Per Serving	389.0	13.0	26.6	25.9	9.3	101.3

Ham Patties Aloha

1½-lb. cooked smoked ham, trimmed of fat and ground
1 tsp. grated onion
1 tbsp. chopped parsley
1 tbsp. prepared mustard
1 egg, beaten
8 pineapple slices (unsweetened, juice-packed) drained reserving 2 tbsp. juice
8 tbsp. crushed cornflakes

Mix the ham with the onion, parsley, mustard, egg, and the 2 tablespoons pineapple juice. Shape the meat into 8 patties and roll in the crushed cornflakes. Arrange the pineapple slices in a shallow baking dish. Place 1 patty on each pineapple slice. Bake in a preheated 375° oven for 25 to 30 minutes. *Makes 8 servings*

	Calories	Carbo-hydrate (gm)	Protein (gm)	Total Fat (gm)	Saturated Fat (gm)	Choles-terol (mg)
Total	2390.5	107.6	151.0	158.0	58.0	860.0
Per Serving	298.8	13.5	18.9	19.8	7.3	107.5

gm = grams; mg = milligrams. Nutritional figures are approximate. Figures are based on findings of U.S. Department of Agriculture.

Pineapple-Ham Stir Fry

1 tbsp. diet margarine
1½ lb. lean cooked smoked ham, trimmed of fat and cut in 1-in. strips
2 large onions, sliced
2 large green peppers, sliced

2 cups unsweetened pineapple chunks, juice packed
2 tbsp. cornstarch
¾ tsp. salt
¼ tsp. pepper
1 tbsp. soy sauce

Melt the margarine in a large, nonstick skillet. Add the ham, onions, and green peppers, and sauté over moderate heat until the ham is browned. Drain the pineapple, reserving the juice. Add enough water to the juice to make ¾ of a cup of liquid. Combine the cornstarch, salt, pepper, soy sauce, and pineapple liquid in a bowl. Add this to the ham and vegetables, and continue cooking over low heat, stirring constantly, until the sauce has thickened. Add pineapple chunks.

Makes 6 servings

	Calories	Carbo-hydrate (gm)	Protein (gm)	Total Fat (gm)	Saturated Fat (gm)	Choles-terol (mg)
Total	1954.7	119.3	217.0	70.0	25.0	600.0
Per Serving	325.8	19.9	36.2	11.7	4.2	100.0

Easy Cheesy Casserole

1 tbsp. diet margarine
½ cup finely chopped onions
1 lb. cooked lean ham, trimmed of fat and chopped
1 cup grated American or cheddar cheese

½ cup finely crushed cracker crumbs
1½ cups skim milk
3 eggs, slightly beaten
2 tsp. prepared mustard

Melt the margarine in a nonstick skillet. Sauté the onions in the melted margarine until they are lightly browned. In an oven-safe casserole combine the rest of the ingredients. Mix the onions into this mixture. Bake the casserole in a preheated 350° oven for 30 to 40 minutes — until a knife blade inserted in the center comes out clean.

Makes 6 servings

	Calories	Carbo-hydrate (gm)	Protein (gm)	Total Fat (gm)	Saturated Fat (gm)	Choles-terol (mg)
Total	2445.7	58.1	228.1	139.6	57.0	1387.3
Per Serving	407.6	9.7	38.0	23.3	9.5	231.2

gm = grams; mg = milligrams. Nutritional figures are approximate. Figures are based on findings of U.S. Department of Agriculture.

Everybody Loves Ground Meat

Hamburger is one of America's favorite meats. The typical American eats in excess of 50 pounds of ground meat a year, much of it, unfortunately, calorie-contaminated with excess fat. Most prepackaged ground meat contains close to the legal limit of fat — 30 percent — and weighs in at more than 1600 calories per pound. Fat-trimmed beef, by contrast, is less than 700 calories per pound. You can eliminate more than 50,000 excess calories this year by switching from pre-packaged hamburger to fat-trimmed beef that has been custom-ground to your order. Simply pick out a piece of lean bottom round and ask the butcher to trim away the fat and grind the lean to order. Almost all supermarkets will perform this service for you, especially when you explain that you have to eliminate as much fat as possible from your diet. Rest assured that you won't be the first customer to request custom-ground, fat-trimmed beef. Many heart-smart cholesterol watchers shop for it as a matter of prudence.

Isn't lean hamburger more expensive? The price tag for boneless bottom round is generally at least one-third higher than ready-ground hamburger. But the price difference is really not as great as it appears. Lean hamburger won't shrink the way fatty hamburger will, so one pound will give you four servings, instead of three or less. And the nutritive value is much higher, because the fat in the packaged ground meat is replaced with protein in the lean meat. Here's how fatty hamburger and lean ground compare:

1 Pound, Raw	Fat	Protein	Calories
Hamburger, 29% fat	148 grams	73 grams	1,647
Lean ground round, trimmed of fat	21 grams	98 grams	612

Isn't lean hamburger dry? Only if you overcook it. Like all lean meat, fat-trimmed hamburger can't stand up to blast-furnace temperatures and prolonged cooking times. The best way to broil lean burgers is to mix the meat with crushed ice, season it, and broil it only until it is well browned on the outside. The inside should remain pink and juicy.

You can do anything with lean hamburger that you can do with fatty hamburger. Meat loaf and casserole dishes are particularly well suited to lean meat since a casserole dish made with fatty hamburger will be greasy and undigestible (as well as fattening) because the fat has nowhere to escape. Meat loaf made with lean meat is delicious hot or cold, while fatty meat loaf is unpleasantly greasy when chilled.

Other Ground Meats

Any meat can be fat-trimmed and ground to order. Try pork, lamb, or veal for a change. If you're fortunate enough to live in an area where the stores stock and sell raw ground turkeyburger, be sure to take advantage of this nonfattening treat — only 736 calories a pound! If freshly ground turkey is unavailable, buy large forzen turkey thighs. Defrost them, remove the meat from the bones (discarding the skin) and put the meat through a grinder. Three large thighs equals about 2 pounds of ground meat.

Recipes

Succulent Burgers

2 lb. lean ground round steak
2 tbsp. snipped chives
¼ cup crushed ice
1 tsp. bitters

Combine all the ingredients and mix well. Shape into 8 patties and place them on a rack in the broiler, 4 inches from the heat source. Broil about 10 minutes, turning once. *Makes 8 servings*

	Calories	Carbo-hydrate (gm)	Protein (gm)	Total Fat (gm)	Saturated Fat (gm)	Choles-terol (mg)
Total	1488.3	1.5	284.4	35.6	11.9	841.4
Per Serving	186.0	0.2	35.6	4.5	1.5	105.2

Saucy-but-Slimming Hamburger Steak

1 lb. lean ground round steak
½ cup high-protein cereal, unsweetened
½ tsp. salt
¼ tsp. pepper
8-oz. can tomato sauce
1 tbsp. chopped green onion
1 tsp. Worcester shire sauce
1 tsp. prepared mustard
1 tsp. dried savory

Mix the ground steak, cereal, salt, and pepper together, and shape the mixture into 4 patties. Brown the patties slowly in a nonstick skillet. Do not add any fat to the pan; if you cook the meat slowly, enough of its own inner fat will be released. Drain the fat from the skillet. In a separate bowl blend together the tomato sauce, onion, Worcestershire sauce, mustard, and savory, and pour this mixture over the patties. Cover and simmer 10 minutes. *Makes 4 servings*

	Calories	Carbo-hydrate (gm)	Protein (gm)	Total Fat (gm)	Saturated Fat (gm)	Choles-terol (mg)
Total	898.2	35.1	147.9	18.3	5.9	421.0
Per Serving	224.6	8.8	37.0	4.6	1.5	105.3

Meat Loaf for Diet Watchers

2 lb. lean ground round steak
2 tsp. salt or garlic salt
¼ tsp. pepper
2 eggs
½ cup high-protein cereal, unsweetened
½ cup skim milk
¼ cup chopped onion
¼ tsp. dried sage

Mix all of the ingredients together thoroughly and form the meat into a loaf in a shallow baking pan. Bake in a preheated 350° oven for about 1 hour, basting occasionally with juices. *Makes 8 servings*

Diet hint: The calorie-wise cook can save a whopping 100 calories (that's 12½ per serving) by using 4 egg whites instead of 2 whole eggs. Egg whites have hardly a trace of saturated fat or cholesterol.

	Calories	Carbo-hydrate (gm)	Protein (gm)	Total Fat (gm)	Saturated Fat (gm)	Choles-terol (mg)
Total	1739.9	16.8	303.7	47.7	15.9	1347.9
Per Serving	217.5	2.1	38.0	6.0	2.0	168.5

Chopped Steak Suey

2 lb. lean ground round steak
1 onion, cut in eighths
2 beef bouillon cubes
½ cup hot water
4-oz. can whole mushrooms, drained reserving liquid
⅓ cup soy sauce
2 tbsp. cornstarch
5- to 6½-oz. can water chestnuts, drained and halved
16-oz. can bean sprouts, drained
16-oz. can Chinese vegetables, drained
¼ cup pimiento strips

Brown the ground meat in a large nonstick skillet. Do not add any oil to the pan because the meat will release enough of its own fat. Add the onion to the browned meat and continue to cook over low heat for 5 minutes. Before going any further, pour off all the fat that has accumulated in the pan. Dissolve bouillon cubes in hot water. Then combine the liquid from the mushrooms with the bouillon and add this to the meat along with the soy sauce and cornstarch. Bring the liquid to a boil, then reduce the heat and simmer, stirring constantly, until the mixture thickens. Stir in the mushrooms, water chestnuts, bean sprouts, and Chinese vegetables, cooking just until they are heated through. Stir in the pimiento strips just before serving.

Makes 8 servings

	Calories	Carbo-hydrate (gm)	Protein (gm)	Total Fat (gm)	Saturated Fat (gm)	Choles-terol (mg)
Total	1964.4	95.4	312.9	36.1	11.9	847.4
Per Serving	245.6	11.9	39.1	4.5	1.5	105.9

gm = grams; mg = milligrams. Nutritional figures are approximate. Figures are based on findings of U.S. Department of Agriculture.

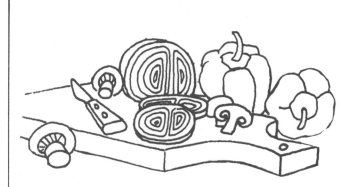

To assemble, combine all the filling ingredients and spoon a little of the mixture onto each crepe. Roll up and arrange the crepes in a single layer in a shallow nonstick baking dish. Pour the sauce over the rolled crepes. Bake in a preheated 350° oven 20 minutes.

Makes 6 servings

	Calories	Carbo-hydrate (gm)	Protein (gm)	Total Fat (gm)	Saturated Fat (gm)	Choles-terol (mg)
Total	1915.6	118.9	147.7	74.7	32.8	1375.8
Per Serving	319.3	19.8	24.6	12.5	5.5	229.3

Italian Steak Sausage

2½ lb. lean ground round steak
½ tsp. coriander
1 tsp. oregano
1 tsp. basil
1 tsp. sage
1 tsp. meat tenderizer
½ tsp. thyme
½ tsp. marjoram

Mix all of the ingredients together lightly. Shape the mixture into small flat patties, using 1 heaping tablespoon for each sausage. Place the patties on a rack in a broiler pan and broil about 4 inches from the heat source for about 3 minutes on each side.

Makes 20 sausages

	Calories	Carbo-hydrate (gm)	Protein (gm)	Total Fat (gm)	Saturated Fat (gm)	Choles-terol (mg)
Total	2165.8	0.0	349.9	66.6	33.3	1032.9
Per Serving	108.3	0.0	17.5	3.3	1.7	51.6

Manicotti

12 High-Protein Egg Crepes (see index)

Sauce:
¾ lb. lean ground beef round
2 onions, chopped
2 cloves garlic, minced. or ¼ tsp. garlic powder
6-oz. can tomato paste
16-oz. can tomatoes, broken up
2 cups water
3 tbsp. chopped fresh parsley
1 tbsp. dried oregano

½ tsp. salt
⅛ tsp. pepper

Filling:
12 oz. 99% fat-free pot-style cottage cheese
1 egg
3 tbsp. grated extra-sharp Romano cheese
2 tbsp. chopped parsley
¼ tsp. salt

Prepare crepes using the recipe and method given in this book. Spread meat in nonstick skillet (add no oil). Heat over moderate flame. Cook until the underside of the meat is brown. Break the meat into chunks and turn to brown evenly. Pour off any fat that accumulates. Add the remaining ingredients, cover and simmer 30 minutes. Uncover and continue simmering another 15 to 20 minutes, stirring ooccasionally, until the sauce is thick.

Italian Meatball Casserole

1 lb. lean beef round, trimmed of fat and ground to order
½ lb. lean ground veal
1 tsp. garlic salt
⅛ tsp. pepper
⅓ cup skim milk
1 medium eggplant, pared
2 cups plain tomato sauce

2-oz. can mushrooms, stems and pieces, drained
½ tsp. dried oregano
6 tbsp. grated Romano cheese
2 tbsp. Italian-seasoned bread crumbs

Combine the beef, veal, garlic salt, pepper and milk. Shape into 1-inch meatballs and brown under the broiler. Cut the eggplant into 1-inch cubes. Combine all the ingredients except the bread crumbs in an ovenproof casserole. Sprinkle the top with bread crumbs. Bake in a preheated 350° oven for 30 minutes or longer until the eggplant is tender.

Makes 8 servings

	Calories	Carbo-hydrate (g)	Protein (gm)	Total Fat (gm)	Saturated Fat (gm)	Choles-terol (mg)
Total	1605.2	56.6	214.5	49.4	24.7	607.2
Per Serving	200.7	7.1	26.8	6.2	3.1	75.9

Turkey Chili

1 tbsp. diet margarine
1¼ lb. fresh ground turkey
1 cup chopped onion
½ cup chopped green pepper
½ cup chopped red pepper

16-oz. can chopped tomatoes, undrained
2 tsp. salt
1 tsp. chili powder
½ tsp. black pepper
¼ tsp. red pepper

Melt the margarine in a heavy nonstick skillet. Add the turkey, onion, and peppers, and brown them slowly. Then add the tomatoes (with the juice) and the seasonings. Cover and simmer the mixture for about 15 minutes.

Makes 6 servings

	Calories	Carbo-hydrate (gm)	Protein (gm)	Total Fat (gm)	Saturated Fat (gm)	Choles-terol (mg)
Total	1293.9	34.5	189.7	42.3	13.4	508.2
Per Serving	215.6	5.8	31.6	7.1	2.2	84.7

gm = grams; mg = milligrams. Nutritional figures are approximate. Figures are based on findings of U.S. Department of Agriculture.

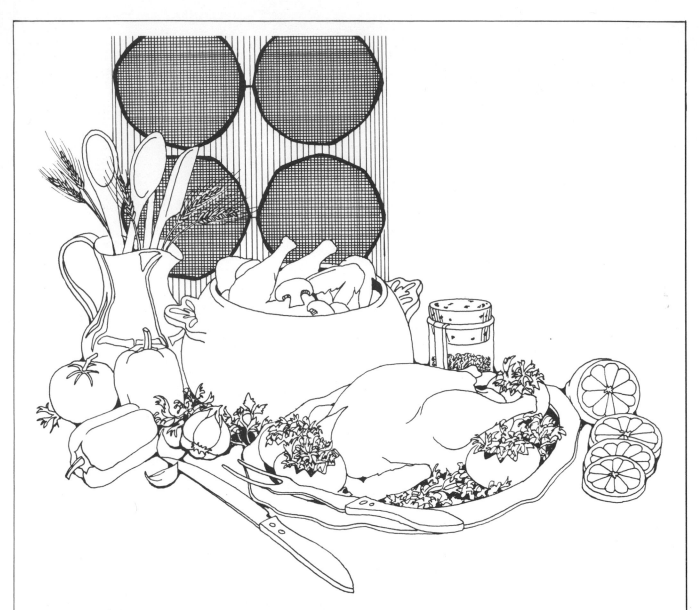

Glamorizing Chicken

Of all the main course choices available to dieters, chicken is the unchallenged champion in terms of popularity, availability, versatility, and affordability. Chicken is lower in calories than any other meat. It's also cholesterol-wise because of its relative lack of saturated fat.

The popularity of chicken and its congenial calorie count are due to modern farming methods that make young spring chickens the least expensive and most available. These prize broiler-fryer chickens are also the prime choice nutritionally. As you will see in the following chart, young frying chickens offer the most protein and the least fat and calories per pound of the four types.

CHICKEN COMPARISONS PER POUND

	Fat	Protein	Calories
Fryers 9 weeks	15 grams	57 grams	382
Roasters 12 weeks	59 grams	43 grams	564
Hens 1½ years	82 grams	41 grams	703
Capons	53 grams	50 grams	668

Although it is clear that you will get the most nutritional value and least calories from a young frying chicken over an older roasting chicken, you can give yourself even greater control over the calories you eat by choosing the leanest parts of the chicken to eat. As the following chart shows, chicken breasts are a nutrition bargain. They are only 21 percent bones; the rest is meat. No other part of the chicken is as meaty. And in all that meat, there are only 7 grams of fat and a giant 75 grams of protein, which makes them a calorie bargain, too.

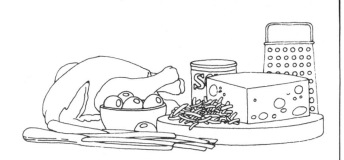

YOUNG FRYING CHICKEN PARTS

	Bones	Fat	Protein
Back	46%	24 grams	40 grams
Breast	21%	7 grams	75 grams
Drumstick	40%	11 grams	51 grams
Neck	52%	21 grams	34 grams
Rib	49%	13 grams	41 grams
Thigh	25%	19 grams	62 grams
Wing	51%	17 grams	41 grams

How to Cook a Chicken

Broiling. Because of the fat in chicken skin, broiler-fryer chickens can be broiled without additional fat.

1. Sprinkle the chicken halves, quarters, or pieces with salt, pepper, lemon juice, and an herb such as tarragon, thyme, or basil.

2. Place the pieces skin side down on a broiler rack. In the broiler of a gas range, the chicken should be 3 to 6 inches from the heat source; in an electric range, the distance should be 6 to 9 inches.

3. Broil the chicken for 20 to 25 minutes. Then turn it and broil 15 to 20 minutes longer.

4. If you like, you can baste the chicken with barbecue sauce near the end of the cooking time.

Frying. One of the most popular ways to cook chicken is to fry it. It's also the most fattening way. What makes frying so fattening, of course, is the oil used in the frying process. So a simple way of decalorizing fried chicken is to eliminate the oil.

1. Cut a broiler-fryer chicken into serving pieces — or buy one that is already cut up. A 2-pound chicken will serve 4 people.

2. In a paper bag, mix 3 tablespoons flour with 1 teaspoon salt, ½ teaspoon pepper, and 1 teaspoon paprika.

3. Add the chicken, a few pieces at a time, to the bag, and shake them until the chicken is coated.

4. Place the chicken in a nonstick baking dish, skin side down.

5. Bake the chicken for about 25 minutes at 400°.

6. Turn the chicken over and bake 20 to 25 minutes more, until it is tender, brown and crisp.

7. Before serving, blot the chicken with paper toweling.

Simmering. Chicken simmered in water and seasonings makes a great beginning for other dishes.

1. Use a broiler-fryer chicken, whole or cut into serving pieces.

2. Put the chicken in a kettle and add 2 cups of water, 1 small sliced onion, 3 celery tops, 1 teaspoon salt and ½ teaspoon pepper.

3. Bring the water to a boil.

4. Cover the kettle, reduce the heat, and simmer the chicken for about 1 hour until it's tender.

5. Strain the broth

6. Refrigerate the chicken and broth in separate containers.

7. When the chicken is cool, remove the meat from the skin and bones, and cut it into chunks.

8. Skim the fat from the surface of the broth.

Roasting. Another healthy and low-calorie way of preparing chicken is roasting it. In this dry-heat method, the chicken is cooked to juicy tenderness while the bird's excess fat is melted away.

1. Even though it may seem more appropriate to use a roasting chicken, buy a broiler-fryer. It is lower in calories and faster to cook.

2. Sprinkle the neck and body cavities with 1 teaspoon salt.

3. If you like, stuff the body cavity with your favorite stuffing. (Several stuffing recipes are in this chapter.)

4. Hook the wing tips onto the chicken's back to hold the neck skin. Tie the legs together, then tie them to the tail.

5. Place the chicken in a shallow roasting pan. Do not brush the chicken with fat.

6. Roast the chicken according to the following timetable.

Weight	Time per Pound	Temperature	Approx. Amt. Stuffing	Approx. Total Time*
1½ lb.	40 min.	400°	¾ cup	1 hour
2 lb.	35 min.	400°	1 cup	1 hr. 10 min.
2½ lb.	30 min.	375°	1¼ cups	1 hr. 15 min.
3 lb.	30 min.	375°	1½ cups	1 hr. 30 min.
3½ lb.	30 min.	375°	1¾ cups	1 hr. 45 min.
4 lb.	30 min.	375°	2 cups	2 hours
4½ lb.	30 min.	375°	2¼ cups	2 hrs. 15 min.
5 lb.	30 min.	375°	2½ cups	2 hrs. 30 min.

*If the chicken is stuffed, add 15 min. to the total roasting time.

7. When the chicken is done, the drumstick meat will feel soft when pressed between your fingers, and the leg will twist easily out of the thigh joint. Another way of testing the chicken for doneness is to pierce the skin of the breast with a fork. If the liquid that seeps out is clear, not yellow, the chicken is done.

8. Let the chicken stand about 10 minutes before carving.

Recipes

Chicken Philippine

2 lb. broiler-fryer chicken pieces	¾ cup unsweetened orange juice
1 tsp. salt	⅛ tsp. cinnamon
8-oz. can unsweetened pineapple chunks, juice packed	⅛ tsp. ground cloves
	1 tbsp. cornstarch
	1 tbsp. water

Season the chicken with the salt. Heat a large nonstick skillet over moderate heat. Add chicken pieces, and brown on both sides for about 20 minutes, turning once. Pour off any fat that accumulates. Drain pineapple, reserving ¼ cup juice. Mix together the reserved pineapple juice and the orange juice; add this mixture to the chicken. Stir in cinnamon and ground cloves. Cover and simmer about 30 minutes until chicken is tender. Remove chicken from the skillet and place it on a platter and keep warm in the oven.

Add the pineapple chunks to skillet. In a cup, blend the cornstarch with 1 tablespoon water; add this mixture to the skillet, stirring rapidly. Cook the pineapple, stirring constantly, until the liquid has thickened and comes to a boil. To serve, spoon some of the sauce over the chicken on the platter and pass the remaining sauce. *Makes 4 servings*

	Calories	Carbo-hydrate (gm)	Protein (gm)	Total Fat (gm)	Saturated Fat (gm)	Choles-terol (mg)
Total	1123.2	64.7	132.8	35.1	13.7	555.7
Per Serving	280.8	16.2	33.2	8.8	3.4	138.9

Chicken Sangria

2 tbsp. flour	2 lb. broiler-fryer chicken pieces
1 tsp. salt	4 seedless oranges
Dash pepper	White sangria
½ tsp. cinnamon	1 tbsp. soy sauce
½ tsp. ground cloves	

Combine the flour, salt, pepper, cinnamon, and cloves in a paper bag. Add the chicken, a few pieces at a time and shake until the chicken is coated. Place the chicken, skin side up, in a nonstick baking pan. Bake in a preheated 450° oven just until the chicken is brown. Before going any further, pour off all the fat that has accumulated in the pan. Peel the oranges and cut them into wedges. Save any juice that accumulates. Add enough sangria to the juice to make ½ cup liquid. Combine this with the soy sauce and orange wedges and pour the entire mixture over the chicken. Cover and continue to bake the chicken for 20 or 30 minutes longer — until the fleshiest part of the chicken is fork-tender. *Makes 4 servings*

	Calories	Carbo-hydrate (gm)	Protein (gm)	Total Fat (gm)	Saturated Fat (gm)	Choles-terol (mg)
Total	1365.3	99.4	137.8	34.5	13.7	555.7
Per Serving	341.3	24.9	34.5	8.6	3.4	138.9

Easy Chicken L'Orange

2 lb. broiler-fryer chicken pieces	1 tsp. garlic salt
	¾ cup unsweetened orange juice

Place the chicken pieces, skin side up, in a nonstick baking dish. Season with garlic salt. Pour the orange juice over the chicken, cover and bake about 1 hour in a preheated 350° oven until it is very tender. *Makes 4 servings*

	Calories	Carbo-hydrate (gm)	Protein (gm)	Total Fat (gm)	Saturated Fat (gm)	Choles-terol (mg)
Total	946.9	19.5	131.8	35.1	13.7	555.7
Per Serving	236.7	4.9	33.0	8.8	3.4	138.9

Chili con Pollo

2 lb. broiler-fryer chicken pieces	3 cups canned tomatoes
2 tsp. salt	2 cups canned kidney beans, drained
¼ tsp. pepper	
1 onion, chopped	1½ tsp. chili powder
1 green pepper, chopped	

Arrange the chicken, skin side up, in a baking pan. Season with the salt and pepper. Brown in a preheated 350° oven for about 30 minutes. Pour off the fat that has accumulated in the pan before going any further. Then add the rest of the ingredients. Cover the pan and continue baking 30 minutes until chicken is tender. *Makes 6 servings*

	Calories	Carbo-hydrate (gm)	Protein (gm)	Total Fat (gm)	Saturated Fat (gm)	Choles-terol (mg)
Total	1529.4	128.0	169.3	39.3	13.7	555.7
Per Serving	254.9	21.3	28.2	6.6	2.3	92.6

Chicken Cacciatore

2 lb. broiler-fryer chicken pieces	1 tsp. oregano
2 tsp. salt	1 tsp. garlic salt
¼ tsp. pepper	4 cups canned tomatoes
1 tbsp. parsley	

Place the chicken in a nonstick skillet. Beginning with skin side down, brown the chicken over medium heat about 15 minutes on each side. Do not add oil to the pan; the chicken will release enough of its own fat for frying. When the chicken is brown, add the remaining ingredients to the pan. Cover and simmer about 30 minutes until the chicken is tender. *Makes 4 servings*

	Calories	Carbo-hydrate (gm)	Protein (gm)	Total Fat (gm)	Saturated Fat (gm)	Choles-terol (mg)
Total	1065.4	40.0	138.3	38.3	13.7	555.7
Per Serving	266.4	10.0	34.6	9.6	3.4	138.9

gm = grams; mg = milligrams. Nutritional figures are approximate. Figures are based on findings of U.S. Department of Agriculture.

The Glorious Main Dish Gallery of Photos

Slim-but-saucy is the theme of the well-seasoned main dishes featured in this section, proving you can cut calories without cutting flavor. Foreign accents abound: Bul Kogi (Korean Beef), Manicotti, Veal Provencal Petite, Chinese Pork. Shown below is Cote d'Azur Steak en Brochette (recipe on page 91), made with marinated beef, zucchini and tomatoes.

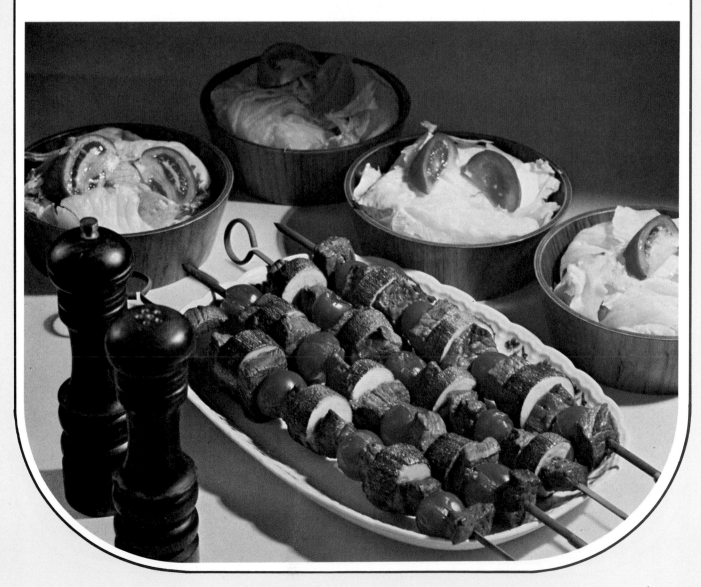

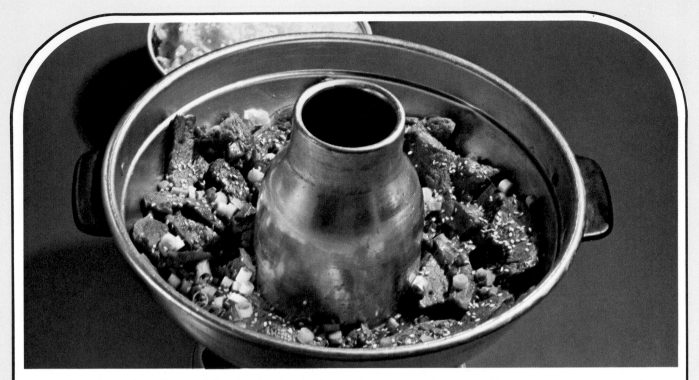

Above, thin slices of flank steak marinate in a potent concoction of soy sauce and sherry to make Bul Kogi (Korean Beef) (recipe on page 88). Below, Browned Turkey Wings simmer in white wine and tomatoes for Turkey Marengo (recipe on page 70).

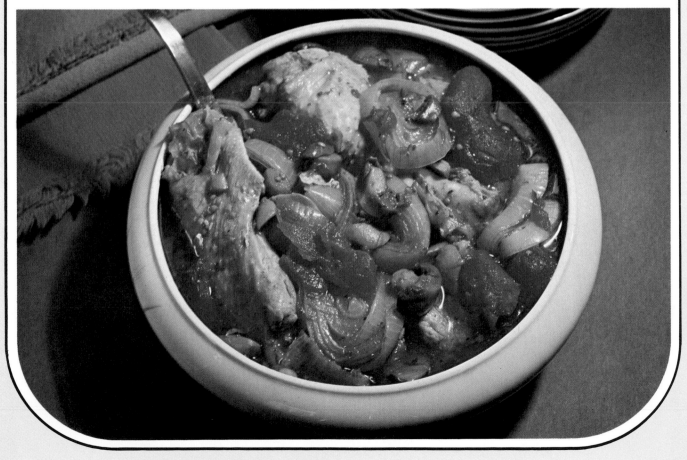

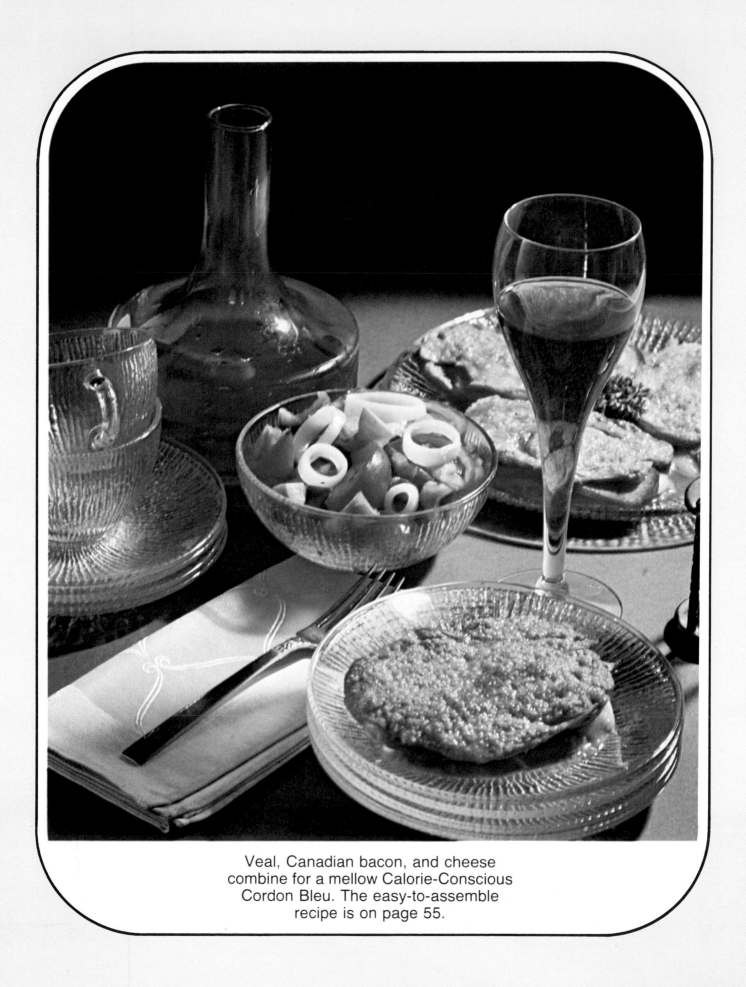

Veal, Canadian bacon, and cheese
combine for a mellow Calorie-Conscious
Cordon Bleu. The easy-to-assemble
recipe is on page 55.

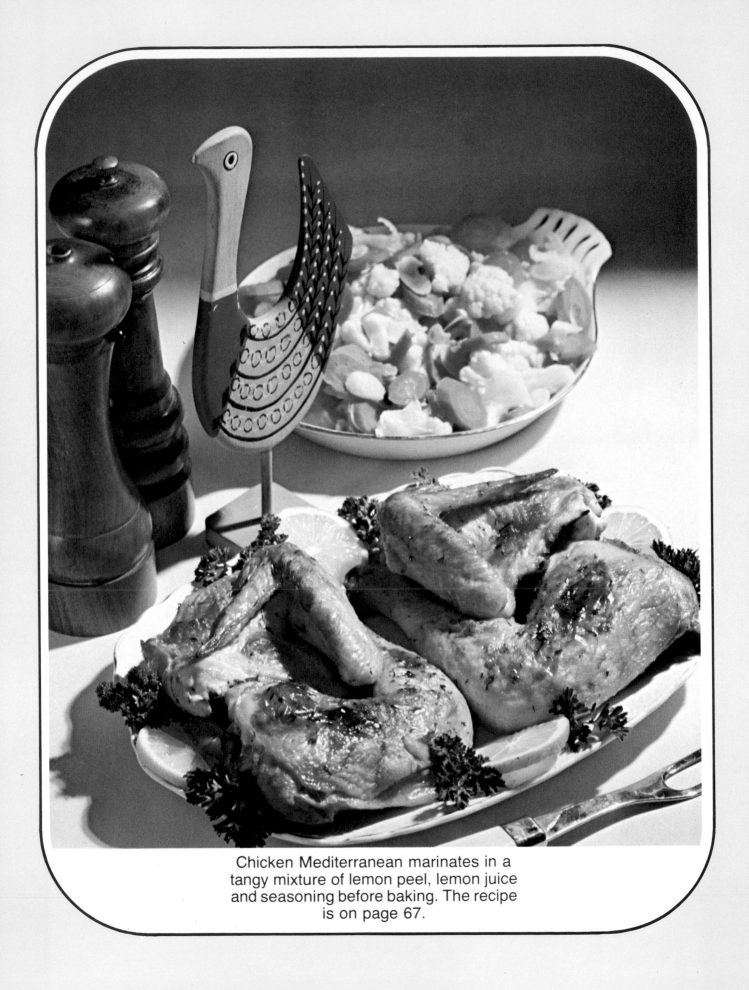

Chicken Mediterranean marinates in a tangy mixture of lemon peel, lemon juice and seasoning before baking. The recipe is on page 67.

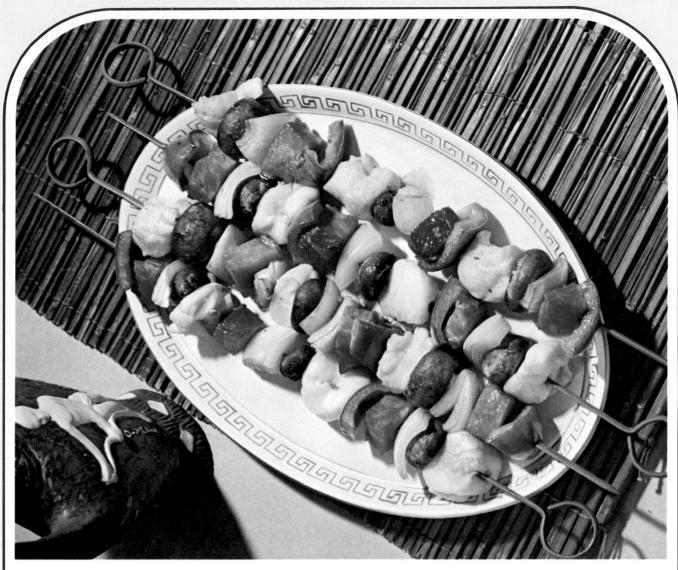

Above, Skewered Scallops with Canadian Bacon (recipe on page 78) make a colorful entree. Below, sliced green peppers and pimento simmer with thin steak strips for a savory Steak Oriental (recipe on page 51).

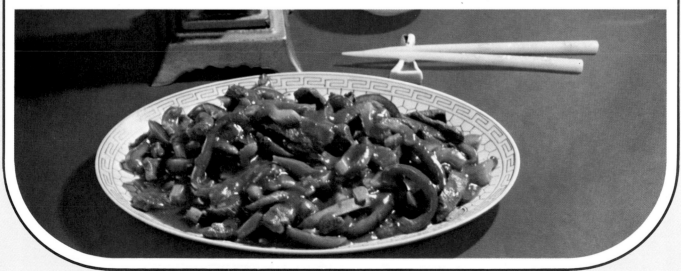

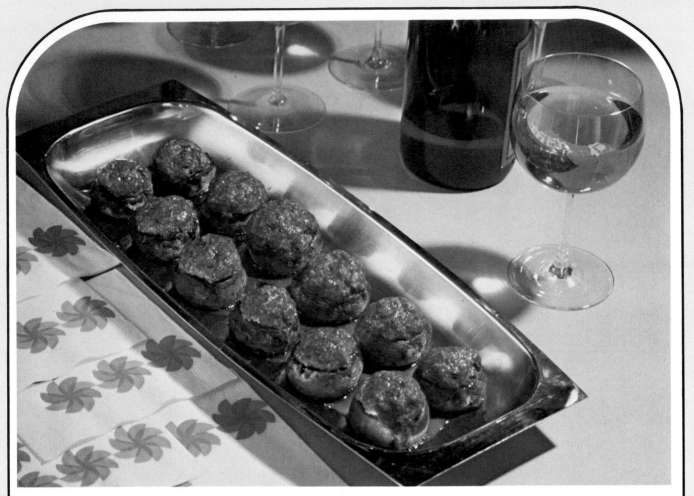

Above, Steak-Stuffed Mushrooms are delicious appetizers. The recipe, on page 86, calls for prepared horseradish to give the stuffing character. Below, Shrimp Bisque (recipe on page 79) tastes super-rich and smooth.

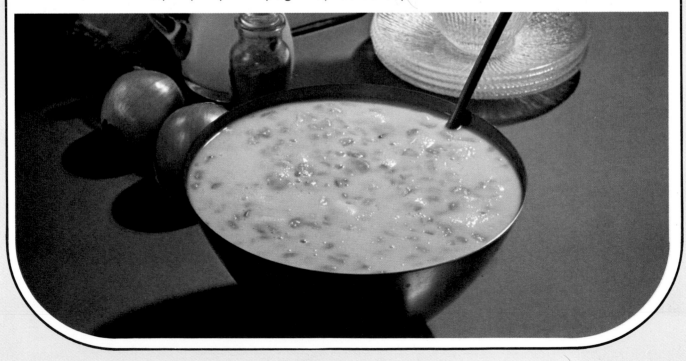

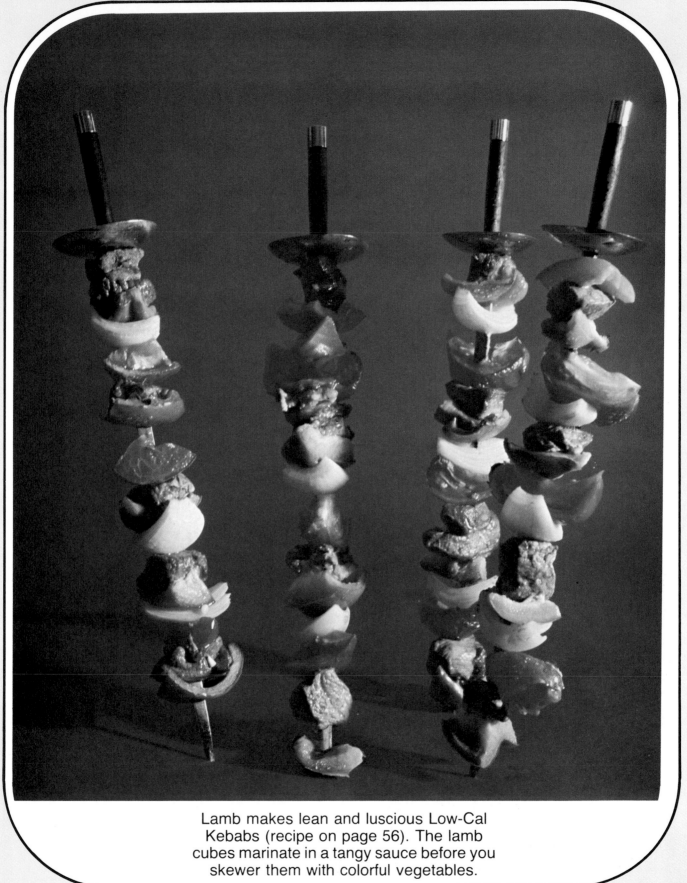

Lamb makes lean and luscious Low-Cal Kebabs (recipe on page 56). The lamb cubes marinate in a tangy sauce before you skewer them with colorful vegetables.

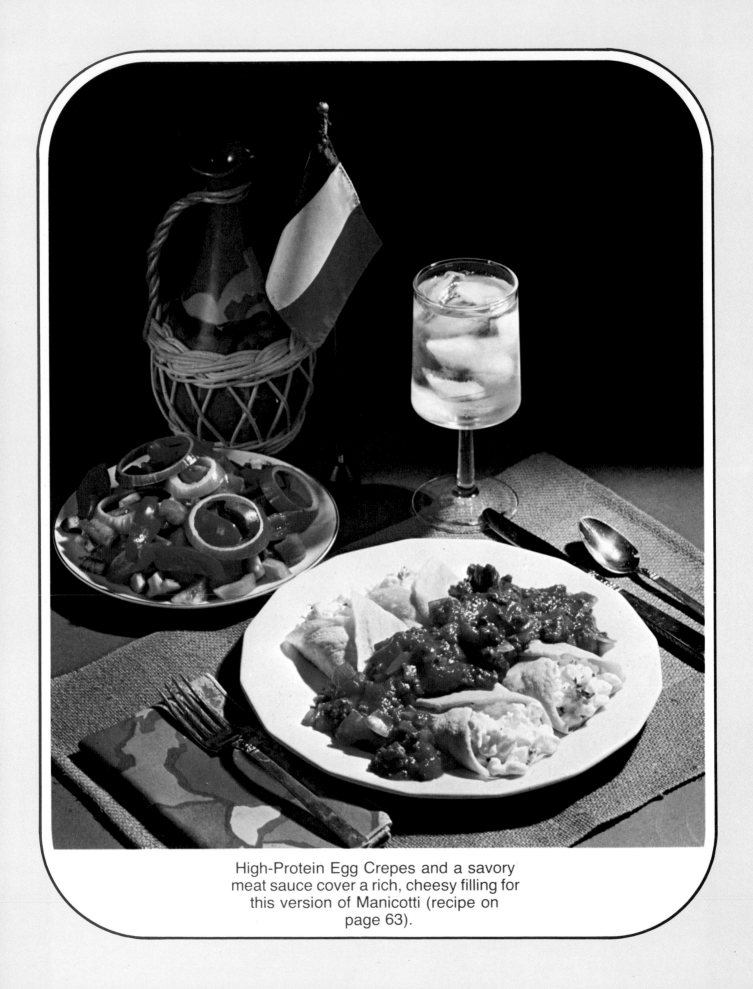

High-Protein Egg Crepes and a savory
meat sauce cover a rich, cheesy filling for
this version of Manicotti (recipe on
page 63).

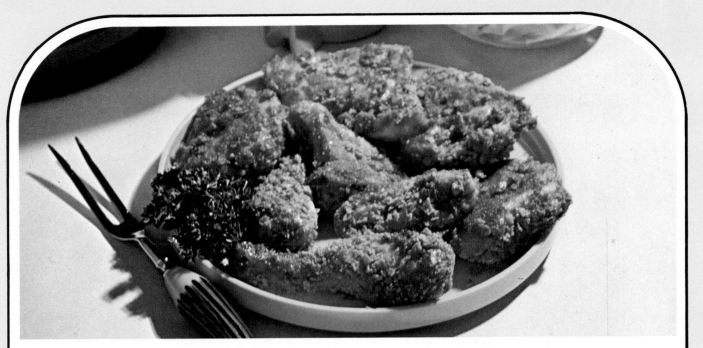

Chicken with a crisp, crunch crust and piquant ribs are two favorite foods usually forbidden to dieters. But, Oven Fried Chicken, above, and Tangy Veal Spareribs, below, have been deliciously decalorized. The recipes appear on pages 68 (chicken) and 53 (ribs).

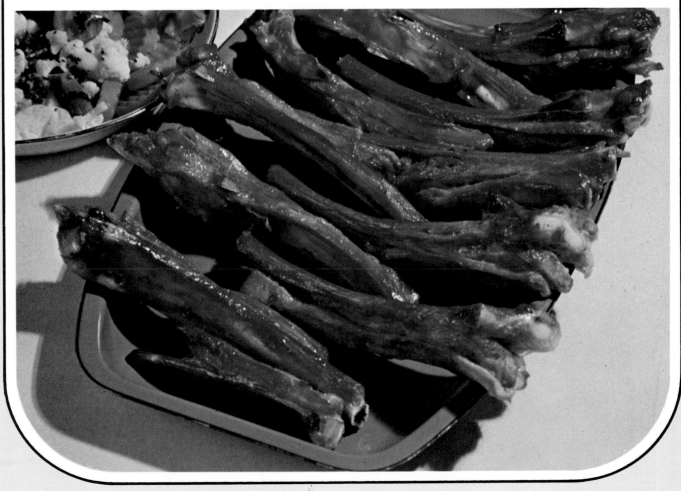

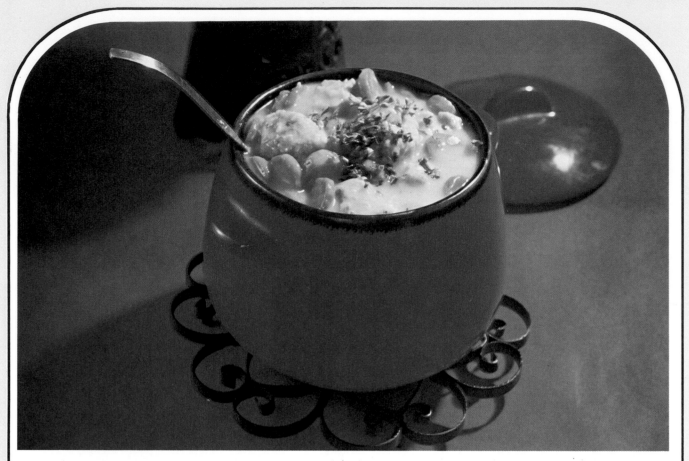

Above, French Turkey Ragout (recipe on page 71) uses boned turkey thigh browned the low-cal way. Below, Chinese Pork (recipe on page 60) is chock full of delicious goodies like mandarin oranges and water chestnuts.

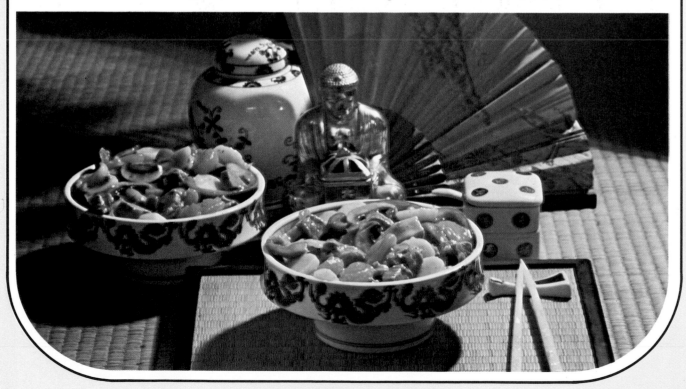

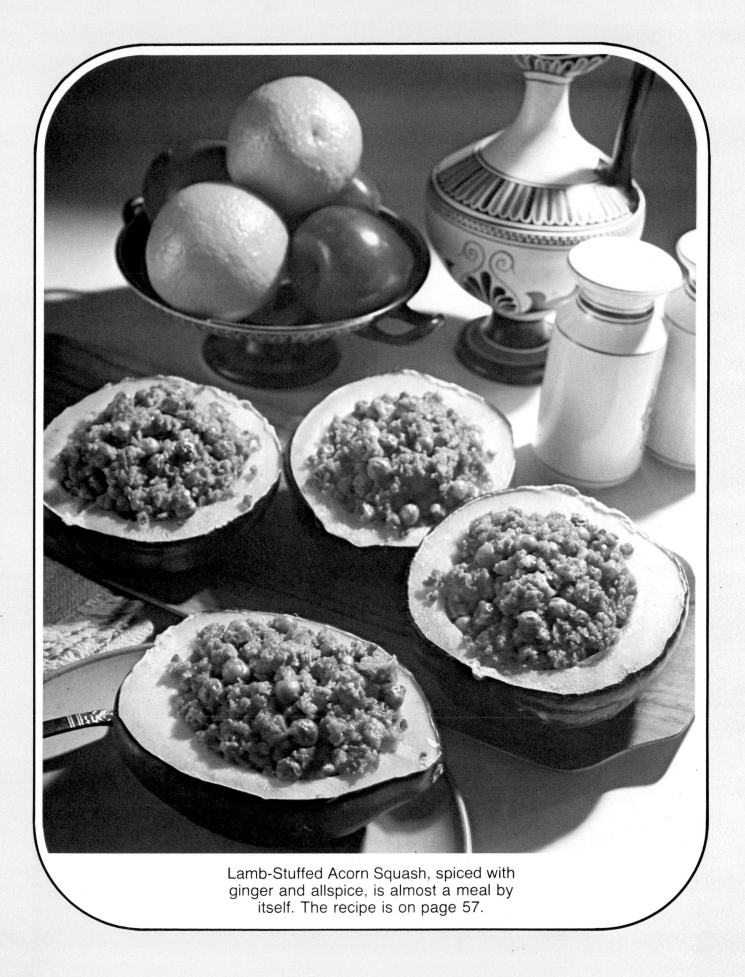

Lamb-Stuffed Acorn Squash, spiced with ginger and allspice, is almost a meal by itself. The recipe is on page 57.

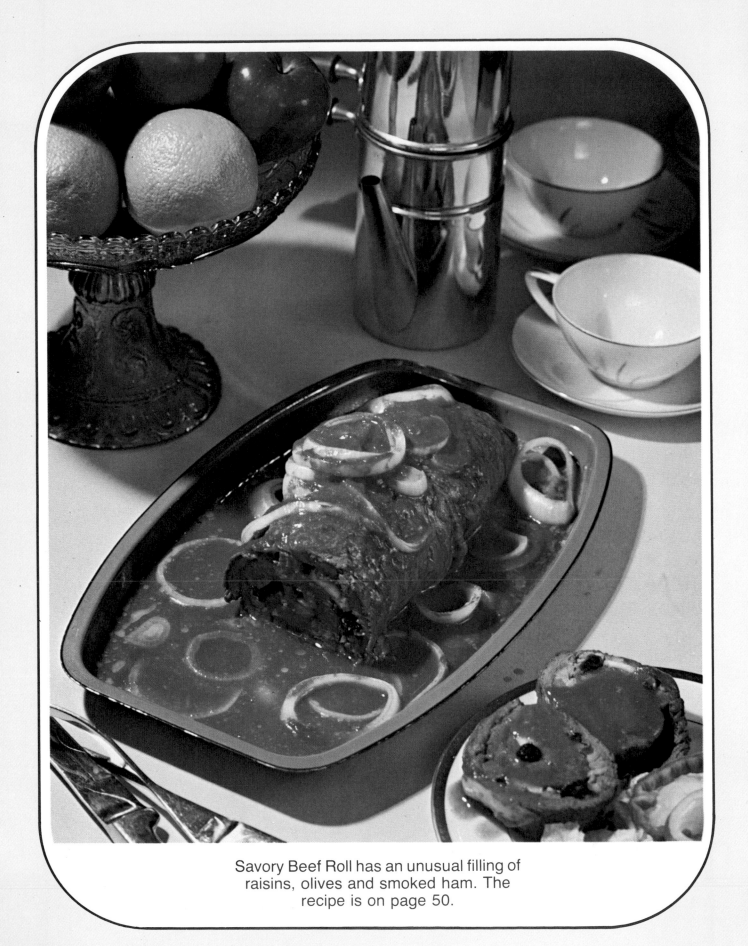

Savory Beef Roll has an unusual filling of
raisins, olives and smoked ham. The
recipe is on page 50.

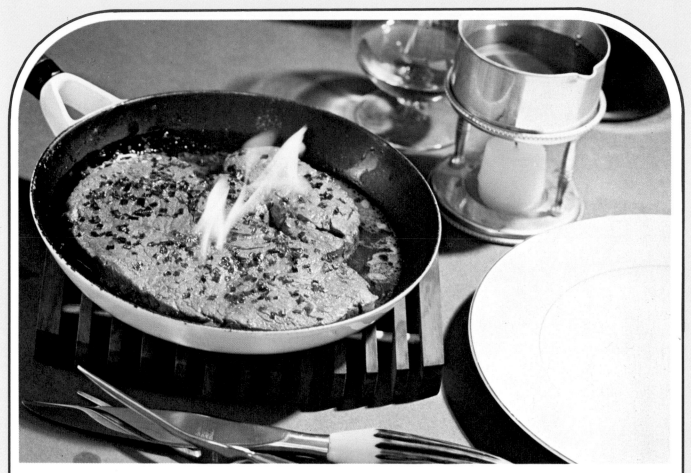

Above, Slim-Down Steak Diane (recipe on page 50) is a showy main dish when you flame it at the table. Below, Pork Steak Viennese (recipe on page 60) is baked on a bed of sauerkraut, tomatoes and onions.

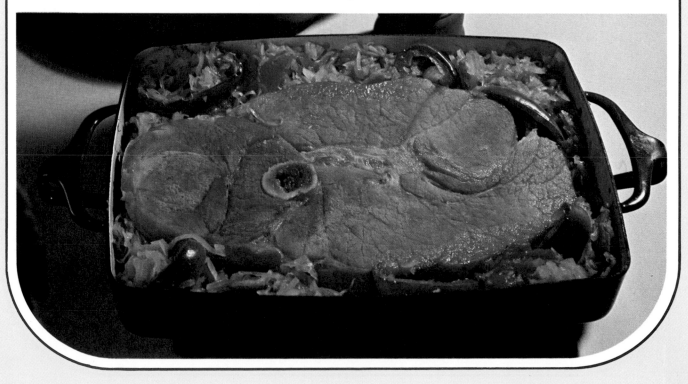

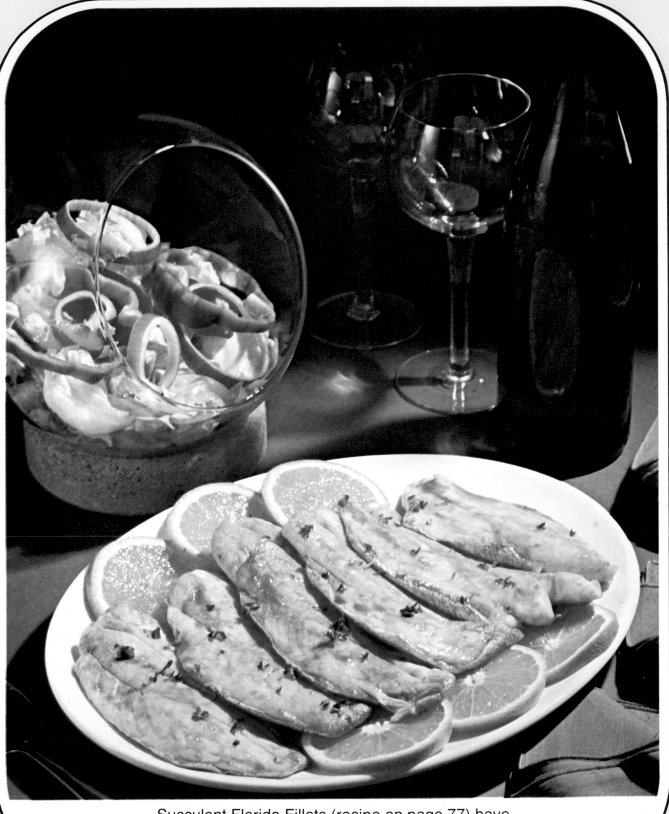

Succulent Florida Fillets (recipe on page 77) have
a mere 156 calories per serving. The fillets
marinate in a sweet-sour mixture of orange juice
and soy sauce before being broiled.

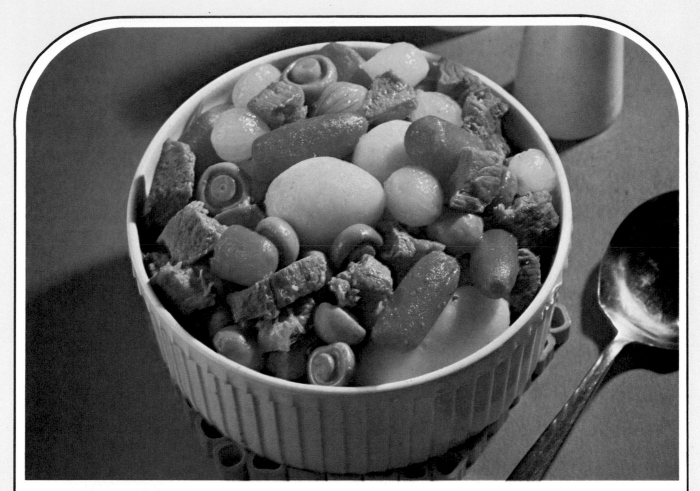

A quick version of a French classic, Veal Provencal Petite (recipe on page 54), above, makes an instantly elegant supper. Below, Chicken with Snow Peas (recipe on page 89) is a spicy version of a Chinese classic.

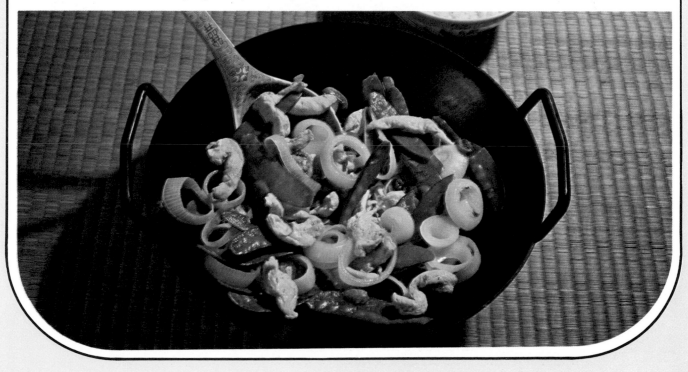

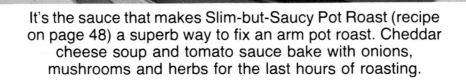

It's the sauce that makes Slim-but-Saucy Pot Roast (recipe on page 48) a superb way to fix an arm pot roast. Cheddar cheese soup and tomato sauce bake with onions, mushrooms and herbs for the last hours of roasting.

Arroz con Pollo

2 lb. broiler-fryer
  chicken pieces
1 medium onion,
  chopped
1 cup uncooked rice

Pinch saffron
4 cups stewed
  tomatoes
1 green pepper,
  chopped
1 tsp. salt

Place the chicken in a baking pan and bake it un-covered in a preheated 450° oven for 30 minutes. Pour off all the fat that accumulates in the pan. Arrange the chicken with the onion in a 3-quart casserole. Sprinkle the rice and saffron around the chicken. Then add the tomatoes, green pepper, and salt. Cover tightly and bake at 350° for 1 hour. *Makes 6 servings*

	Calories	Carbo-hydrate (gm)	Protein (gm)	Total Fat (gm)	Saturated Fat (gm)	Choles-terol (mg)
Total	1789.4	203.0	153.3	39.3	13.7	555.7
Per Serving	298.2	33.8	25.6	6.6	2.3	92.6

Chicken Mediterranean

1 tbsp. grated lemon
  peel
1/2 cup water
1/4 cup lemon juice
1 tsp. thyme
1 tsp. garlic salt

1/2 tsp. black pepper
2-lb. broiler-fryer
  chicken,
  quartered
1 lemon, sliced
1/4 cup chopped
  parsley

Combine the grated lemon peel, water, lemon juice, thyme, garlic salt, and pepper. Spoon this mixture over the chicken, coating it well. Refrigerate 3 to 4 hours, turning chicken in the marinade several times.

Arrange the chicken in a single layer in a shallow baking dish. Save the marinade. Bake the chicken, un-covered, in a preheated 425° oven for 25 minutes. Pour off the fat that accumulates in the pan. Lower the heat to 350°. Brush the chicken with the reserved marinade and bake for an additional 25 to 35 minutes until tender and brown. Garnish with lemon slices and parsley. *Makes 4 servings*

	Calories	Carbo-hydrate (gm)	Protein (gm)	Total Fat (gm)	Saturated Fat (gm)	Choles-terol (mg)
Total	886.6	5.8	130.7	34.3	13.7	555.7
Per Serving	221.7	1.5	32.7	8.6	3.4	138.9

Lemony Chicken

1 lb. broiler-fryer
  chicken pieces
1/2 tsp. salt
1/2 tsp. onion salt
1/2 tsp. crushed thyme
1/2 tsp. crushed
  marjoram

2 tsp. grated lemon
  peel
1/3 cup fresh lemon
  juice
1/2 cup water
1 lemon, quartered
Dash paprika
Snipped parsley

Season the chicken with salt and place in a nonstick baking pan, skin side down. Combine the seasonings, lemon peel, and lemon juice with 1/2 cup water and pour over the chicken. Bake, uncovered, in a pre-heated 350° oven about 30 minutes, basting once or twice with the pan liquid. Then turn the chicken over, and continue basting with the pan liquid until the chicken is done and the skin is crispy. Remove the chicken to a heated platter. Garnish with lemon quar-ters, paprika, and parsley. *Makes 4 servings*

	Calories	Carbo-hydrate (gm)	Protein (gm)	Total Fat (gm)	Saturated Fat (gm)	Choles-terol (mg)
Total	886.8	7.2	130.7	34.3	13.7	555.7
Per Serving	221.7	1.8	32.7	8.6	3.4	138.9

Herbed Chicken

1 tsp. salt
3 tbsp. lemon juice
2 tbsp. water
1 tsp. rosemary
1 tsp. thyme

2 tsp. dried tarragon
  leaves
1-lb. broiler-fryer
  chicken, split in
  half lengthwise

Make a basting sauce by combining all the ingredients except the chicken. Place the chicken on a broiler rack, skin side up, and brush it with the basting sauce. Broil the chicken 8 to 10 inches from the heat source for approximately 45 minutes, until tender, basting it as needed. *Makes 4 servings*

	Calories	Carbo-hydrate (gm)	Protein (gm)	Total Fat (gm)	Saturated Fat (gm)	Choles-terol (mg)
Total	857.8	3.8	130.5	34.3	13.7	555.7
Per Serving	219.0	1.0	32.6	8.6	3.4	138.9

Baked Chicken with Mushrooms

2 (2 lb. each) broiler-
  fryer chickens,
  quartered
1 1/2 tsp. salt
1 tsp. celery seed

1/2 tsp. dried
  marjoram
8-oz. can
  mushrooms,
  drained
  reserving liquid

Sprinkle the chicken quarters with salt and place skin side up in a shallow baking dish. Season them with celery seed and marjoram. Add the liquid from the mushrooms and bake the chicken in a preheated 350° oven for 30 minutes, occasionally spooning the liquid over the meat. Then add the mushrooms to the pan and continue baking 20 or 30 minutes longer until the chicken is tender. Drain the liquid from the pan. Using a bulb-type baster, skim the fat from the liquid so the liquid can be used as a gravy. *Makes 8 servings*

	Calories	Carbo-hydrate (gm)	Protein (gm)	Total Fat (gm)	Saturated Fat (gm)	Choles-terol (mg)
Total	1767.5	6.0	265.5	68.6	27.4	1110.5
Per Serving	220.9	0.8	33.2	8.6	3.4	138.8

gm = grams; mg = milligrams. Nutritional figures are approximate. Figures are based on findings of U.S. Department of Agriculture.

Chicken Parmigiana

1 egg
2 tbsp. safflower oil
3 whole chicken
 breasts, boned,
 skinned, halved

½ cup Italian-
 flavored bread
 crumbs
3 oz. part-skim
 mozzarella
 cheese, sliced

Whip the egg and oil together in a shallow dish. Dip the chicken first into the egg mixture, then into the bread crumbs, to coat lightly. Place the coated chicken in a single layer on a shallow nonstick baking tray or cookie sheet. Bake in a preheated 450° oven for 20 minutes, turning the pieces once. Then top each piece with a slice of cheese and return to the oven just until the cheese begins to melt. Serve the chicken as it is or with Jiffy Tomato Sauce (see index).

Makes 6 servings

	Calories	Carbo-hydrate (gm)	Protein (gm)	Total Fat (gm)	Saturated Fat (gm)	Choles-terol (mg)
Total	1260.0	38.1	153.5	63.5	13.5	614.0
Per Serving	210.0	6.4	25.6	10.6	2.3	102.3

Chicken Kiev

4 whole chicken
 breasts (about 1 lb.
 each), boned,
 skinned, halved
1 tbsp. freeze-dried
 chives
1 tsp. butter-flavored
 salt
½ tsp. thyme

½ tsp. marjoram
¼ tsp. ground black
 pepper
4 oz. Neufchatel
 cheese, cut in 8
 slices
2 eggs
2 tbsp. safflower oil
8 tbsp. seasoned
 bread crumbs

Pound the chicken breasts halves with a rolling pin until they are about ¼ inch thick. Sprinkle with the chives and seasonings. Place 1 cheese slice on the edge of each piece of chicken and roll up tightly, tucking in the sides to enclose the cheese completely. Secure the rolls with toothpicks. Beat the eggs with the oil in a shallow dish. Place the bread crumbs in another shallow dish. Dip the chicken rolls in the egg mixture, and then roll in the bread crumbs. Arrange the chicken in a single layer in a baking pan. Bake in a preheated oven at 450° for 20 minutes. *Makes 8 servings*

	Calories	Carbo-hydrate (gm)	Protein (gm)	Total Fat (gm)	Saturated Fat (gm)	Choles-terol (mg)
Total	2381.2	41.3	311.1	102.0	40.3	1496.8
Per Serving	297.7	5.2	38.9	12.8	5.0	187.1

Oven-Fried Chicken

1 cup crushed high-
 protein cereal,
 unsweetened
2 tsp. salt
¼ tsp. pepper

2 lb. broiler-fryer
 chicken pieces
½ cup evaporated
 skim milk

Mix the crushed cereal, salt, and pepper together on a flat plate. Dip the chicken pieces into the milk, and then roll them in the cereal mixture. Place them, skin side down, on a nonstick cookie sheet and bake 30 minutes in a preheated 350° oven. Turn and bake on the other side for another 30 minutes.

Makes 4 servings

	Calories	Carbo-hydrate (gm)	Protein (gm)	Total Fat (gm)	Saturated Fat (gm)	Choles-terol (mg)
Total	1124.1	28.6	143.9	44.5	19.2	594.7
Per Serving	281.0	7.2	36.0	11.1	4.8	148.7

Chicken Pizza

2 lbs. chicken breasts,
 boned and skinned
 (2½ lbs. with bone
 will yield 2 lbs.
 boned)
1 tsp. onion salt
½ tsp. pepper
8 oz. can tomato sauce

½ tsp. oregano
4 oz. can
 mushrooms,
 undrained
1 cup shredded part-
 skim mozzarella
 cheese (4 oz.)

Season the chicken breasts with the onion salt and pepper, and arrange them in a shallow baking dish. Combine the tomato sauce, mushrooms, liquid, and oregano in a bowl; then pour this over the chicken. Bake the chicken, uncovered at 350° for 35 minutes or more until it is tender. Sprinkle the cheese over the top of the chicken, and return it to the oven for about 5 minutes, until the cheese is melted and bubbly.

Makes 8 servings

	Calories	Carbo-hydrate (gm)	Protein (gm)	Total Fat (gm)	Saturated Fat (gm)	Choles-terol (mg)
Total	1625.4	18.6	278.9	52.4	14.7	786.2
Per Serving	203.2	2.3	34.9	6.6	1.8	98.3

Mushroom Poultry Stuffing

½ lb. fresh mushrooms
 finely chopped
1 cup shredded carrots
1 cup diced celery
¾ cup diced onion
½ cup nonfat dry milk
1 tsp. salt

1 tbsp. chopped
 parsley
¼ tsp. ground sage
⅛ tsp. ground
 marjoram
Dash ground red
 pepper

Combine all of the ingredients in a medium saucepan. Place the pan over low heat, and cook the stuffing for about 5 minutes, until liquid appears in the pan. Then cover and simmer 30 minutes, stirring occasionally. The stuffing may be served hot, as is, or placed in the cavity of a chicken before roasting. This recipe makes about 2 cups of stuffing, which is enough for a 4-pound chicken. *Makes 8 servings*

	Calories	Carbo-hydrate (gm)	Protein (gm)	Total Fat (gm)	Saturated Fat (gm)	Choles-terol (mg)
Total	378.5	68.5	33.0	2.5	0.0	7.5
Per Serving	47.3	8.6	4.1	0.3	0.0	0.9

gm = grams; mg = milligrams. Nutritional figures are approximate. Figures are based on findings of U.S. Department of Agriculture.

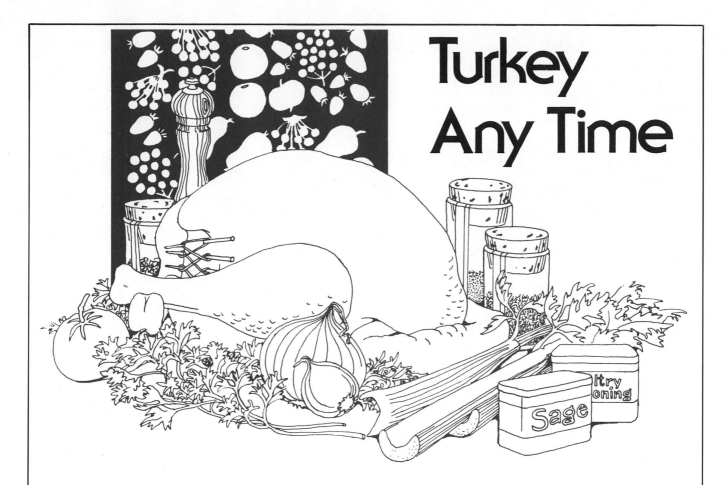

Turkey Any Time

If the turkey is only a holiday visitor at your house, you are missing out on one of America's best buys in cost, calories and nutrition. Like chicken, turkey is a lean and low-cal choice for figure-watchers and heart-smart cooks. With the increasing availability of smaller birds, boneless roast, turkey-in-parts, and such recent innovations as turkey steaks, turkey cutlets, ground turkey meat, and even turkey sausage, there's no reason why turkey can't make a frequent appearance at the family dinner table.

Nowadays, most turkey comes to market relatively young, and that's good news. It's not only more convenient to cook and store a smaller bird, but the calorie-protein-fat ratio is more in keeping with the dieter's aims. Moreover, the old idea that big old birds offer more meat and less waste just isn't true, as the following chart shows. The figures are per pound of ready-to-cook turkey.

	Waste	Fat	Protein	Calories
Young (under 24 weeks)	27%	20 gm	71 gm	480
Medium (up to 32 weeks)	27%	52 gm	66 gm	752
Mature (over 32 weeks)	27%	97 gm	61 gm	1136

How to Roast a Turkey

1. Most turkeys are bought frozen, so the first thing you must do is defrost it. When defrosting, leave the turkey in its original wrapper and use one of the following methods:
   - **No Hurry.** Place the turkey on a tray and keep it in the refrigerator for 3 to 4 days.
   - **Faster.** Place the turkey on a tray and leave it out at room temperature. This will take 1 hour per pound of turkey.
   - **Fastest.** Place the turkey in the sink and cover it with cold water. Change the water occasionally. This will take 1/2 hour per pound of turkey.
2. The turkey should be refrigerated or roasted as soon as it has thawed. If you plan to stuff the turkey, don't do it until just before you are ready to roast it. If the turkey has been commercially stuffed, follow the directions on the turkey wrapper, but omit the fat.
3. When you are ready to roast the turkey, remove the plastic wrapper. Remove the neck and giblets from the bird's cavity.
4. Rinse the turkey and wipe it dry.
5. Simmer the neck and giblets to make a broth for flavoring the stuffing or as a base for giblet gravy.
6. If you wish to stuff your turkey, follow your favorite stuffing recipe. (Several stuffing recipes are suggested in this chapter). To stuff the turkey loosely, you will need 3/4 cup stuffing per pound of oven-ready weight.

7. If you do not stuff the turkey, rub the cavity generously with salt. If you like, insert pieces of celery, carrot, onion and parsley for added flavor. Unstuffed turkeys require about 1/2 hour less roasting time.

8. Fasten down the bird's legs either by tying them together or by sticking them under the skin band. The neck skin should be skewered to the bird's back, and the wings should be twisted akimbo.

9. Place the turkey breast-side-up on a rack in a shallow roasting pan. Don't brush it with any butter or oil.

10. If you like, insert a meat thermometer into the thickest part of the thigh. Make certain that the tip of the thermometer (the bulb) doesn't touch the bone.

11. A tent of foil placed loosely over the turkey will eliminate the need for basting, although the turkey may be basted if you like. If you use foil, remove it for the last 1/2 hour of roasting so the bird gets nicely browned.

12. Or, if the turkey isn't too heavy for convenient handling, it can be roasted upside-down (using a V rack) for the first half of roasting time. In that case, don't insert the thermometer until the turkey has been turned over. This upside-down method results in juicier white meat.

13. Roast the turkey in a preheated 325° oven according to the following time chart, or until the meat thermometer registers 180° to 185°. If you're not using a thermometer, you can tell that the turkey is done if the drumstick feels soft when pressed with your thumb and forefinger, and when the drumstick and thigh move easily.

TURKEY ROASTING TIMETABLE

Ready-to-Cook Weight	Approximate Cooking Time*
6 to 8 lb.	3 - 3½ hours
8 to 12 lb.	3½ - 4½ hours
12 to 16 lb.	4½ - 5½ hours
16 to 20 lb.	5½ - 6½ hours
20 to 24 lb.	6½ - 7 hours

*If the turkey is stuffed, add ½ hour to the total cooking time.

14. Let the roast stand 10 minutes before carving.

How to Roast a Boneless Turkey Breast

The boneless turkey breast roast offers the same economical goodness and high nutritive value of a whole turkey, but it has the added advantage of coming in smaller sizes. A turkey roast is just the right size for the family's dinner or as an entree for a small dinner party.

The breast roast is particularly good for the weight-conscious person. Each average serving of white meat (3½ ounces) costs only 176 calories. It also has the least cholesterol of all the popular meats. Yet it provides high-quality protein and generous amounts of the B vitamins, riboflavin, and niacin.

1. To thaw a turkey roast, leave it sealed in its plastic wrap and place it on a tray in the refrigerator overnight. For quicker thawing, submerge the wrapped roast in cold water, changing the water occasionally. This will take ½ hour per pound of turkey.

2. After the roast has thawed, unwrap it, rinse it in cool water, drain it, and pat it dry.

3. Skewer the turkey's skin to the meat along the cut edges of the roast. This will prevent the skin from shrinking during the roasting time.

4. Rub the cavity of the roast lightly with salt.

5. If the wings are still attached, lay them flat over the breast and tie a string around the breast end to hold the wings down.

6. Insert a meat thermometer into the roast so that the tip of the thermometer (the bulb) is in the center of the meat.

7. Place the roast on a rack, skin side up, in a shallow roasting pan.

8. If you like, you may place a tent of foil loosely over the turkey. This will eliminate the need for basting, although the turkey may be basted if you wish. If you use foil, remove it for the last ½ hour of roasting, so that the turkey gets nicely browned.

9. Roast the turkey in a 325° oven according to the following timetable. The meat is done when the thermometer reads 180° to 185°.

TURKEY BREAST ROASTING TIMETABLE

Ready-to-Cook Weight	Total Roasting Time
5 to 8 lb.	2½ - 3½ hours
8 to 10 lb.	3½ - 4 hours
10 to 12 lb.	4 - 4½ hours

10. Let the turkey stand for 10 minutes before carving it.

Recipes

Turkey Marengo

3 lb. turkey wings, tips removed	1-lb. can tomatoes
1 cup sliced onions	½ cup dry white wine
4-oz. can sliced mushrooms, undrained	2 cups water
	1 tsp. salt
	½ tsp. pepper
	1 tsp. oregano

Separate the wing sections and place in a nonstick Dutch oven. Brown them without adding any oil to the pot. After the turkey has browned, add all of the remaining ingredients. Cover the pot and simmer over low heat for 2 hours. Refrigerate until serving time.

Just before serving, remove the pot from the refrigerator. The fat will have floated to the top and congealed. Lift off the fat and discard it. Then reheat the turkey, uncovered, simmering it for 10 or 15 minutes, until most of the liquid has evaporated.

Makes 6 servings

	Calories	Carbo-hydrate (gm)	Protein (gm)	Total Fat (gm)	Saturated Fat (gm)	Choles-terol (mg)
Total	2059.8	37.6	193.6	111.7	27.4	719.8
Per Serving	343.2	6.3	32.3	18.6	4.6	120.0

gm = grams; mg = milligrams. Nutritional figures are approximate. Figures are based on findings of U.S. Department of Agriculture.

French Turkey Ragout

1¼ lb. turkey thighs	1 garlic clove,
2 tbsp. water	minced
2 cups water	1 bay leaf
2 medium white	1 lb. small carrots,
potatoes, peeled	fresh or frozen
and halved	½ tsp. salt
1 cup tomato juice	¼ tsp. pepper
2 onions, chopped	2 tbsp. flour
	¼ cup cold water

With a sharp knife, strip the turkey meat from the bone, and cut it into 1½-inch cubes. Put the turkey, skin side down, in a heavy nonstick Dutch oven and add 2 tablespoons water. Cover and cook over high heat until the water evaporates and the turkey cubes begin to brown in their own melted fat. Then lower the heat, uncover the pot, and continue to cook the turkey until it is brown on all sides. Before going any further, drain the accumulated fat from the pot. Then add 2 cups water and all the remaining ingredients, except the flour and ¼ cup water. Cover the pot and simmer the contents over low heat for 35 to 45 minutes — until the turkey is tender. Then combine the flour with ¼ cup cold water and stir this mixture into the pot. Continue to cook and stir until the gravy has thickened. *Makes 4 servings*

	Calories	Carbo-hydrate (gm)	Protein (gm)	Total Fat (gm)	Saturated Fat (gm)	Choles-terol (mg)
Total	1407.3	112.4	155.7	36.7	13.7	461.6
Per Serving	351.8	28.1	38.9	9.2	3.4	115.4

Hearty Turkey Chowder

8 cups turkey or	6 medium-sized
chicken broth	carrots, pared
1 lb. fresh ground	and sliced
turkey	½ cup water
2 tbsp. flour	¼ cup flour
1 tsp. salt	2 tbsp. fresh lemon
⅛ tsp. pepper	juice
2 eggs	2 tbsp. chopped
1 tbsp. grated onion	parsley
½ cup skim milk	

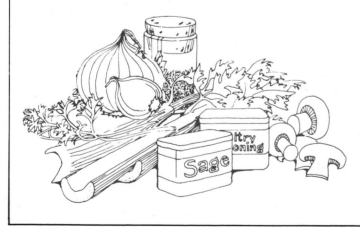

Skim the fat from the broth by chilling it until the fat floats to the top and can be whisked away. Combine the turkey with the flour, salt, pepper, eggs, onion, and milk in a bowl. Shape the mixture into 36 small balls. In a stock pot, bring the broth to a boil. Add the meatballs, cover and simmer 10 minutes. Remove the meatballs from the broth and set them aside. Then add the carrots to the broth and cook them in the same way for 20 minutes. In a cup combine the water and flour. Add the mixture to the broth and carrots, and continue cooking about 2 minutes until it is bubbly. Then add the lemon juice and meatballs. Serve the chowder garnished with chopped parsley. *Makes 10 servings*

	Calories	Carbo-hydrate (gm)	Protein (gm)	Total Fat (gm)	Saturated Fat (gm)	Choles-terol (mg)
Total	1577.2	96.1	198.5	39.8	13.1	1025.2
Per Serving	157.7	9.6	19.9	4.0	1.3	102.5

Apple-Bacon Poultry Stuffing

6 apples, peeled and	¼ cup chopped
chopped	parsley
2 cups cubed protein	1 tsp. salt
bread, lightly	¼ tsp. pepper
toasted	1 tsp. poultry
½ cup chopped onion	seasoning
½ cup cubed Canadian	½ cup hot giblet
bacon	stock or boiling
1 cup minced celery	water

Combine all the ingredients, mixing them lightly. Loosely fill the cavity of a turkey, chicken, or rock Cornish hen. The stuffing can also be baked in a 1½-quart casserole in a preheated 350° oven for 45 minutes. *Makes 12 servings (4 cups)*

	Calories	Carbo-hydrate (gm)	Protein (gm)	Total Fat (gm)	Saturated Fat (gm)	Choles-terol (mg)
Total	797.1	147.1	26.3	14.3	3.7	61.2
Per Serving	66.4	12.3	2.2	1.2	0.3	5.1

High-Fiber Stuffing

1 cup chicken broth	20 slices dry whole
2 cups minced celery	wheat or other
2 cups minced onion	high-fiber bread,
2 tsp. poultry seasoning	cubed

Skim the fat from the broth by using a bulb-type baster or by chilling it until the fat floats to the top and can be lifted off. Add the rest of the ingredients to the skimmed broth and mix them lightly. Loosely fill the cavity of a large turkey with the stuffing, or spoon it into a 1½-quart casserole. If you use a casserole, bake the stuffing in a preheated 350° oven for 45 minutes. *Makes 12 servings. (4 cups)*

	Calories	Carbo-hydrate (gm)	Protein (gm)	Total Fat (gm)	Saturated Fat (gm)	Choles-terol (mg)
Total	1227.0	258.0	48.0	12.0	4.0	28.0
Per Serving	102.3	21.5	4.0	1.0	0.3	2.3

gm = grams; mg = milligrams. Nutritional figures are approximate. Figures are based on findings of U.S. Department of Agriculture.

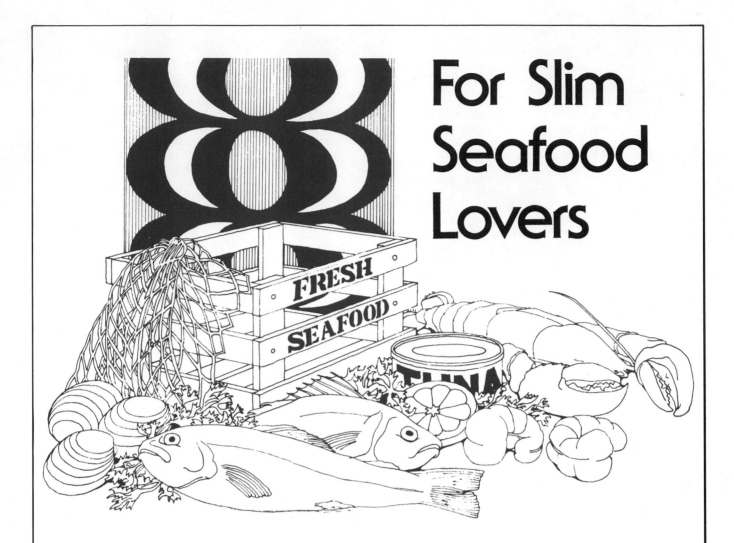

For Slim Seafood Lovers

If you are now a seafood fan, this section is for you. If you are *not* . . . then this section is *especially* for you. It's quite possible that most overweights who claim to dislike fish have never really had it — good fish, that is.

If your seafood-sampling history is limited to frozen fish sticks, diner-fried fish fillets of indeterminate species, or the Friday fish special dished up in the company or school cafeteria, then you should count yourself among the vast number of Americans who have never had really good fish.

What is good fish? To begin with, it must be absolutely fresh. Fish that smells fishy isn't fresh — because really fresh fish has no odor. The admonition that fish must be fresh doesn't mean you have to catch you own or barter with a charter boat operator down at the docks. And it doesn't mean that you must limit your marketing to fancy fish stores. Perfectly good fresh fish is available bargain-priced in your supermarket freezer case. Yes, frozen fish can be the freshest of all — if it has been properly handled. Frozen fish is frequently processed right on the commercial vessel on which it is caught. However, partial thawing or careless handling anywhere along the distribution route can result in subquality seafood when you thaw it out

at home. If frozen seafood shows signs of mishandling when you thaw it out, simply wrap it in plastic and return it to the store for a refund.

Good seafood is also properly cooked. And here's where lots of perfectly fine fish winds up a culinary casuality. Unlike meat, fish doesn't need cooking to make it tender. The purpose of cooking fish is to develop its fine flavor. Overcooking — either too much or for too long — only results in toughness, dryness, and unpleasant flavor. Fish that has been overfloured and carelessly tossed into a skillet full of fat is not only fattening, it is unappetizing in taste, texture, and appearance. If that's the sort of seafood you've been exposed to, it is time to give fish a fighting chance.

Why the Emphasis on Fish for Slimming?

Anyone who has a nodding acquaintance with dieting knows that seafood turns up with sometimes monotonous frequency on most lose-weight plans. The reason is that seafood is the slimmest of all main course choices, the one that's highest in protein and lowest in fat.

All fish, even so-called fatty fish, is low calorie when

compared with most meat. Flounder, a lean fish, is only 308 calories a pound compared with 1,818 calories for rib roast, with a comparable protein content. Mackerel, which is a fat fish, has only 866 calories a pound and *more* protein that rib roast. To see how other popular species of seafood compare, check the following list.

FISH CALORIE COMPARISONS
Calories per Pound*

Beef, rib	1,818
Bass, striped	476
Bluefish	530
Butterfish	522
Carp	522
Catfish	467
Clams	363
Cod	354
Crabmeat	422
Flounder	308
Haddock	358
Halibut	453
Lake Trout	1,093
Lobster	413
Mackerel	866
Oysters	299
Perch	431
Pompano	753
Porgy	508
Pike	408
Red Snapper	422
Rockfish	440
Salmon	939
Sole	308
Sardines canned in tomato sauce	893
Scallops	367
Smelt	445
Shrimp	412
Swordfish	535
Tuna canned in oil	1,306
Tuna canned in water	576
Whitefish	703

Meat only. Raw, except for canned seafood

Buying Fresh Fish

Here is the advice of the National Marine Fisheries Service* on selecting the freshest fish. Look for these qualities:

Flesh: Firm flesh, not separating from the bones, indicates fish are fresh and have been handled carefully.

Odor: Fresh and mild. A fish just taken from the water has practically no fishy odor. The fishy odor becomes more pronounced with passage of time, but it should not be disagreeably strong when the fish is bought.

Eyes: Bright, clear, and full. The eyes of fresh fish are bright and transparent; as the fish becomes stale, the eyes become cloudy and often turn pink. When fish are fresh, the eyes often protrude, but with increasing staleness, the eyes tend to become sunken.

*"Let's Cook Fish: A Complete Guide to Fish Cookery." *Fishery Market Development Series No. 8*. U.S. Department of Interior, Fish and Wildlife Service, Bureau of Commercial Fisheries, U.S. Govt. Printing Office, 60 cents.

Gills: Red and free from slime. The color gradually fades with age to a light pink, then gray, and finally brownish or greenish.

Skin: Shiny, with color unfaded. When first taken from the water, most fish have an irridescent appearance. Each species has its characteristic markings and colors that fade and become less pronounced as the fish loses freshness.

Fresh fillets, steaks, and chunks have the following characteristics:

Flesh: Fresh-cut in appearance. It should be firm in texture without traces of browning or drying around the edges,

Odor: Fresh and mild.

Wrapping: If the fillets, steaks, or chunks are wrapped, the wrapping should be a moisture/vapor-proof material. There should be little or no airspace between the fish and the wrapping.

Buying Frozen Fish

High-quality frozen fish that are properly processed, packaged, and held at 0° or below will remain in good condition for relatively long periods of time. Frozen fish of good quality have the following characteristics:

Flesh: The flesh should be solidly frozen when bought. The flesh should have no discoloration or freezer burn. Virtually all deterioration in quality is prevented when fish are properly held in the frozen state. Frozen fish that have been thawed and then refrozen are poorer in quality.

Odor: Frozen fish should have little or no odor. A strong fish odor means poor quality.

Wrapping: Most frozen fillets, steaks, chunks, portions, and sticks are wrapped either individually or in packages of various weights. The wrapping should be of moisture/vapor-proof material. There should be little or no airspace between the fish and the wrapping.

How Much Fish Should You Buy?

Whole: This is fish as it comes from the water. Before cooking, the fish must be scaled and gutted. Usually the head, tail and fins are removed. The fish may then be cooked, filleted, or cut into steaks or chunks. Allow 2/3 to 3/4 pound per serving.

Dressed: This is fish with scales and entrails removed. Usually the head, tail, and fins are also removed. The fish may then be cooked whole, filleted, or cut into steaks or chunks. (The smaller size fish are called pan-dressed and are ready to cook as purchased). About 1/3 to 1/2 pound equals one serving.

Fillets: The flesh of the fish cut lengthwise away from the backbone. They are boneless, usually skinless and ready to cook as purchased. Allow 1/4 pound per serving.

Steaks: These are cross-section slices from large dressed fish cut 1/2 to 1 inch thick. A cross-section of the backbone is the only bone in a steak. They are ready to cook as purchased. Allow 1/4 to 1/3 pound per serving.

Chunks: These are cross-sections of large dressed fish. A cross-section of the backbone is the only bone in a chunk. They are ready to cook as purchased. Allow 1/3 to 1/4 pound per serving.

TIMETABLE FOR COOKING FISH

Method of Cooking	Market Form	Cooking Temp.	Approx. Cooking Time
Baking	Dressed	350°	45 to 60 min.
	Pan-dressed	350°	25 to 30 min.
	Fillets or steaks	350°	20 to 25 min.
Broiling	Pan-dressed	3 to 4 inches from heat	10 to 16 min. turning once
	Fillets or steaks		10 to 15 min.
	Frozen fried fish		10 to 15 min.
	Frozen fried fish sticks		10 to 15 min.
Charcoal Broiling	Pan-dressed	Moderate	10 to 16 min. turning once
	Fillets or steaks	Moderate	10 to 16 min.
Oven-Frying	Pan-dressed	500°	15 to 20 min.
	Fillets or steaks	500°	10 to 12 min.
Pan-Frying	Pan-dressed	Moderate	8 to 10 min. turning once
	Fillets or steaks	Moderate	8 to 10 min.
Poaching	Whole Fish	Simmer	30 to 60 min.
	Fillets or steaks	Simmer	5 to 10 min.
Steaming	Fillets or steaks	Boil	5 to 10 min.

What Dieters Should Avoid

Although fish is the best calorie and nutrition bargain you can buy, there are some types of frozen fish that dieters should stay away from. Fish is often frozen already breaded as a "convenience" to busy homemakers. What you get when you pay for already-breaded fish is a lot of breading and not much fish. You also get a lot of extra calories.

Raw breaded fish portions: These are portions cut from frozen fish blocks, coated with a batter, breaded, packaged, and frozen. Raw breaded fish portions generally contain only 75 percent fish.

Fried fish sticks: These are cut from frozen fish blocks. They are coated with a batter, then fried in fat, and frozen. Fried fish sticks are only 60 percent fish.

Recipes

Hollandaise Cod

2 tbsp. sliced almonds
6 cod or other fish steaks (1½ lb.)
½ cold skim milk
2 tbsp. flour
½ tsp. salt
Dash pepper
2 tbsp. lemon juice
2 egg yolks, beaten

Toast the almonds by spreading them out on a cookie sheet and baking them at 350° until they are lightly browned.

Place the fish steaks in a small skillet or saucepan and add just enough water to cover. Cover the pot and simmer the fish 8 to 10 minutes until it flakes easily. Drain the liquid from the pan, reserving 1 cup. In another saucepan, stir the cold milk and flour together over low heat until the mixture thickens. Add the reserved liquid from cooking the fish, and the salt and pepper. Cook and stir the mixture until it is bubbly. Then stir in the lemon juice. Stir a small amount of this hot mixture into the beaten egg yolks; then stir the egg yolk mixture back into the saucepan. Cook the sauce over low heat, stirring constantly, about 1 minute until it has thickened. (If you accidentally overcook it and the egg curdles, simply beat it smooth again in your blender.) Pour the hot sauce over the poached fish steaks and sprinkle with the toasted almonds.

Makes 6 servings

	Calories	Carbo-hydrate (gm)	Protein (gm)	Total Fat (gm)	Saturated Fat (gm)	Choles-terol (mg)
Total	1488.0	23.2	207.1	59.3	12.7	1058.1
Per Serving	248.0	3.9	34.5	9.9	2.1	176.4

gm = grams; mg = milligrams. Nutritional figures are approximate. Figures are based on findings of U.S. Department of Agriculture.

Paella

10½-oz. can chicken broth
2-lb. broiler-fryer
  chicken, cut in
  small pieces
2 tbsp. instant minced
  onion
1½ tsp. garlic salt
¼ tsp. pepper
⅛ tsp. powdered saffron
1½ cups uncooked
  converted rice

1 lb. medium shrimp,
  shelled and
  deveined
12 small clams (in
  shell)
10-oz. pkg. frozen
  peas, partially
  defrosted
1 whole pimiento,
  cut in strips

Skim the broth of fat by chilling it until the fat rises to the top and can be whisked away. Arrange the chicken pieces, skin side up, in a large nonstick baking pan. Bake them, uncovered, in a preheated 450° oven for about 20 minutes until they are brown. Remove the pan from the oven. Pour off all the fat that has accumulated in the pan. Lower the oven to 350°. Add enough water to the broth to make 3 cups. Pour 1 cup of the broth mixture into the pan with the chicken. Then stir in the onion, garlic salt, pepper, and saffron. Cover the pan with foil and bake 25 minutes. Sprinkle the rice into the pan and pour in the remaining broth. Arrange the shrimp and clams over this mixture and sprinkle the peas over all. Cover the pan again, and return it to the oven for about 25 minutes, until the rice is cooked and the liquid is absorbed. Garnish with the pimiento and serve right from the pan.   *Makes 10 servings*

	Calories	Carbo-hydrate (gm)	Protein (gm)	Total Fat (gm)	Saturated Fat (gm)	Choles-terol (mg)
Total	2691.3	278.8	273.3	43.6	13.7	1360.7
Per Serving	269.1	27.9	27.3	4.4	1.4	136.1

Crabmeat Supreme

15-oz. can artichoke
  hearts, drained and
  halved
4-oz. can sliced
  mushrooms,
  drained
1 lb. crabmeat, fresh or
  thawed
1 cup evaporated skim
  milk
2½ tbsp. flour
½ tsp. butter-flavored
  salt

Dash cayenne
2 tbsp. dry sherry
2 tbsp. crushed
  high-protein
  cereal,
  unsweetened
1 tbsp. grated
  Parmesan
  cheese
Dash paprika

Spray a shallow 1½-quart casserole with vegetable coating. Place the artichokes in the casserole and cover them with the mushrooms and crabmeat. In a saucepan, combine the milk, flour, and seasonings. Cook this mixture slowly, stirring constantly, until it is thick. Then stir in the sherry. Pour the sauce over the crabmeat. Combine the cereal crumbs and cheese, and sprinkle them over the sauce. Sprinkle paprika

over all. Bake the casserole in a preheated 450° oven 12 to 15 minutes until it is bubbly.   *Makes 6 servings*

	Calories	Carbo-hydrate (gm)	Protein (gm)	Total Fat (gm)	Saturated Fat (gm)	Choles-terol (mg)
Total	1098.4	79.8	123.1	36.4	14.0	547.3
Per Serving	183.1	13.3	20.5	6.1	2.3	91.2

Tuna Stroganoff

13½-oz. can chicken broth
¼ cup flour
2 (7-oz.) cans water-
  packed tuna,
  drained, reserving
  liquid
8-oz. can tomato sauce

¼ cup instant
  chopped onions
4-oz. can
  mushrooms,
  undrained
1 tsp. parsley flakes
1 cup plain low-fat
  yogurt

Skim the fat from the chicken broth by chilling it until the fat floats to the top and can be whisked away. Combine the flour with the liquid from the tuna in a saucepan. Gradually stir in the broth and cook over low heat, stirring constantly, until it has thickened. Stir in the tomato sauce, onions, mushrooms, parsley, and tuna. Cover the pot and simmer until heated through. Stir in the yogurt, and continue cooking just until hot — do not boil.   *Makes 8 servings*

	Calories	Carbo-hydrate (gm)	Protein (gm)	Total Fat (gm)	Saturated Fat (gm)	Choles-terol (mg)
Total	930.2	72.9	134.6	8.6	2.0	306.7
Per Serving	116.3	9.1	16.8	1.1	0.3	38.3

Tuna with Grapes

⅔ cup water
½ cup instant rice
1 vegetable bouillon
  cube
¼ cup finely chopped
  celery
2 tbsp. snipped parsley
2 tbsp. all-purpose flour
½ tsp. salt
1 cup evaporated
  skim milk

7-oz. can water-
  packed tuna,
  drained and
  broken into
  chunks
½ cup seedless
  green grapes,
  halved
2 tbsp. dry white
  wine
1 tbsp. lemon juice

Bring the ⅔ cup water to a boil in a saucepan. Add the rice, bouillon, celery, and parsley, and cook for 2 minutes. Spray 4 individual casseroles with vegetable coating and spoon the rice mixture into them. Then, combine the flour, salt, and evaporated milk in a saucepan. Cook over low heat, stirring constantly, until the mixture is thick and bubbly. Remove the pot from the heat and stir in the remaining ingredients. Spoon this mixture into the casseroles over the rice. Bake in a preheated 350° oven for 20 minutes.

Makes 4 servings

	Calories	Carbo-hydrate (gm)	Protein (gm)	Total Fat (gm)	Saturated Fat (gm)	Choles-terol (mg)
Total	1076.3	134.2	94.9	30.3	13.2	204.0
Per Serving	269.1	33.6	23.7	7.6	3.3	51.0

gm = grams; mg = milligrams. Nutritional figures are approximate. Figures are based on findings of U.S. Department of Agriculture.

Italian Oven-Fried Sea Cutlets

1 egg	6 tbsp. Italian-
2 tbsp. corn or safflower	seasoned bread
oil	crumbs
5 tbsp. freshly grated	4 fish fillets (1 lb.)
Romano cheese	Dash paprika
	1/4 tsp. salt
	Dash pepper

Beat the egg and oil together. Sprinkle the cheese on a plate. Sprinkle the bread crumbs on another plate. Dip each fillet lightly in the egg-oil mixture, then in the cheese, then in the crumbs, coating both sides lightly and evenly. Sprinkle with paprika. Arrange in a single layer on a nonstick cookie tin or shallow baking pan sprayed with vegetable coating. Sprinkle with salt and pepper. Bake in a preheated 450° oven for 5 to 6 minutes. Turn the steaks over and continue baking another 3 to 4 minutes. *Makes 4 servings*

	Calories	Carbo-hydrate (gm)	Protein (gm)	Total Fat (gm)	Saturated Fat (gm)	Choles-terol (mg)
Total	1148.3	30.6	192.6	105.6	33.1	761.5
Per Serving	287.1	7.7	48.2	26.4	8.3	190.4

Seafood Parmesan

8 skinless flounder or	4 tbsp. diet
other fish fillets (2	mayonnaise
lb.)	3 tbsp. chopped
2 tbsp. fresh lemon	green onion
juice	1/4 tsp. salt
5 tbsp. grated	Dash hot pepper
Parmesan cheese	sauce

Spray a bake-and-serve platter with vegetable coating. Arrange the fillets in a single layer on the platter. Brush fillets with lemon juice and let them stand for 10 minutes.

Combine the remaining ingredients in a bowl. Broil the fillets about 4 inches from the heat source for 5 to 6 minutes. Remove them from the broiler and spread the cheese mixture over them. Return the fillets to the broiler and continue broiling 3 to 4 minutes longer until fillets are lightly browned. *Makes 8 servings*

	Calories	Carbo-hydrate (gm)	Protein (gm)	Total Fat (gm)	Saturated Fat (gm)	Choles-terol (mg)
Total	2318.3	11.3	313.7	109.6	36.3	933.8
Per Serving	289.8	1.4	39.2	13.7	4.5	116.7

Barbecued Fish

1/4 cup chopped onion	2 tbsp. fresh lemon
2 tbsp. chopped green	juice
pepper	1 tbsp. Worcester-
1 garlic clove, finely	shire sauce
chopped	2 tsp. salt
8-oz. can tomato sauce	1/4 tsp. pepper
3/4 cup unsweetened	8 fish fillets or
apple cider	steaks (2 lb.)

Combine all the ingredients except the fish in a saucepan and cook over moderate heat 5 minutes, stir-ring occasionally. Allow this sauce to cool. Arrange the fish in a single layer in a shallow baking dish. Pour the sauce over the fish and let it stand at room temperature for 30 minutes, turning the fish once. Then remove the fish from the baking dish and save the sauce for basting. Place the fish in a well-oiled, hinged wire grill. Place the grill about 4 inches from moderately hot coals and cook the fish for 5 to 8 minutes. Baste it with the sauce. Turn the fish over and cook it 5 to 8 minutes longer or until the fish flakes easily when tested with a fork. *Makes 8 servings*

	Calories	Carbo-hydrate (gm)	Protein (gm)	Total Fat (gm)	Saturated Fat (gm)	Choles-terol (mg)
Total	1725.5	43.9	228.0	64.4	21.3	543.7
Per Serving	215.7	5.5	28.5	8.1	2.7	68.0

Oven-Fried Fish Fillets I

1 egg	1/2 cup seasoned
2 tbsp. corn or safflower	bread crumbs
oil	4 fish fillets (1 lb.)

Whip the egg and oil together with a fork. Pour this mixture onto a plate. Place the bread crumbs on another plate. Dip the fillets first into the egg mixture and then into the bread crumbs so they are lightly coated. Place the breaded fillets on a nonstick cookie sheet or other shallow pan with nonstick coating and bake them in a preheated 450° oven for 10 to 12 minutes, until they are golden and cooked through. *Makes 4 servings*

	Calories	Carbo-hydrate (gm)	Protein (gm)	Total Fat (gm)	Saturated Fat (gm)	Choles-terol (mg)
Total	1441.8	36.5	151.1	73.8	15.2	664.9
Per Serving	360.5	9.1	37.7	18.5	3.8	166.2

Oven-Fried Fish Fillets II

4 fish fillets (1 lb.)	1/2 cup unseasoned
1/2 cup French or Italian	bread crumbs
salad dressing	
(regular, not diet)	

Marinate the fish fillets in the dressing for 15 minutes, turning frequently. Spray a nonstick cookie sheet or shallow baking pan with vegetable coating for no-fat frying. Sprinkle the crumbs on a shallow plate. Press each well-moistened fillet in the crumbs, coating both sides lightly. Then arrange in a single layer on the cookie sheet. Bake in a preheated 450° oven for 5 to 6 minutes. Carefully turn fillets with a spatula and continue baking another 5 to 6 minutes. *Makes 4 servings*

	Calories	Carbo-hydrate (gm)	Protein (gm)	Total Fat (gm)	Saturated Fat (gm)	Choles-terol (mg)
Total	1227.9	48.5	134.4	53.2	9.8	370.3
Per Serving	307.00	12.1	33.6	13.3	2.5	92.6

gm = grams; mg = milligrams. Nutritional figures are approximate. Figures are based on findings of U.S. Department of Agriculture.

Florida Fillets

8 skinless snapper or other fish fillets (2 lb.)
½ cup frozen unsweetened orange juice concentrate, thawed
1 tbsp. corn or safflower oil
¼ cup soy sauce
¼ cup cider vinegar
½ tsp. salt
Chopped parsley
Orange slices (optional)

Spray a 15x10x1-inch baking pan with vegetable coating for no-fat cooking. Arrange the fish, skinned side up, in a single layer. In a bowl, combine the orange juice, oil, soy sauce, vinegar, and salt. Brush the fish with this sauce. Broil the fish about 4 inches from the heat source for 5 minutes. Turn the fish carefully and brush it again with the sauce. Continue to broil another 5 to 7 minutes, until the fish is lightly browned and flakes easily when tested with a fork. Sprinkle chopped parsley over the top. Garnish with orange slices if you like. *Makes 8 servings*

	Calories	Carbo-hydrate (gm)	Protein (gm)	Total Fat (gm)	Saturated Fat (gm)	Choles-terol (mg)
Total	1252.3	66.3	188.6	24.7	1.0	501.0
Per Serving	156.5	8.3	23.6	3.1	0.1	62.6

Sole alla Mozzarella

8 skinless sole or other fish fillets (2 lb.)
2 tbsp. grated onion
1½ tsp. garlic salt
⅛ tsp. pepper
½ tsp. oregano
2 large tomatoes, cut in pieces
1 cup shredded part-skim mozzarella cheese

Spray a bake-and-serve platter with vegetable coating for no-fat, no-stick cooking. Arrange the fillets in a single layer on the platter and sprinkle them with the grated onion, salt, pepper, and oregano. Then cover the fillets with the tomato pieces. Broil the fish about 4 inches from the heat source for 10 to 12 minutes or until the fillets flake easily when tested with a fork. Sprinkle the cheese over the fish, and continue broiling 2 to 3 minutes until the cheese melts. *Makes 8 servings*

	Calories	Carbo-hydrate (gm)	Protein (gm)	Total Fat (gm)	Saturated Fat (gm)	Choles-terol (mg)
Total	2226.7	21.5	341.5	94.6	25.3	892.8
Per Serving	278.3	2.7	42.7	11.8	3.2	111.6

Curried Fish I

6 fish fillets (1½ lb.)
1½ tbsp. fresh lemon juice
½ tsp. butter-flavored salt
¼ tsp. pepper
10½-oz. can condensed cream of celery soup
¼ cup skim milk
1 tsp. curry powder (or more to taste)

Arrange the fish in a single layer in a baking dish. Season with the lemon juice, salt, and pepper, and bake uncovered in a preheated 425° oven for 12 minutes. While the fish is baking, heat the condensed soup in a saucepan. Stir in the milk, a little at a time. When the sauce is smooth, add the curry powder. To serve, place the baked fillets on a platter and spoon the sauce over the fish. *Makes 6 servings*

	Calories	Carbo-hydrate (gm)	Protein (gm)	Total Fat (gm)	Saturated Fat (gm)	Choles-terol (mg)
Total	1328.7	26.7	183.6	45.2	0.0	499.7
Per Serving	221.5	4.5	30.6	7.5	0.0	83.3

Curried Fish II

¾ cup water
¾ tsp. salt
4 fish fillets (1 lb.)
2 tbsp. flour
1 tsp. curry powder
1 tbsp. onion flakes
Dash ground ginger
¾ cup skim milk

In a skillet, bring the water and ½ teaspoon of the salt to a boil. Lower the heat, add the fish, and cover the pan. Simmer the fish 6 to 10 minutes until it flakes easily when tested with a fork. Drain the liquid from the pan, reserving ¼ cup. Remove the fillets, and break them into 2-inch pieces. Combine the flour, curry powder, onion flakes, ¼ teaspoon salt, ginger, milk, and reserved liquid in the now-empty skillet. Heat this mixture to boiling, stirring constantly, and boil and stir for 1 minute. Then stir in the fish and heat it through. *Makes 4 servings*

	Calories	Carbo-hydrate (gm)	Protein (gm)	Total Fat (gm)	Saturated Fat (gm)	Choles-terol (mg)
Total	1049.4	22.9	147.3	37.4	10.7	414.2
Per Serving	262.4	5.7	36.8	9.4	2.7	103.6

Fish Broil Maui

8 skinless fish fillets (2 lb.)
¼ cup low-calorie French dressing
3 tbsp. soy sauce
¾ tsp. ground ginger
8 lemon slices

Spray a bake-and-serve platter with vegetable coating, and arrange the fillets on it in a single layer. Combine the French dressing, soy sauce and ginger, and pour this mixture over the fish. Let the fish stand for 10 minutes. Broil the fillets about 4 inches from the heat source 10 to 15 minutes, until they flake easily when tested with a fork. Baste once during the broiling time with the sauce in the platter. To serve, garnish the fish with lemon slices. *Makes 8 servings*

	Calories	Carbo-hydrate (gm)	Protein (gm)	Total Fat (gm)	Saturated Fat (gm)	Choles-terol (mg)
Total	1867.5	3.0	280.2	74.6	21.3	820.8
Per Serving	233.4	0.4	35.0	9.3	2.7	102.6

gm = grams; mg = milligrams. Nutritional figures are approximate. Figures are based on findings of U.S. Department of Agriculture.

Ramekins of Crab and Shrimp

1 tbsp. diet margarine
1/3 cup sliced green
 onions
1/4 cup flour
1 tsp. salt
1/8 tsp. white pepper
13-oz. can evaporated
 skim milk
6-oz. pkg. frozen
 king crabmeat,
 thawed
7 oz. cooked Pacific
 pink shrimp
2 tbsp. fresh lemon
 juice
6-oz. can sliced
 water chestnuts,
 drained
2 1/2 cups cooked rice
2 tbsp. diced
 pimiento
1/2 cup shredded
 cheddar cheese

Melt the margarine in a small nonstick skillet. Sauté the green onions in the margarine until they are tender. In a large saucepan, blend together the flour, salt, and pepper; then add the milk. Cook this mixture over low heat, stirring constantly, until it is thick and smooth. Then stir in the crabmeat, shrimp, lemon juice, water chestnuts, cooked rice, pimiento, and sautéed green onions. Spoon the entire mixture into 6 individual-size ramekins, top with cheese and bake in a preheated 350° oven for about 25 minutes until the mixture is hot and bubbly. *Makes 6 servings*

	Calories	Carbo-hydrate (gm)	Protein (gm)	Total Fat (gm)	Saturated Fat (gm)	Choles-terol (mg)
Total	2364.6	234.6	145.4	90.6	44.1	735.8
Per Serving	394.1	39.1	24.2	15.1	7.4	122.6

Crab-Filled Green Peppers

4 medium green
 peppers, halved
 and seeded
8 oz. crabmeat, flaked
1 cup cooked rice
2 eggs, slightly beaten
2 tbsp. lemon juice
1 tbsp. chopped
 onion
1/2 tsp. curry
1/4 tsp. salt
Dash cayenne
1/2 cup crushed rice
 cereal
1 tbsp. diet
 margarine

Cook the peppers in boiling salted water for 5 minutes and then drain.
 Combine the crabmeat with the rice, beaten eggs, lemon juice, onion, curry, salt and cayenne. Fill the pepper halves with the crab mixture. Then combine the crushed cereal with the margarine and sprinkle this over the crab mixture. Place the stuffed green peppers on a baking sheet and bake in a preheated 400° oven for 15 minutes. *Makes 4 servings*

	Calories	Carbo-hydrate (gm)	Protein (gm)	Total Fat (gm)	Saturated Fat (gm)	Choles-terol (mg)
Total	745.5	71.5	60.8	23.3	5.0	731.0
Per Serving	186.4	17.9	15.2	5.8	1.3	182.8

Savory Rock Lobster Tails

1/4 cup chicken bouillon
2 to 3 drops butter
 flavoring
1 tbsp. fresh lemon
 juice
1/8 tsp. bitters
1/8 tsp. ground ginger
1/8 tsp. chili powder
4 rock lobster tails (5
 oz. each)

Combine the bouillon, butter flavoring, lemon juice, bitters, ginger, and chili powder in a bowl. (For the bouillon, you may use canned bouillon undiluted or a bouillon cube mixed with 1/4 cup water.) Cut through the lobster shells lengthwise to keep the tails from curling during cooking. Place the lobster tails on a broiler rack, meat side up, and brush the meat with the bouillon mixture. Broil about 4 inches from the heat source 8 to 10 minutes. *Makes 4 servings*

	Calories	Carbo-hydrate (gm)	Protein (gm)	Total Fat (gm)	Saturated Fat (gm)	Choles-terol (mg)
Total	554.9	2.2	108.3	6.7	0.0	487.2
Per Serving	138.7	0.6	27.1	1.7	0.0	121.8

Cheddar Chowder

7-oz. can minced clams,
 undrained
1 tbsp. finely chopped
 onion
10 3/4-oz. can condensed
 cheddar cheese
 soup
1/2 cup skim milk
16-oz. can tomatoes,
 undrained

Combine all the ingredients, including the liquid from the cans of tomatoes and clams, in a large saucepan. Simmer the mixture, covered, 10 to 12 minutes. *Makes 4 servings*

	Calories	Carbo-hydrate (gm)	Protein (gm)	Total Fat (gm)	Saturated Fat (gm)	Choles-terol (mg)
Total	630.3	56.5	37.5	29.5	12.6	128.4
Per Serving	157.6	14.1	9.4	7.4	3.2	32.1

Skewered Scallops with Canadian Bacon

1 lb. small scallops,
 rinsed and drained
1/2 lb. Canadian bacon,
 cubed
1 large onion in chunks
2 green peppers in
 chunks
1/2 lb. fresh
 mushrooms
1 tbsp. corn or
 safflower oil
2 tbsp. soy sauce
1/4 tsp. garlic salt
Dash of cayenne

Thread the scallops on 6 skewers, alternating them with the bacon cubes and vegetable chunks. Combine the oil, soy sauce, and seasonings in a shallow plate. Rotate the skewers in this mixture to coat the scallops and vegetables evenly. Place the skewers 3 or 4 inches over hot coals for 15 minutes, turning them frequently and basting with remaining marinade. Or place the skewers on a shallow nonstick roasting pan or cookie sheet. Pour on the remaining sauce. Bake them in a preheated 450° oven for 15 minutes, turning them once or twice during the cooking. *Makes 6 servings*

	Calories	Carbo-hydrate (gm)	Protein (gm)	Total Fat (gm)	Saturated Fat (gm)	Choles-terol (mg)
Total	1548.7	73.5	193.5	61.9	11.7	429.5
Per Serving	258.1	12.3	32.3	10.3	2.0	71.6

gm = grams; mg = milligrams. Nutritional figures are approximate. Figures are based on findings of U.S. Department of Agriculture.

Scallop Sauté

2 tbsp. diet margarine	2 tomatoes, cut in
2 lb. scallops, rinsed	eighths
and drained	1/4 cup water
7-oz. pkg. frozen pea	2 tbsp. cornstarch
pods, thawed and	1 tbsp. soy sauce
drained	1/2 tsp. salt
	1/8 tsp. pepper

Melt the margarine in a 10-inch nonstick skillet. Add the scallops, and sauté over low heat for 3 or 4 minutes. Then add the pea pods and tomatoes. In a cup, combine the water, cornstarch, soy sauce, salt, and pepper. Add this mixture to the skillet and cook, stirring constantly, until the sauce is thick.

Makes 6 servings

	Calories	Carbo-hydrate (gm)	Protein (gm)	Total Fat (gm)	Saturated Fat (gm)	Choles-terol (mg)
Total	1357.4	89.3	218.2	22.7	2.0	479.7
Per Serving	226.2	14.9	36.4	3.8	0.3	80.0

Cioppino

2 cups sliced onion	1/2 tsp. oregano
2 garlic cloves, finely	1/4 tsp. pepper
minced	1 1/2 lb. halibut, ling
1-lb. 12-oz. can Italian	cod, rockfish or
tomatoes,	sea bass, cut into
undrained	1 1/2-in. chunks
8-oz. can tomato sauce	1 doz. clams in shell
1 cup water	1 cup cooked
1/4 cup chopped parsley	shrimp, peeled
2 tsp. salt	and deveined
1 tsp. basil	

Combine all the ingredients except the fish, clams, and shrimp in a Dutch oven. Cover and simmer gently 30 minutes. Add the fish chunks and continue to simmer, covered, about 15 minutes. Then add the clams in their shells and the shrimp. Cover the pot and continue simmering about 10 minutes or until the fish chunks flake easily when tested with a fork.   *Makes 8 servings*

	Calories	Carbo-hydrate (gm)	Protein (gm)	Total Fat (gm)	Saturated Fat (gm)	Choles-terol (mg)
Total	1723.8	76.8	224.2	55.2	16.0	664.2
Per Serving	215.5	9.6	28.0	6.9	2.0	83.0

Skinny Scampi

1 lb. sea scallops or	1/2 tsp. salt or butter-
raw shrimp (peeled	flavored salt
and deveined)	1/8 tsp. freshly ground
2 tbsp. soft butter	pepper
(margarine may be	Dash paprika
substituted)	(optional)
2 tbsp. dry white wine or	1 tbsp. chopped
lemon juice	parsley
2 cloves garlic,	(optional)
finely minced	

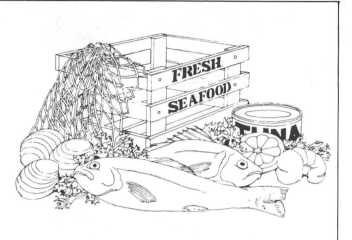

Arrange seafood in a single layer in a shallow broiling pan or 4 individual flameproof servers. Dot lightly with the butter. Add the wine or lemon juice and minced garlic. Sprinkle with salt and pepper. Broil 3 or 4 inches from the heat, turning frequently, until seafood is cooked through, 3 to 6 minutes. Sprinkle with paprika and garnish with parsley, if desired.

Makes 4 servings

	Calories	Carbo-hydrate (gm)	Protein (gm)	Total Fat (gm)	Saturated Fat (gm)	Choles-terol (mg)
Total	660.5	7.8	80.3	28.3	12.8	753.6
Per Serving	165.1	2.0	20.1	7.1	3.2	188.4

Shrimp Bisque

1/4 cup finely chopped	1 tsp. butter-flavored
onion	salt
1/4 cup finely chopped	1/4 tsp. paprika
celery	Dash white pepper
1/4 cup water	4 cups skim milk
2 tbsp. flour	14 oz. cooked shrimp,
	coarsely
	chopped

Place the onion, celery, and water in a nonstick skillet. Cook until the vegetables are tender. Stir in the flour and seasonings. Add the milk to the skillet and cook the entire mixture over low heat, stirring constantly, until it is thick. Fold in the shrimp. Continue cooking just until the shrimp is heated through; serve it at once.

Makes 6 servings

	Calories	Carbo-hydrate (gm)	Protein (gm)	Total Fat (gm)	Saturated Fat (gm)	Choles-terol (mg)
Total	787.2	63.4	108.0	4.8	0.0	616.5
Per Serving	131.2	10.6	18.0	0.8	0.0	102.7

gm = grams; mg = milligrams. Nutritional figures are approximate. Figures are based on findings of U.S. Department of Agriculture.

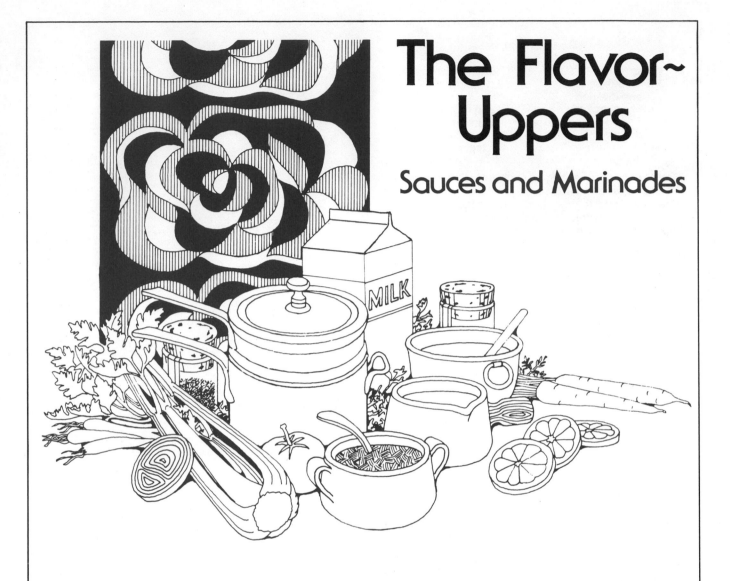

The Flavor~Uppers

Sauces and Marinades

Most diet plans warn the would-be slimmer to stay away from sauces and gravies — and with good reason. Most sauces are calorie-rich. But thickeners aren't the main source of a sauce's calories. The real culprit is hidden fat in the form of butter, cream, margarine, oil, or meat fat. Without the fat calories, sauces and gravies can serve as savory toppings for lean meat, fish and poultry, or as replacement for butter or margarine on top of vegetables.

How to Make Low-Fat Gravy

Fat is not a necessary ingredient in gravy. You can subtract 100 calories for every tablespoon of meat fat you skim from pan drippings.

1. The easy way to do this is to drain the drippings into a cup and quick-chill it in your freezer until the fat rises to the surface and hardens. Then, simply lift the fat off and discard it. If you're in a real rush, pour the hot drippings in a tall narrow heat-proof container and wait a minute or two until the fat reaches the surface.

Then *zoop* it up with a bulb-type baster.

2. Measure the stock and heat it to boiling.

3. For each cup of stock, combine 2 tablespoons flour and ¼ cup cold water in a small cup. Stir until smooth and lump-free, then stir the flour mixture into the simmering stock to thicken it. (Never add flour directly to a hot liquid or it will lump.)

4. Simmer the gravy over very low heat until it is the desired thickness. If it gets too thick, thin it with a little water.

5. For a darker gravy, stir in a little soy sauce or brown gravy coloring. Season the gravy to your taste with salt, pepper, onion powder, or herbs.

Canned beef broth or chicken broth can be used in place of meat drippings for gravy-making. When you open the can, be sure to remove any globules of grease floating on the surface. Use condensed products straight, without diluting. But do not use canned cream soups for sauces because these contain unneeded fat. A can of cream of chicken soup , for example, is 245 calories.

How to Make Cream Sauce

Cream sauce, or white sauce, doesn't need cream or butter for a dairy-rich flavor. Canned evaporated skim milk is an ideal stand-in for cream. It has only a fraction of the fat and calories and it's much higher in protein.

1. For a medium cream sauce, combine one 13-ounce can of evaporated skim milk with 4 tablespoons flour in a nonstick saucepan over very low heat. Cook and stir until the sauce begins to bubble. Simmer two minutes.

2. Season to taste with chopped parsley, a pinch of nutmeg, white pepper, and butter-flavored salt (or bottled butter flavoring).

3. Increase or decrease the amount of flour for a thick or thin white sauce.

This sauce can be used in any favorite recipe that calls for white sauce as a base:

Wine sauce. Add 3 tablespoons dry white wine. Simmer 2 minutes.

Cheese sauce. Add 6 tablespoons shredded cheese. Stir until melted.

Curry sauce. Add 1 (or more) teaspoon curry powder.

Bechamel sauce. Omit salt, add 2 chicken bouillon cubes.

Recipes

Smooth Cream Sauce for Vegetables

1/4 cup flour	1/8 tsp. pepper
2 cups skim milk	Dash nutmeg
3/4 tsp. butter-flavored salt	Dash cayenne

Blend the ingredients in a nonstick saucepan over moderate heat, stirring constantly until the sauce is thick and smooth. *Makes 2 cups (8 servings)*

	Calories	Carbo-hydrate (gm)	Protein (gm)	Total Fat (gm)	Saturated Fat (gm)	Choles-terol (mg)
Total	293.8	47.8	21.3	0.3	0.0	10.0
Per Serving	36.7	6.0	2.7	0.0	0.0	1.3

Jiffy Tartar Sauce

1/2 cup diet mayonnaise	1/4 cup pickle relish, drained

Combine the ingredients well and serve with fish.
Makes 3/4 cup (6 servings)

Hint: If you like spice in your life, add 1/2 teaspoon horseradish and 1 teaspoon Worcestershire sauce.

	Calories	Carbo-hydrate (gm)	Protein (gm)	Total Fat (gm)	Saturated Fat (gm)	Choles-terol (mg)
Total	240.0	28.0	0.0	16.0	0.0	64.0
Per Serving	40.0	4.7	0.0	2.7	0.0	10.7

Lemony Egg Sauce for Fish

2 tbsp. flour	1 tbsp. fresh lemon juice
1/2 tsp. butter-flavored salt	2 hard-cooked eggs
Dash white pepper	2 tbsp. diced pimiento (optional)
13-oz. can evaporated skim milk	

In a saucepan, stir together the flour, salt, pepper and milk. Cook this mixture slowly, stirring constantly, until it has become thick and smooth. Then fold in the lemon juice, chopped eggs, and pimiento. Continue to cook the sauce just until it is heated through. Serve over baked fish or vegetables.

Makes 2 cups (8 servings)

	Calories	Carbo-hydrate (gm)	Protein (gm)	Total Fat (gm)	Saturated Fat (gm)	Choles-terol (mg)
Total	777.1	51.5	42.9	44.5	21.8	630.4
Per Serving	97.1	6.4	5.4	5.6	2.7	78.8

Low-Calorie Hollandaise Sauce

3/4 cup diet mayonnaise	Dash white pepper
3 tbsp. skim milk	1 tbsp. lemon juice
1/4 tsp. salt	1 tbsp. grated lemon peel

Combine the mayonnaise, milk, salt, and pepper in a saucepan and heat very slowly, stirring constantly, until the mixture is warm. Then stir in the lemon juice and grated lemon peel. Serve with cooked vegetables or fish. *Makes 16 tablespoons (8 servings)*

	Calories	Carbo-hydrate (gm)	Protein (gm)	Total Fat (gm)	Saturated Fat (gm)	Choles-terol (mg)
Total	261.1	13.7	1.7	20.0	0.0	10.0
Per Serving	32.6	1.7	0.2	2.5	0.0	1.3

Jiffy Tomato Sauce

1 tsp. diet margarine	2 tsp. instant bouillon (or 2 bouillon cubes)
1/4 cup finely chopped onion	
2 cups coarsely chopped tomatoes (1-lb. can)	

Melt the margarine in a nonstick skillet, and sauté the onions until they are tender. Then stir in the tomatoes and bouillon. Simmer the mixture, uncovered, about 15 minutes until the sauce is thick and well blended.
Makes 1 1/2 cups (6 servings)

	Calories	Carbo-hydrate (gm)	Protein (gm)	Total Fat (gm)	Saturated Fat (gm)	Choles-terol (mg)
Total	136.5	22.5	6.5	4.0	0.3	6.0
Per Serving	22.8	3.8	1.1	0.7	0.1	1.0

gm = grams; mg = milligrams. Nutritional figures are approximate. Figures are based on findings of U.S. Department of Agriculture.

Sugarless Blender Catsup

16-oz. can unsweetened
    juice-packed
    pineapple,
    undrained
6-oz. can tomato paste
1/3 cup cider vinegar

1 tsp. onion powder
1/4 tsp. liquid hot
    pepper sauce
1/2 tsp. salt
1/2 tsp. dry mustard
1/4 tsp. cinnamon

Combine all of the ingredients in a covered blender and blend until smooth. Spoon into 2 plastic squeeze catsup containers and refrigerate.

Makes about 3 cups (48 servings)

	Calories	Carbo-hydrate (gm)	Protein (gm)	Total Fat (gm)	Saturated Fat (gm)	Choles-terol (mg)
Total	366.6	95.8	5.9	0.4	0.0	0.0
Per Serving	7.6	2.0	0.1	0.0	0.0	0.0

Sweet 'n' Sour Sauce

6-oz. can tomato paste
2 cups unsweetened
    pineapple juice
3 tbsp. lemon juice or
    vinegar

1/2 tsp. salt (or onion
    or garlic salt)
1/8 tsp. pepper (or
    dash hot pepper)
Parsley or herbs to
    taste

Stir all the ingredients together in a small saucepan until well-blended. Simmer, uncovered, 5 minutes. Serve over meat, poultry, seafood or vegetables, or use as a cooking sauce.

Makes 2 1/2 cups (10 servings)

	Calories	Carbo-hydrate (gm)	Protein (gm)	Total Fat (gm)	Saturated Fat (gm)	Choles-terol (mg)
Total	410.4	101.6	6.9	0.0	0.0	0.0
Per Serving	41.0	10.2	0.7	0.0	0.0	0.0

Mustard Sauce

1/2 cup plain low-fat
    yogurt
1 1/2 tbsp. prepared
    mustard

1/2 tsp. parsley flakes
1/8 tsp. butter-flavored
    salt

Combine all of the ingredients in a saucepan. Heat the mixture slowly, stirring occasionally, but don't let it boil. Serve with fish or cooked vegetables.

Makes 10 tablespoons (5 servings)

	Calories	Carbo-hydrate (gm)	Protein (gm)	Total Fat (gm)	Saturated Fat (gm)	Choles-terol (mg)
Total	236.5	50.0	4.0	2.0	1.0	10.0
Per Serving	47.3	10.0	0.8	0.4	0.2	2.0

Lean Luau Sauce

7 3/4-oz. jar baby food
    peaches or apricots
5 tbsp. tomato paste
2 tbsp. honey

1/3 cup cider vinegar
1 tbsp. soy sauce
1 tsp. ground ginger
1/8 tsp. garlic powder

Bring all of the ingredients to a boil in a small saucepan, stirring frequently. Serve with broiled pork or chicken.

Makes 1 1/2 cups (5 servings)

	Calories	Carbo-hydrate (gm)	Protein (gm)	Total Fat (gm)	Saturated Fat (gm)	Choles-terol (mg)
Total	387.8	101.5	5.2	0.0	0.0	0.0
Per Serving	77.6	20.3	1.0	0.0	0.0	0.0

Curry in a Hurry Sauce

2 tsp. instant chicken
    bouillon or 2
    chicken bouillon
    cubes
1 cup dry skim milk
    powder

1/4 cup all-purpose
    flour
3/4 tsp. curry powder
    (or more to taste)
2 cups cold water

Combine all of the ingredients in a saucepan. Cook the mixture over moderate heat, stirring constantly, until it thickens and boils. Serve the sauce hot over cooked vegetables or fish.

Makes 2 1/2 cups (10 servings)

	Calories	Carbo-hydrate (gm)	Protein (gm)	Total Fat (gm)	Saturated Fat (gm)	Choles-terol (mg)
Total	391.0	99.6	47.2	14.3	4.0	15.0
Per Serving	39.1	10.0	4.7	1.4	0.4	1.5

Quick Hot Curry Sauce

2 tsp. instant chicken or
    beef bouillon or 2
    bouillon cubes
6-oz. can tomato paste
2 cups unsweetened
    apple juice
2 tbsp. raisins

1 tsp. apple pie or
    pumpkin pie
    spice
1 tsp. curry powder
    (or more to taste)
Few drops hot
    pepper sauce (or
    more to taste)

Combine all the ingredients in a saucepan. Cook and stir over moderate heat until mixture is thick and bubbling. Serve over cooked meat, seafood or poultry, or on vegetables or rice.

Makes 2 3/4 cups (11 servings)

	Calories	Carbo-hydrate (gm)	Protein (gm)	Total Fat (gm)	Saturated Fat (gm)	Choles-terol (mg)
Total	436.2	140.1	24.1	14.0	4.0	0.0
Per Serving	39.7	12.7	2.2	1.3	0.4	0.0

Applesauce Glaze

1 cup unsweetened
    applesauce

1/8 tsp. allspice

Combine the applesauce and allspice and brush on meat during cooking.

Makes 1 cup (4 servings)

	Calories	Carbo-hydrate (gm)	Protein (gm)	Total Fat (gm)	Saturated Fat (gm)	Choles-terol (mg)
Total	100.0	26.0	1.0	0.0	0.0	0.0
Per Serving	25.0	6.5	0.3	0.0	0.0	0.0

gm = grams; mg = milligrams. Nutritional figures are approximate. Figures are based on findings of U.S. Department of Agriculture.

Pineapple Tenderizing Marinade

1 cup fresh or defrosted (not canned) unsweetened pineapple juice

2 tbsp. soy sauce

Mix the ingredients together. To use the marinade, puncture 1 pound lean meat deeply in several places with a fork. Place the meat in a glass or plastic bowl, or in a plastic bag set in a bowl. Cover meat with the marinade. Cover the container and marinate at room temperature 1 hour; or refrigerate several hours or overnight. The enzyme in the fresh juice will help to break down meat fibers. Baste the meat with the remaining marinade as it cooks.

Makes about 1 cup (4 servings)

	Calories	Carbo-hydrate (gm)	Protein (gm)	Total Fat (gm)	Saturated Fat (gm)	Choles-terol (mg)
Total	526.7	127.0	6.0	0.0	0.0	0.0
Per Serving	131.8	31.8	1.5	0.0	0.0	0.0

Seasoned Tenderizing Marinade

½ cup bottled Italian low-calorie salad dressing

1 tsp. instant meat tenderizer
½ cup warm water (or more, to cover)

Combine the ingredients. To use, puncture 1 pound lean meat deeply with a fork in several places. Place the meat in a glass or plastic bowl, or in a plastic bag set in a bowl. Cover the meat with marinade. Cover the container and marinate 1 hour at room temperature; or refrigerate several hours or overnight. Baste the meat with the remaining marinade during cooking.

Makes 1 cup (4 servings)

	Calories	Carbo-hydrate (gm)	Protein (gm)	Total Fat (gm)	Saturated Fat (gm)	Choles-terol (mg)
Total	144.0	8.0	0.0	16.0	0.0	0.0
Per Serving	38.0	2.0	0.0	4.0	0.0	0.0

French Tenderizing Marinade

½ cup low-calorie French dressing

½ cup dry white wine
1 tsp. instant meat tenderizer

Combine the ingredients. To use, puncture 1 pound meat deeply with a fork in several places. Place the meat in a glass or plastic bowl, or in a plastic bag set in a bowl. Cover the meat with marinade. Cover the container and marinate 1 hour at room temperature; or refrigerate for several hours or overnight. Baste the meat with the remaining marinade during cooking.

Makes 1 cup (4 servings)

	Calories	Carbo-hydrate (gm)	Protein (gm)	Total Fat (gm)	Saturated Fat (gm)	Choles-terol (mg)
Total	252.2	16.4	0.0	12.0	0.0	0.0
Per Serving	63.0	4.1	0.0	3.0	0.0	0.0

Italian Wine Marinade

½ cup low-calorie Italian salad dressing

½ cup dry red wine
1 tsp. instant meat tenderizer

Combine the ingredients. To use, puncture 1 pound lean meat deeply with a fork in several places. Place the meat in a glass or plastic bowl, or in a plastic bag set in a bowl. Cover the meat with marinade. Cover the container and marinate 1 hour at room temperature; or refrigerate for several hours or overnight. Baste the meat with the remaining marinade during cooking.

Makes 1 cup (4 servings)

	Calories	Carbo-hydrate (gm)	Protein (gm)	Total Fat (gm)	Saturated Fat (gm)	Choles-terol (mg)
Total	239.2	12.4	0.0	16.0	0.0	0.0
Per Serving	59.8	3.1	0.0	4.0	0.0	0.0

Mandarin Marinade

1 cup soy sauce
1 cup unsweetened orange juice

2 cloves garlic, minced
1 tsp. ground ginger
¼ tsp. pepper

Combine all of the ingredients well. To use, puncture 2 pounds lean meat deeply in several places with a fork. Place the meat in a glass or plastic bowl, or in a plastic bag set in a bowl. Pour the marinade over the meat. Cover and marinate at room temperature 1 hour; or refrigerate several hours or overnight. Baste the meat with the remaining marinade during cooking.

Makes 2 cups (8 servings)

	Calories	Carbo-hydrate (gm)	Protein (gm)	Total Fat (gm)	Saturated Fat (gm)	Choles-terol (mg)
Total	270.0	42.0	18.0	1.0	0.0	0.0
Per Serving	33.8	5.3	2.3	0.1	0.0	0.0

Yogurt Marinade

½ cup plain low-fat yogurt
2 tbsp. lemon juice
¼ cup chopped onion

1 tbsp. dry mustard
½ tsp. garlic salt
½ tsp. salt
⅛ tsp. pepper

Combine all of the ingredients well. To use, puncture 1 pound lean meat deeply in several places with a fork. Place the meat in a glass or plastic bowl, or in a plastic bag set in a bowl. Pour the marinade over the meat. Cover and let the mixture stand at room temperature 1 hour; or refrigerate several hours or overnight. Brush the meat with remaining marinade during cooking.

Makes ⅞ cup (4 servings)

	Calories	Carbo-hydrate (gm)	Protein (gm)	Total Fat (gm)	Saturated Fat (gm)	Choles-terol (mg)
Total	80.3	11.6	4.6	2.0	1.0	10.0
Per Serving	20.1	2.9	1.2	0.5	0.3	2.5

gm = grams; mg = milligrams. Nutritional figures are approximate. Figures are based on findings of U.S. Department of Agriculture.

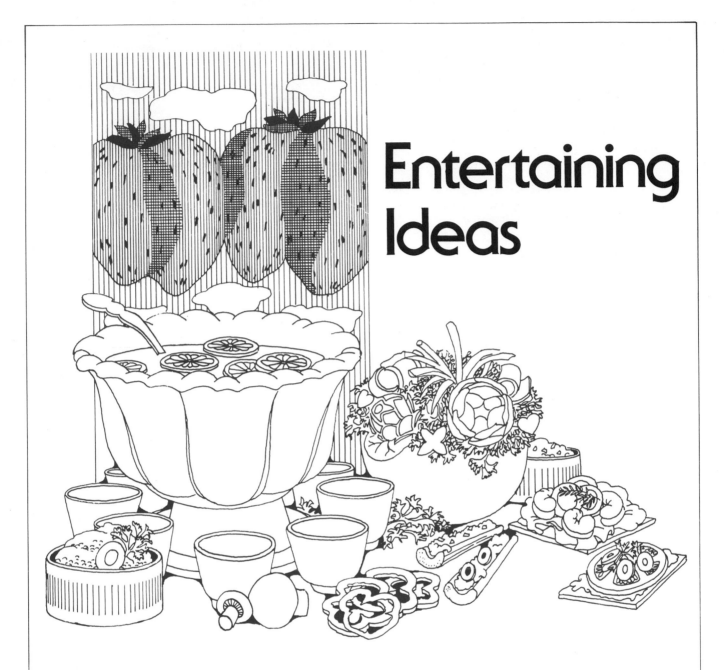

Entertaining Ideas

You do not have to sit on the sidelines when it's time to celebrate. Festive foods needn't be fattening. In fact, skinny stuff is standard fare at parties where the beautiful people circulate. How else would they keep their fashionable forms? Keeping nibbles trimming as well as tantalizing is easy to do. All it takes is a little imagination and some artful substituting of low-calorie ingredients for the fat-makers dips and spreads usually contain.

Most dips from packaged mixes pack a weighty wallop of calories. But it is not the mix that makes them fattening; it is what they're mixed with. Most packaged mixes add only 50 calories, but the directions call for a base of sour cream (485 calories a cupful) or cream cheese (850 calories in an 8-ounce package). You can cut calories dramatically by substituting plain low-fat yogurt for sour cream (only around 125 calories) or the low-calorie, low-fat imitation cream cheese (only 416 calories).

The prettiest — and most sophisticated — party trays start out at the vegetable stand. Dippers needn't be greasy kid stuff. Here are some crisp and tasty ones that make diet sense.

red and green pepper rings
cucumber slices
scallions
celery scoops
raw mushroom caps
canned water chestnut slices
seedless orange sections
fresh pineapple tidbits

melon cubes
zucchini strips
cauliflower buds
radish roses
raw turnip wedges
tiny pickles

Recipes

Zippity Dip

2 cups 99% fat-free
   cottage cheese
2 tsp. grated onion
1 tsp. celery salt

1/4 tsp. Worcester-
   shire sauce
1 1/2 cups (6 oz.)
   shredded extra-
   sharp cheddar
   cheese

Combine cottage cheese, onion, celery salt and Worcestershire sauce. Using the highest speed of your mixer or blender, beat until smooth. Gradually add 1 cup of shredded cheese and continue beating at high speed until the mixture is smooth. Fold in the remaining cheese. Serve immediately. *Makes 3 cups*

	Calories	Carbo-hydrate (gm)	Protein (gm)	Total Fat (gm)	Saturated Fat (gm)	Choles-terol (mg)
Total	1051.6	18.4	102.1	58.0	32.4	206.8
Per 1/2 cup	175.3	3.1	17.0	9.7	5.4	34.5

Spanish Olive Dip

1 1/4 cups 99% fat-free
   cottage cheese
1/4 cup skim milk
1 tbsp. instant minced
   onion

1/8 to 1/4 tsp. crushed
   red pepper
   flakes
1/4 cup chopped
   pimiento-stuffed
   olives

In a blender or mixer, blend the cottage cheese and milk until smooth. Stir in the remaining ingredients and chill until 30 minutes before serving time. *Makes 1 1/2 cups*

	Calories	Carbo-hydrate (gm)	Protein (gm)	Total Fat (gm)	Saturated Fat (gm)	Choles-terol (mg)
Total	273.5	10.6	36.2	8.3	1.4	23.1
Per 1/2 cup	91.2	3.5	12.1	2.8	0.5	7.7

Curried Apple Dip

2 cups 99% fat-free
   cottage cheese
1 tsp. curry
1/2 tsp. garlic salt

8-oz. can juice-
   packed
   unsweetened
   crushed
   pineapple, well-
   drained
2/3 cup chopped
   unpeeled red
   apple

Using the highest speed of your mixer or blender, beat together the cottage cheese, curry and garlic salt until they are smooth. Stir in the pineapple and apple. Cover and chill before serving. *Makes 3 cups*

	Calories	Carbo-hydrate (gm)	Protein (gm)	Total Fat (gm)	Saturated Fat (gm)	Choles-terol (mg)
Total	541.8	58.0	61.0	4.0	1.2	19.4
Per 1/2 cup	90.3	9.7	10.2	0.7	0.2	3.2

Chive Dip

1 cup 99% fat-free
   cottage cheese
2 tsp. chicken bouillon
4 tbsp. water

1 tbsp. finely
   chopped parsley
1 tbsp. chopped
   chives
1/2 tsp. dill

Whip the cottage cheese, bouillon, and water in a blender until they are creamy. Stir in the remaining ingredients. Chill at least 1 hour before serving. *Makes 1 cup*

	Calories	Carbo-hydrate (gm)	Protein (gm)	Total Fat (gm)	Saturated Fat (gm)	Choles-terol (mg)
Total	191.5	25.3	40.2	9.0	3.2	19.4
Per 1/2 cup	95.8	12.7	20.0	4.5	1.6	9.7

Avocado Dip

1 cup 99% fat-free
   cottage cheese
2 tsp. grated onion
1 tsp. fresh lemon juice
1 crushed garlic clove
3/4 tsp. salt

1/8 tsp. pepper
1 ripe avocado,
   mashed
1 medium-size ripe
   tomato, peeled
   and minced

Combine the cottage cheese, onion, lemon juice, garlic, salt and pepper. Beat with the highest speed of your mixer or blender until smooth. Fold in the avocado and tomato. Cover and chill before serving. *Makes 2 cups*

	Calories	Carbo-hydrate (gm)	Protein (gm)	Total Fat (gm)	Saturated Fat (gm)	Choles-terol (mg)
Total	612.0	42.8	36.1	35.0	8.2	19.4
Per 1/2 cup	153.0	10.7	9.0	8.8	2.1	4.9

Savory Bleu Cheese Dip

2 cups 99% fat-free
   cottage cheese
1 cup (4 oz.) crumbled
   bleu cheese
2 tbsp. chopped green
   onion
1/4 tsp. garlic salt

1 tsp. Worcester-
   shire sauce
2 tbsp. fresh lemon
   juice
1 cup plain low-fat
   yogurt

Mix the cottage cheese and bleu cheese using the highest speed of your blender or mixer. Then beat in the onion, garlic salt, Worcestershire sauce, and lemon juice. Fold in the yogurt. Cover and chill before serving. *Makes 4 cups*

Special hint: The dip can also be used as a salad dressing or served on baked potatoes.

	Calories	Carbo-hydrate (gm)	Protein (gm)	Total Fat (gm)	Saturated Fat (gm)	Choles-terol (mg)
Total	917.0	32.9	92.4	44.0	24.4	154.8
Per 1/2 cup	114.6	4.1	11.6	5.5	3.1	19.4

gm = grams; mg = milligrams. Nutritional figures are approximate. Figures are based on findings of U.S. Department of Agriculture.

Danish Dilly Dip

1 cup plain low-fat
   yogurt
1 tsp. fresh lemon juice
1 tsp. grated onion or
   onion juice

½ tsp. salt
½ tsp. dry mustard
¼ tsp. dill weed

Combine all of the ingredients and mix well. Chill before serving.   *Makes 1 cup*

	Calories	Carbo-hydrate (gm)	Protein (gm)	Total Fat (gm)	Saturated Fat (gm)	Choles-terol (mg)
Total	127.0	13.6	8.0	4.0	2.0	20.0
Per ½ cup	63.5	6.8	4.0	2.0	1.0	10.0

New Delhi Dip

1 cup plain low-fat
   yogurt

2 tsp. instant onion
¼ tsp. curry

Blend all of the ingredients together and refrigerate until ready to serve.   *Makes 1 cup*

	Calories	Carbo-hydrate (gm)	Protein (gm)	Total Fat (gm)	Saturated Fat (gm)	Choles-terol (mg)
Total	125.8	13.2	8.0	4.0	2.0	20.0
Per ½ cup	62.9	6.6	4.0	2.0	1.0	10.0

Tuna Cheese Dip

8-oz. pkg. low-calorie
   cream cheese
3-oz. can water-packed
   tuna, drained and
   flaked

1 tsp. onion flakes
2 tsp. chicken
   bouillon
   granules
2 tbsp. water

Allow the cream cheese to reach room temperature. Combine the cream cheese, tuna, onion, and bouillon granules in a mixing bowl. Mix well. Blend in the water. Cover the dip and chill at least 1 hour. Serve with fresh vegetables.   *Makes 1⅓ cups*

	Calories	Carbo-hydrate (gm)	Protein (gm)	Total Fat (gm)	Saturated Fat (gm)	Choles-terol (mg)
Total	685.5	45.8	59.6	62.9	36.0	222.2
Per ⅓ cup	171.3	11.5	14.9	15.7	9.0	55.6

Tangy Horseradish Dip

1 cup 99% fat-free
   cottage cheese
1 tbsp. horseradish
¼ tsp. dry mustard

2 drops Worcester-
   shire sauce
2 drops hot pepper
   sauce

Combine all the ingredients. Using the high speed of your mixer or blender, beat until smooth. Chill the dip before serving.   *Makes 1 cup*

	Calories	Carbo-hydrate (gm)	Protein (gm)	Total Fat (gm)	Saturated Fat (gm)	Choles-terol (mg)
Total	186.0	7.0	30.0	2.0	1.2	19.4
Per ½ cup	93.0	3.5	15.0	1.0	0.6	9.7

Deviled Eggs

6 hard-cooked eggs
¼ cup plain low-fat
   yogurt
1 tsp. fresh lemon juice
½ tsp. Worcestershire
   sauce

¼ tsp. dry mustard
Paprika
6 pitted black olives,
   sliced

Peel the eggs and slice them in half lengthwise. Remove the yolks and mash them with all the remaining ingredients except the paprika and olives. Spoon the egg yolk mixture back into the egg white halves. Refrigerate the eggs until ready to serve. Sprinkle them with paprika and garnish with the olive slices.   *Makes 12 servings*

	Calories	Carbo-hydrate (gm)	Protein (gm)	Total Fat (gm)	Saturated Fat (gm)	Choles-terol (mg)
Total	558.7	4.1	38.0	43.0	12.5	1517.0
Per Serving	46.6	0.3	3.2	3.6	1.0	126.4

Steak-Stuffed Mushrooms

1 lb. lean ground round
   steak
2 tsp. prepared
   horseradish
1 tsp. chopped chives

½ tsp. garlic salt
Coarse-ground
   pepper to taste
1 lb. mushrooms
   (about 18)
⅔ cup dry white wine

Mix the beef, horseradish, chives, garlic salt, and pepper together. Remove the stems from the mushrooms and stuff the mushrooms caps with the beef mixture. Place the stuffed mushrooms in a shallow baking dish and pour the wine over them. Bake in a preheated 350° oven about 20 minutes until the meat is browned.   *Makes 18 servings*

	Calories	Carbo-hydrate (gm)	Protein (gm)	Total Fat (gm)	Saturated Fat (gm)	Choles-terol (mg)
Total	1339.3	61.9	175.0	31.6	13.3	412.9
Per Serving	74.4	3.4	9.7	1.8	0.7	22.9

Pickled Fresh Mushrooms

4 cups tiny fresh
   mushrooms
1 onion, sliced, in rings
¾ cup tarragon vinegar
¼ cup water
3 tbsp. corn or safflower
   oil

1 garlic clove,
   minced
1½ tsp. salt
¼ tsp. pepper
⅛ tsp. cayenne
   pepper

Combine all the ingredients in a bowl. Cover and refrigerate 24 hours. Drain before serving.   *Makes 8 servings*

	Calories	Carbo-hydrate (gm)	Protein (gm)	Total Fat (gm)	Saturated Fat (gm)	Choles-terol (mg)
Total	698.9	65.9	30.0	46.0	3.0	0.0
Per Serving	87.4	8.2	3.8	5.8	0.4	0.0

gm = grams; mg = milligrams. Nutritional figures are approximate. Figures are based on findings of U.S. Department of Agriculture.

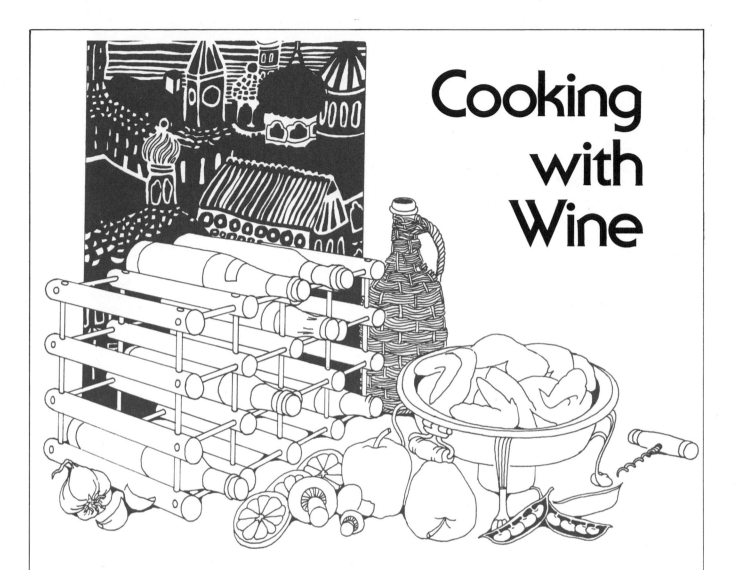

Cooking with Wine

Dieters are always cautioned against the overuse of alcohol. And with good reason, since alcohol adds nothing to nutrition but calories. But there is one way a dieter can enjoy liquor without paying the price and that's cooking with it. Alcohol evaporates when it cooks and leaves little in the way of calories but lots in the way of flavor.

Sweet wines, of course, will leave behind sugar calories, so the calorie-cautious cook should choose only the driest table wines for cooking. Beer used in cooking will also give up its alcohol calories but the carbohydrate calories will remain. Low-calorie beers that are also low-carboyhdrate are a good alternative in recipes calling for beer. Distilled spirits like scotch, bourbon, plain brandy, and rum have no carbohydrate calories to remain after cooking. Neither does vodka, but since vodka has no flavor, there is little point in using it in cooking.

Of course, liquor that is used in uncooked recipes still retains all its alcohol and alcohol calories — rum or brandy in an unbaked refrigerator pie filling, for example.

Recipes

Tenderloin with Gourmet Wine Sauce

2-lb. beef tenderloin, trimmed of fat	1 cup dry red wine
1½ tsp. salt (or garlic salt or onion salt)	2 tsp. arrowroot or cornstarch
1 tsp. coarse ground pepper	4-oz. can sliced mushrooms, drained reserving liquid

Season the meat with salt and pepper. Insert a meat thermometer so that the tip is in the center of the roast. (By all means, do not forget to use a thermometer; tenderloin is too expensive to ruin by overcooking). Place the roast on a rack in a nonstick roasting pan and roast it in a preheated 450° oven 30 to 35 minutes, until

gm = grams; mg = milligrams. Nutritional figures are approximate. Figures are based on findings of U.S. Department of Agriculture.

the thermometer reads 125°. Baste every 10 minutes with the wine. Remove the roast to a platter.

Using a bulb-type baster, skim all the fat from the pan juices. In a cup, combine the arrowroot with the juice from the mushrooms. Then stir this into the roasting pan, scraping well. Cook the sauce over moderate heat until it thickens and simmers. Then add the mushrooms. Slice the roast thinly, and serve it with the sauce.   *Makes 8 servings*

	Calories	Carbo-hydrate (gm)	Protein (gm)	Total Fat (gm)	Saturated Fat (gm)	Choles-terol (mg)
Total	2082.8	18.1	291.8	64.0	32.0	816.0
Per Serving	260.4	2.3	36.5	8.0	4.0	102.0

Bul Kogi (Korean Beef)

1½-lb. flank steak	1 tbsp. corn or
⅓ cup soy sauce	safflower oil
3 tbsp. cream sherry	¼ cup sliced green
2 tbsp. onion flakes	onions
1 tsp. garlic powder	3 tsp. toasted
	sesame seeds

Have the steak partially frozen for easier handling. Slice it in thirds, lengthwise. Then slice each third across the grain into ¼-inch slices. Combine the meat, soy sauce, sherry, onion, and garlic powder in a bowl. Cover and refrigerate for several hours.

Heat the oil over high heat in a large nonstick skillet. Add the steak strips and stir-fry them quickly until they are seared. Be careful not to overcook. Place the meat on a platter and sprinkle with the green onions and toasted sesame seeds.   *Makes 6 servings*

Hint: Sesame seeds can be toasted by stirring them quickly over medium heat in a nonstick skillet. Or place them on a cookie sheet in a preheated 350° oven until they are golden. They must be watched carefully or they will burn.

	Calories	Carbo-hydrate (gm)	Protein (gm)	Total Fat (gm)	Saturated Fat (gm)	Choles-terol (mg)
Total	1596.6	16.4	218.0	58.5	21.6	620.0
Per Serving	266.1	2.7	36.3	9.8	3.6	103.3

Kyoto-Style Lamb Skewers

2 lb. lean boneless	2 tbsp. vinegar
lamb	2 tbsp. cocktail
1 cup beef broth or	sherry
bouillon	2 garlic cloves,
¼ cup soy sauce	crushed
2 tbsp. frozen	¼ tsp. ground ginger
unsweetened apple	
juice concentrate,	
defrosted but not	
diluted	

Trim the lamb of fat and slice across the grain into thin 3-inch strips. If beef broth is used, skim off fat with a bulb-type baster; or chill it until the fat rises and can be lifted off. Combine the remaining ingredients and

pour the mixture over the meat. Turn the meat to coat it well and let it stand, uncovered, for 1 hour at room temperature, or cover it and refrigerate overnight. Turn the meat occasionally so it gets seasoned evenly.

Weave the meat onto skewers. Broil them about 4 inches from the heat source for about 2 minutes on each side.   *Makes 8 servings*

	Calories	Carbo-hydrate (gm)	Protein (gm)	Total Fat (gm)	Saturated Fat (gm)	Choles-terol (mg)
Total	1973.8	25.6	246.8	83.6	41.8	920.8
Per Serving	246.7	3.2	30.9	10.5	5.2	115.1

Elegant Veal

1 tbsp. diet margarine	¼ tsp. coarse-ground
2 lb. lean veal shoulder,	pepper
trimmed of fat,	1 lb. fresh
cubed	mushrooms,
½ cup sliced onion	sliced
¾ cup sherry	2 tbsp. chopped
1½ tsp. garlic salt	fresh parsley

Melt the margarine in a large, nonstick skillet. Add the meat and brown it over moderate heat. Then add the onion, sherry, garlic salt, and pepper. Cover the pan, and simmer the contents for 45 minutes or until the veal is almost tender. Add the mushrooms, cover and simmer 15 minutes longer. Just before serving, stir in the parsley.   *Makes 6 servings*

	Calories	Carbo-hydrate (gm)	Protein (gm)	Total Fat (gm)	Saturated Fat (gm)	Choles-terol (mg)
Total	1741.8	66.8	217.4	53.7	22.3	640.2
Per Serving	290.3	11.1	36.2	9.0	3.7	106.7

Hunter's Chicken

2 lb. broiler-fryer	1 small garlic clove,
chicken pieces	minced
8 small white onions	10½-oz. can condensed
1 medium green	tomato soup
pepper, cut in strips	½ cup water
4-oz. can sliced	2 tbsp. dry white
mushrooms,	wine
drained	½ tsp. oregano

Arrange the chicken pieces in a single layer in a casserole. Bake the chicken, uncovered, in a preheated 450° oven for 30 minutes. Pour off the fat that accumulates in the casserole. Then add the onions, green pepper, mushrooms, and garlic. Blend together the tomato soup, water, wine, and oregano in a bowl. Pour this mixture over the chicken and vegetables. Bake the casserole, uncovered, at 350° for about 30 minutes.   *Makes 6 servings.*

	Calories	Carbo-hydrate (gm)	Protein (gm)	Total Fat (gm)	Saturated Fat (gm)	Choles-terol (mg)
Total	1323.8	90.8	147.5	42.2	13.7	555.7
Per Serving	220.6	15.1	24.6	7.0	2.3	92.6

gm = grams; mg = milligrams. Nutritional figures are approximate. Figures are based on findings of U.S. Department of Agriculture.

Chicken with Snow Peas

2 large whole chicken breasts	1 tbsp. corn or safflower oil
2 tbsp. soy sauce	1 cup sliced onions
2 tbsp. sherry	1 cup sliced mushrooms
1 tsp. ground ginger	7-oz. pkg. frozen snow peas, defrosted
1 clove garlic, crushed	

Bone and skin the chicken breasts. Cut the meat into bite-size strips. Blend the soy sauce, sherry, ginger, and garlic together in a bowl. Add the chicken to the bowl and let the mixture sit, uncovered, at room temperature for 30 minutes.

Heat the oil in a nonstick skillet, rotating the pan to spread it evenly. Add the chicken, onions, mushrooms, and snow peas. Sauté the chicken and vegetables about 5 minutes, stirring constantly, until the chicken is tender and the vegetables are crisp.

Makes 4 servings

	Calories	Carbo-hydrate (gm)	Protein (gm)	Total Fat (gm)	Saturated Fat (gm)	Choles-terol (mg)
Total	746.7	47.4	84.8	23.0	5.0	204.0
Per Serving	186.7	11.9	21.2	5.8	1.3	51.0

Canadian Chicken

2 whole chicken breasts	½ cup chopped green pepper
1 cup chicken broth	¼ cup flour
½ lb. Canadian bacon, cubed	13 oz. evaporated skim milk
1 tbsp. diet margarine	⅓ cup dry white wine
½ lb. fresh mushrooms, sliced	½ tsp. salt
	¼ tsp. white pepper
	¼ tsp. nutmeg

Simmer the chicken breasts according to the directions in How to Cook Chicken (see index). When the chicken has cooled, remove the skin and bones and dice the meat. Skim the chicken broth of fat by using a bulb-type baster, or by chilling the broth until the fat rises to the surface and can be lifted off.

Combine the diced chicken and Canadian bacon. Melt the margarine in a nonstick skillet and sauté the mushrooms and peppers for 5 minutes. Add the mushrooms and peppers to the meat. Blend the flour with the chicken broth and milk in a saucepan. Bring this mixture to a boil, stirring to keep it smooth. Add the meat and vegetables to the saucepan along with the wine, salt, pepper, and nutmeg. Simmer the entire mixture for 3 minutes. *Makes 6 servings*

Note: Use the water in which you simmer the chicken as your broth. Or you may use canned bouillon undiluted, or 2 chicken bouillon cubes mixed with 1 cup water.

	Calories	Carbo-hydrate (gm)	Protein (gm)	Total Fat (gm)	Saturated Fat (gm)	Choles-terol (mg)
Total	1972.0	101.2	179.5	89.5	33.6	534.7
Per Serving	328.7	16.9	29.9	14.9	5.6	89.1

Coq Au Vin Rouge

1 cup chicken broth	1 bay leaf
3 lb. broiler-fryer chicken pieces	1 large garlic clove, minced
½ cup Burgundy or other dry red wine	¼ tsp. poultry seasoning
1 lb. (about 16) small white onions	¼ tsp. salt
4-oz. can sliced mushrooms, drained	2 tbsp. flour

Skim the fat from the broth by chilling it until the fat rises to the top and can be whisked off.

Brown the chicken skin side down in a large, heavy nonstick skillet. Add no oil to the pan; the chicken will release enough of its own fat for frying. Pour off the fat that accumulates in the pan. Then add ⅔ cup of the broth, the wine, onions, mushrooms, and seasonings to the skillet. Turn the chicken pieces. Cover and cook over low heat about 45 minutes until the chicken is tender. Blend the other ⅓ cup broth with the flour in a cup until it is smooth. Then slowly stir this mixture into the sauce. Continue cooking and stirring until the sauce has thickened. *Makes 8 servings*

	Calories	Carbo-hydrate (gm)	Protein (gm)	Total Fat (gm)	Saturated Fat (gm)	Choles-terol (mg)
Total	1672.6	65.6	211.0	51.9	20.5	845.0
Per Serving	209.1	8.2	26.4	6.5	2.6	105.6

Chicken Czardas

3 whole chicken breasts	¼ cup sherry or dry white wine
1 tbsp. diet margarine	2 tsp. arrowroot or cornstarch
1½ tsp. salt	2 tbsp. cold water
1 onion, chopped	1 cup plain low-fat yogurt
½ lb. mushrooms, sliced	1½ tsp. paprika

Bone the chicken breasts and remove the skin. Cut the meat into strips. Melt the margarine in a nonstick skillet over medium heat. Add the chicken and season it with the salt. Cook the chicken, stirring constantly, for 3 minutes. Then add the onion and mushrooms and continue cooking and stirring 2 minutes longer. Add the sherry, cover the pan, and cook for an additional 4 minutes. Blend the arrowroot and water together in a cup. Add this to the skillet and continue cooking, stirring rapidly, until the sauce has thickened. Stir in the yogurt and paprika, continuing to cook just until the mixture is heated through. Do not let it boil.

Makes 6 servings

	Calories	Carbo-hydrate (gm)	Protein (gm)	Total Fat (gm)	Saturated Fat (gm)	Choles-terol (mg)
Total	955.6	57.2	123.5	24.5	9.0	326.0
Per Serving	159.3	9.5	20.6	4.1	1.5	54.3

gm = grams; mg = milligrams. Nutritional figures are approximate. Figures are based on findings of U.S. Department of Agriculture.

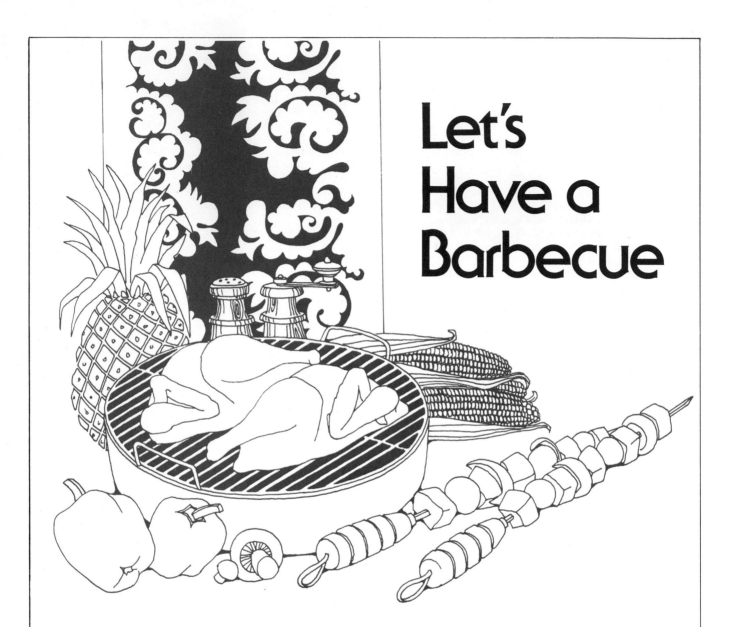

Let's Have a Barbecue

Cooking over the coals can be a calorie-saver or a dietary disaster, depending on your approach. If your backyard repertoire is mainly limited to hot dogs, steaks, spareribs, and sugar-packed sauces, barbecues are bound to be bikini-stretchers.

On the other hand, barbecuing is really just another form of broiling, the most calorie-safe cooking of all. If you choose your ingredients with a sharp eye for calorie counts, there is no reason why your rotisserie or hibachi cannot prove to be an effective weapon in your war against overweight.

The first rule is to expand your horizons. Most backyard chefs limit their choices to steaks and fatty hamburger, with less emphasis on poultry, seafood, and the leaner cuts of meat. And most sauces or bastes, whether bottled or homemade, are generally packed with fats and sugars that add unneeded calories.

Many of the recipes throughout this book call for broiling. In all cases, broiling can be done outside over hot coals for an additional flavor treat.

Recipes

Barbecued Shish Kebab

1½ lb. boneless leg of lamb	12 bay leaves
2 large tomatoes	12 slices lemon peel
2 medium onions	¼ cup diet Italian
2 medium green peppers	salad dressing

Cut the lamb into 1½-inch cubes, trimming off all fat. Cut each tomato and onion into 6 wedges, and each green pepper into 6 pieces. On one set of skewers, alternate the lamb, bay leaves, and lemon peel. On a second set of skewers, arrange the tomatoes. And on a

gm = grams; mg = milligrams. Nutritional figures are approximate. Figures are based on findings of U.S. Department of Agriculture.

third set of skewers, alternate the onion and green pepper. Brush all of the meat and vegetables with the salad dressing. Grill the lamb kebabs and the onion and green pepper kebabs 3 to 5 inches from the hot coals for 5 to 7 minutes on each side, or until the lamb has reached the desired doneness and the onion and pepper are brown and tender. Grill the tomatoes for about 3 minutes on each side. Baste the lamb and vegetables frequently with the salad dressing.

Makes 6 servings

	Calories	Carbo-hydrate (gm)	Protein (gm)	Total Fat (gm)	Saturated Fat (gm)	Choles-terol (mg)
Total	1497.5	52.9	202.9	52.0	28.8	681.6
Per Serving	249.6	8.8	33.8	8.7	4.8	113.6

Chicken Dinner in a Pocket

2 chicken breasts, halved	4 small raw carrots, cut in sticks
4 raw medium-sized white potatoes, peeled	2 tsp. salt
	¼ tsp. pepper
	½ tsp. oregano

Tear off 4 pieces of heavy-duty aluminum foil, approximately 18 inches square. Place 1 piece of chicken, 1 potato, and ¼ of the carrot sticks on each piece of foil. Sprinkle salt, pepper, and oregano over all. Wrap the foil tightly around the food and cook it in a covered grill about 1 hour until the chicken is tender.

Makes 4 servings

	Calories	Carbo-hydrate (gm)	Protein (gm)	Total Fat (gm)	Saturated Fat (gm)	Choles-terol (mg)
Total	776.0	104.0	80.0	8.0	4.0	204.0
Per Serving	194.0	26.0	20.0	2.0	1.0	51.0

Lemon Chicken Cookout

¼ cup soy sauce	½ tsp. paprika
4 tbsp. fresh lemon juice	2-lb. broiler-fryer chicken, split in half lengthwise
½ tsp. salt	
¼ tsp. pepper	

Make a sauce by combining the soy sauce, lemon juice, salt, pepper, and paprika. Place the chicken on a grill, skin side up, and brush with sauce. Broil 10 inches from the coals for about 45 minutes, basting as needed, until chicken is tender. *Makes 4 servings*

	Calories	Carbo-hydrate (gm)	Protein (gm)	Total Fat (gm)	Saturated Fat (gm)	Choles-terol (mg)
Total	975.0	9.0	164.3	24.0	8.0	536.0
Per Serving	243.8	2.3	41.1	6.0	2.0	134.0

Rotisserie Leg of Lamb

4-lb. leg of lamb	5 tbsp. tomato paste
2 tsp. salt	¼ cup coarsely chopped onion
¾ tsp. pepper	
8-oz. can tomato sauce	

Season the lamb with salt and pepper and skewer it onto a rotisserie spit. Insert a meat thermometer so that the tip is in the center of the roast, but make sure it's not touching the spit. Place the spit about 8 inches above grey-hot coals and roast the lamb for 30 minutes. Combine the remaining ingredients in a bowl and brush this mixture on the lamb frequently as the lamb roasts for a total of 25 to 30 minutes per pound, or until the meat thermometer registers 160° to 170° for medium doneness. *Makes 12 servings*

	Calories	Carbo-hydrate (gm)	Protein (gm)	Total Fat (gm)	Saturated Fat (gm)	Choles-terol (mg)
Total	3466.8	30.9	517.7	128.4	76.8	1817.6
Per Serving	288.9	2.6	43.1	10.7	6.4	151.5

Côte d'Azur Steak en Brochette

2 lb. lean top round steak, trimmed of fat and cubed	2 medium zucchini, cut in 1-in. slices
1 cup diet Italian salad dressing	12 cherry tomatoes

Combine the beef cubes and dressing in a bowl, coating the meat thoroughly. Cover the meat tightly and refrigerate 10 hours or overnight, stirring once or twice. Drain the marinade from the meat, but reserve it. Thread 4 metal skewers alternately with the beef cubes, zucchini, and tomatoes. Brush with the marinade. Place the kebabs over hot coals and broil them 12 to 18 minutes, depending upon degree of doneness desired, turning and brushing them with the marinade occasionally. *Makes 8 servings*

	Calories	Carbo-hydrate (gm)	Protein (gm)	Total Fat (gm)	Saturated Fat (gm)	Choles-terol (mg)
Total	2133.3	61.6	294.1	69.3	26.7	826.5
Per Serving	266.7	7.7	36.8	8.7	3.3	103.3

Veal Kebabs

2 lb. lean ground veal	½ tsp. garlic salt
1 small onion, minced	⅛ tsp. pepper
1 small apple, cored, peeled, minced (or ¼ cup unsweetened applesauce)	2 eggs
	Optional: tomato wedges, green pepper slices, mushroom caps, tomato sauce
2 stalks celery, minced	

Combine all of the ingredients except optional ones. Shape into 1½-inch balls. Slip the meatballs onto skewers, alternating them with tomato wedges, green pepper slices, and mushroom caps, if desired. Tomato sauce may be used as a baste if you wish. Broil the kebabs about 10 minutes, turning occasionally.

Makes 8 servings

	Calories	Carbo-hydrate (gm)	Protein (gm)	Total Fat (gm)	Saturated Fat (gm)	Choles-terol (mg)
Total	1463.0	32.0	195.2	54.6	25.3	1143.6
Per Serving	182.9	4.0	24.4	6.8	3.2	143.0

gm = grams; mg = milligrams. Nutritional figures are approximate. Figures are based on findings of U.S. Department of Agriculture.

Spicy Beef en Brochette

2 lb. lean round steak, cut 2-in. thick	3 tbsp. fresh lemon juice
1 1/2 tsp. dry mustard	16 cherry tomatoes
3/4 tsp. ground ginger	16 wedges green
1/8 tsp. ground pepper	pepper
1/8 tsp. garlic powder	16 whole fresh
6 tbsp. soy sauce	mushrooms

Trim the meat of all visible fat and slice it into 1/4-inch strips. Place the strips in a shallow pan or dish. Combine the mustard, ginger, pepper, garlic powder, soy sauce, and lemon juice. Mix these ingredients well and pour over the steak strips. Cover the dish and refrigerate at least 4 hours.

Thread the marinated steak strips on metal skewers, alternating them with the tomatoes, green pepper, and mushrooms. Brush the meat and vegetables with the marinade and broil over hot coals for 3 minutes. Turn, brush with marinade and cook 3 to 4 minutes longer.

Makes 8 servings

	Calories	Carbo-hydrate (gm)	Protein (gm)	Total Fat (gm)	Saturated Fat (gm)	Choles-terol (mg)
Total	2214.8	99.5	310.3	54.1	26.7	826.5
Per Serving	276.9	12.4	38.8	6.8	3.3	103.3

Luau Veal Skewers

1 1/2 lb. lean veal steak, trimmed of fat and cubed	1 tsp. salt
	1/2 tsp. pepper
	1/2 tsp. marjoram
3 tbsp. cider vinegar	16-oz. can juice-packed unsweetened pineapple chunks, drained reserving liquid

Put the veal cubes in a ceramic bowl. Add the vinegar and seasonings. Add just enough drained pineapple juice to cover all the meat. Cover the bowl and marinate the veal in the refrigerator all day or overnight. Drain the meat and thread it on skewers, alternating it with the pineapple chunks. Broil 15 to 20 minutes over hot coals, turning frequently. *Makes 6 servings*

	Calories	Carbo-hydrate (gm)	Protein (gm)	Total Fat (gm)	Saturated Fat (gm)	Choles-terol (mg)
Total	1329.7	70.9	137.7	56.0	24.0	480.0
Per Serving	221.6	11.8	23.0	9.3	4.0	80.0

Turkey Steaks Oriental

6 turkey breast steaks, cut 1 1/2-in. thick	1/2 cup soy sauce
	1 tbsp. corn or safflower oil
1 tsp. grated fresh ginger or ground ginger	3 garlic cloves, minced
1 tsp. dry mustard	

Place the steaks in a bowl. Combine all of the remaining ingredients and pour over the turkey steaks. Cover and refrigerate several hours or overnight. Drain the steaks and cook them quickly on both sides on a barbecue grill, allowing about 8 minutes per side. Brush them occasionally with the marinade, if you like.

Makes 6 servings

Hint: If turkey breast steaks are not available, have a butcher cut a turkey breast crosswise into 1 1/2-inch thick steaks. Frozen breasts can be cut also and thawed when ready to use.

	Calories	Carbo-hydrate (gm)	Protein (gm)	Total Fat (gm)	Saturated Fat (gm)	Choles-terol (mg)
Total	1412.4	8.0	234.4	41.4	7.9	528.2
Per Serving	235.4	1.3	39.1	6.9	1.3	88.0

Apple-Soy Sauce

1/2 cup soy sauce	3/4 cup unsweetened applesauce
1/2 cup sherry	1/2 tsp. instant garlic

Combine all of the ingredients and mix well. The sauce may be used as a marinade or a basting sauce or both with steaks, chops or poultry. To use as a marinade, puncture 1 1/2 pounds of lean meat deeply in several places with a fork. Place the meat in a glass or plastic bowl, or in a plastic bag inside a bowl. Cover the meat with the marinade. Cover the container and marinate the meat at room temperature 1 hour; or cover and refrigerate for several hours or overnight. Baste the meat with the remaining marinade as you broil it.

Makes 1 3/4 cups (7 servings)

	Calories	Carbo-hydrate (gm)	Protein (gm)	Total Fat (gm)	Saturated Fat (gm)	Choles-terol (mg)
Total	250.2	31.9	8.8	0.0	0.0	0.0
Per Serving	35.7	4.6	1.3	0.0	0.0	0.0

Smoke-Seasoned Barbecue Sauce

5 tbsp. white vinegar	1/4 tsp. (or more) Tabasco sauce
3 tbsp. lemon juice	
5 tbsp. tomato paste	2 tsp. prepared mustard
1 tsp. Worchestershire sauce	
	3 tbsp. instant minced onion
2 tsp. liquid smoke seasoning	1/4 tsp. instant garlic
	3/4 tsp. salt

Combine all of the ingredients and mix well. The sauce may be used as a marinade or a basting sauce or both with steaks, chops, or poultry. To use as a marinade, puncture 1 1/2 pounds of lean meat deeply in several places with a fork. Place the meat in a glass or plastic bowl, or in a plastic bag inside a bowl. Cover the meat with the marinade. Cover the container and marinate the meat at room temperature 1 hour; or cover and refrigerate for several hours or overnight. Baste the meat with the remaining marinade as you broil it.

Makes about 1 1/2 cups (6 servings)

	Calories	Carbo-hydrate (gm)	Protein (gm)	Total Fat (gm)	Saturated Fat (gm)	Choles-terol (mg)
Total	183.0	47.7	3.0	0.1	0.0	0.0
Per Serving	30.5	7.8	0.5	0.0	0.0	0.0

gm = grams; mg = milligrams. Nutritional figures are approximate. Figures are based on findings of U.S. Department of Agriculture.

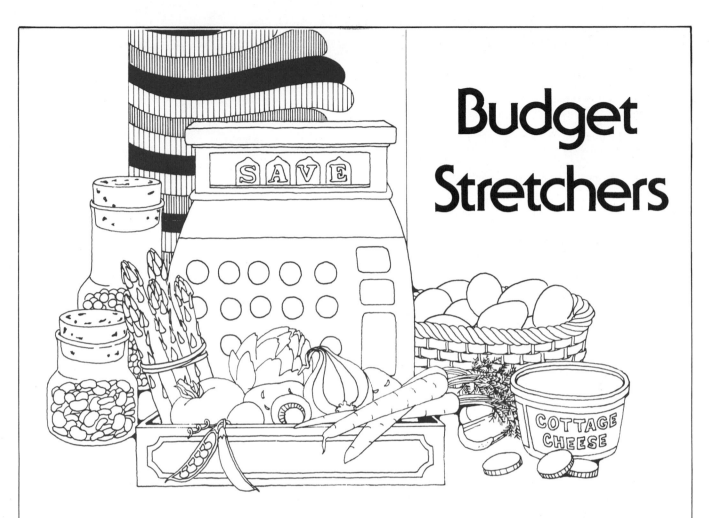

Budget Stretchers

Unfortunately, many packaged casserole mixes, budget recipes, and cafeteria concoctions are starch-laden, nutritionally neutered pound-provokers. They tend to be loaded with fat but stingy on appetite-appeasing protein. Moreover, some packaged hamburger stretchers are not even a bargain, often costing more per pound than the meat they're supposed to replace. But it is possible to eat inexpensively and save calories too. If you have to pinch pennies while counting calories, here are some low-meat and no-meat recipes that will help you tighten your belt, in both senses of the phrase!

Recipes

Meatballs for Slender Swedes

1 cup canned beef broth or bouillon	2 medium onions, chopped
1 lb. lean ground round steak	2 tsp. salt
2 slices day-old or toasted high-fiber bread, cubed	⅛ tsp. pepper
	¼ tsp. nutmeg
	1 tbsp. flour
1 cup skim milk	2 tbsp. cold water
1 egg, well beaten	

If you are using canned broth, chill it until the fat rises to the top, hardens and can be lifted off. Combine the meat with the bread, milk, egg, onions, and seasonings. Mix them together well and form the meat into 1-inch balls. Spray a nonstick skillet with spray-on vegetable coating for no-fat frying. Brown the meatballs over moderate heat. Add the broth to the skillet, stirring and scraping the pan well. In a cup, combine the flour with 2 tablespoons cold water. Mix them together well and then stir into the skillet. Bring to a boil, stirring constantly, until the sauce has thickened. Cover the pan, lower the heat, and simmer the meatballs for about 20 minutes, adding more water if necessary. If you like, you may add a few drops of brown gravy coloring. *Makes 6 servings*

Diet hint: To save an extra 50 calories (about 8 per serving), use 2 egg whites instead of 1 whole egg.

	Calories	Carbo-hydrate (gm)	Protein (gm)	Total Fat (gm)	Saturated Fat (gm)	Choles-terol (mg)
Total	1138.6	56.7	171.1	24.9	7.9	702.0
Per Serving	189.8	9.5	28.5	4.2	1.3	117.0

gm = grams; mg = milligrams. Nutritional figures are approximate. Figures are based on findings of U.S. Department of Agriculture.

Crocked Flank Romanoff

10½-oz. can beef broth
1½-lb. flank steak
2 tsp. tomato paste
2 tsp. Worcestershire sauce
3 tbsp. sherry
4-oz. can mushrooms, undrained
2 onions, thinly sliced
⅛ tsp. instant garlic
1 tbsp. minced fresh parsley, or 1½ tsp. parsley flakes
2 tbsp. flour
¾ cup plain low-fat yogurt
1 tsp. salt
¼ tsp. pepper
⅛ tsp. paprika

Skim the broth of fat by chilling until the fat rises and can be lifted off. Spread the flank steak flat on a cutting board. Slice it against the grain into thin strips. In a slow cooker, combine the steak with half the broth, tomato paste, Worcestershire sauce, sherry, mushrooms, onions, garlic and parsley. Cover, and cook at low setting 6 to 8 hours, until the meat is very tender. Uncover, raise the heat to high. Combine the flour with the remaining beef broth and stir into the slow cooker. Cook and stir until the mixture simmers and thickens. Turn off the heat. When the mixture stops simmering, stir in the yogurt. Season with salt, pepper, paprika. *Makes 6 servings*

	Calories	Carbo- hydrate (gm)	Protein (gm)	Total Fat (gm)	Saturated Fat (gm)	Choles- terol (mg)
Total	1634.4	47.7	230.0	43.1	21.5	666.4
Per Serving	272.4	8.0	38.3	7.2	3.6	111.1

Baked Beef and Noodles

1 lb. lean ground round steak
⅓ cup sliced green onions
⅓ cup chopped green pepper
6-oz. can tomato paste
½ cup plain low-fat yogurt
¼ tsp. salt
8-oz. pkg. medium noodles, cooked and drained
1 cup 99% fat-free cottage cheese
8-oz. can tomato sauce

Brown the meat slowly in a large nonstick skillet. Do not add any oil to the pan; the meat will release enough fat for frying. After the meat is browned, pour off the fat that has accumulated in the pan. Then add the onions and green pepper, and continue cooking until they are tender. Set the meat aside. Stir the tomato paste, yogurt, and salt together in a large bowl; add the noodles and the cottage cheese. Place half the meat mixture in a baking dish. Add the noodle mixture and top with the remaining meat mixture. Pour the tomato sauce over all. Bake the casserole in a preheated 350° oven for 30 to 35 minutes until it is heated through. *Makes 8 servings*

	Calories	Carbo- hydrate (gm)	Protein (gm)	Total Fat (gm)	Saturated Fat (gm)	Choles- terol (mg)
Total	1501.2	119.4	195.8	25.0	9.5	520.4
Per Serving	187.7	14.9	24.5	3.1	1.2	65.1

Lean Lasagna

1 lb. lean ground round steak
1 cup 99% fat-free cottage cheese
1 egg
3 tbsp. extra-sharp grated Romano cheese
1 tsp. garlic salt
¼ tsp. pepper
1 tsp. oregano
2 tbsp. parsley
8 oz. protein-enriched lasagna noodles, cooked rinsed and drained
1½ cups canned tomato sauce
1 tbsp. Italian seasoned bread crumbs

Brown the meat in a nonstick skillet, breaking it up as it cooks. Do not add oil to the pan; the meat will release enough fat for frying. Drain off any accumulated fat after the meat has browned. In a bowl, combine the cottage cheese, egg, Romano cheese, garlic salt, pepper, oregano, and parsley. In a 2-quart shallow baking dish, arrange the meat, noodles, cheese mixture, and tomato sauce in layers. Sprinkle the bread crumbs evenly over the top. Bake the lasagna in a preheated 350° oven for 30 to 45 minutes. *Makes 8 servings*

	Calories	Carbo- hydrate (gm)	Protein (gm)	Total Fat (gm)	Saturated Fat (gm)	Choles- terol (mg)
Total	2118.1	130.9	204.0	83.4	41.5	870.6
Per Serving	264.8	16.4	25.5	10.4	5.2	108.8

Budget Stroganoff

1 lb. lean ground round steak
2 onions, chopped
1 cup water
4 cups tomato juice
2 tsp. garlic salt
¼ tsp. pepper
2 tsp. Worcestershire sauce
6 oz. curly egg noodles
1 cup plain low-fat yogurt

Sauté the beef and onions in a large nonstick skillet. Do not add any oil; the meat will release enough fat for frying. When the meat is brown, add 1 cup water to the skillet and bring it to a boil. Drain all the liquid from the pan. This will remove the remaining fat from the meat. Stir in the tomato juice, garlic salt, pepper, and Worcestershire sauce, and heat until boiling Add the noodles, just a few at a time, so that the mixture continues to boil. When all the noodles have been added, cover the skillet, reduce the heat, and simmer 10 minutes or longer, stirring occasionally, until the noodles are tender. Stir in the yogurt and continue cooking just until the yogurt is heated through but not boiling. *Makes 6 servings*

	Calories	Carbo- hydrate (gm)	Protein (gm)	Total Fat (gm)	Saturated Fat (gm)	Choles- terol (mg)
Total	1501.8	142.6	175.4	27.5	9.7	535.8
Per Serving	250.3	23.8	29.2	4.6	1.6	89.3

gm = grams; mg = milligrams. Nutritional figures are approximate. Figures are based on findings of U.S. Department of Agriculture.

Meatball Goulash

1½ lb. lean ground round
    steak
1 cup high-protein
    cereal,
    unsweetened
1 egg, slightly beaten
1 tsp. salt
⅛ tsp. nutmeg
⅛ tsp. thyme

⅛ tsp. pepper
2 (10¾-oz.) cans
    condensed
    tomato soup
½ cup "V-8" juice
2 cups cooked
    protein-enriched
    macaroni
5 tbsp. shredded
    cheddar cheese

Combine the beef, cereal, egg, and seasonings in a large bowl. Shape the meat mixture into 24 meatballs and set them on a nonstick baking sheet. Place them in an oven preheated to 450° — or under the broiler — just until the meat is brown. Transfer the meatballs to a casserole, and add the soup, "V-8" juice, and macaroni. Bake the casserole in a preheated 400° oven for 35 minutes, stirring occasionally. Then sprinkle the cheese over the top and continue to bake about 5 minutes until the cheese has melted. *Makes 8 servings*

	Calories	Carbo-hydrate (gm)	Protein (gm)	Total Fat (gm)	Saturated Fat (gm)	Choles-terol (mg)
Total	2335.6	171.6	260.9	70.4	21.9	944.8
Per Serving	292.0	21.5	32.6	8.8	2.7	118.1

Turkey and Fruited Rice

4-lb. turkey breast
1½ cups cooked rice
¾ cup fresh cranberries,
    chopped
1 orange, peeled and
    diced

2 tbsp. chives
½ tsp. salt
1 cup unsweetened
    orange juice
¼ cup sweet red wine

Bake the turkey uncovered in a preheated 350° oven approximately 2½ hours until well browned, basting occasionally with pan juices. Skim the fat from the pan drippings. Mix together the rice, cranberries, orange, chives and salt. Heap the mixture around the turkey in pan. Mix the orange juice and wine. Pour over the meat and rice. Cover and bake at 350° 20 minutes more.
Makes 6 servings

	Calories	Carbo-hydrate (gm)	Protein (gm)	Total Fat (gm)	Saturated Fat (gm)	Choles-terol (mg)
Total	2818.0	85.2	457.9	55.9	13.7	1055.7
Per Serving	469.7	14.2	76.3	9.3	2.3	176.0

Spiced Sangria Turkey

2 frozen turkey thighs,
    defrosted (about 1⅞
    lb.)
1 cup unsweetened
    orange juice

½ cup dry red wine
½ tsp. mixed
    pumpkin pie
    spice
½ tsp. salt
⅛ tsp. pepper

Preheat oven to 450°. Arrange the turkey thighs skin side up in a shallow baking pan. Bake, uncovered, 30 minutes until the skin is crisp and well rendered of fat. Pour off the fat and lower the heat to 275°. Combine the orange juice, wine, spice, salt and pepper, and pour over turkey. Bake uncovered, basting occasionally, until the turkey is fork-tender and the sauce has evaporated to a thick glaze (add water if needed).
Makes 6 servings

	Calories	Carbo-hydrate (gm)	Protein (gm)	Total Fat (gm)	Saturated Fat (gm)	Choles-terol (mg)
Total	2126.3	32.4	276.2	85.7	25.7	797.0
Per Serving	354.4	5.4	46.0	14.3	4.3	132.8

Veal-Spinach Timbales

1 small onion, minced
10-oz. pkg. frozen
    chopped spinach
2 lb. lean ground veal
¼ cup parsley, chopped
1 slice high-fiber or diet
    bread, crumbled

1 tsp. salt
¼ tsp. pepper
    Pinch nutmeg
2 eggs
¾ cup skim milk

Add the onion to the spinach in a saucepan and cook according to package directions; drain. Brown the meat and drain the fat. Mix all the ingredients together thoroughly. Spoon into nonstick muffin cups about ⅔ full. Bake in a preheated 350° oven for 30 minutes until set.
Makes 9 servings

	Calories	Carbo-hydrate (gm)	Protein (gm)	Total Fat (gm)	Saturated Fat (gm)	Choles-terol (mg)
Total	1555.8	33.5	213.5	71.6	25.3	1147.4
Per Serving	172.9	3.7	23.7	8.0	2.8	127.5

Fresh Mushroom Cheese Pie

Basic Piecrust (see
    index)
1 cup shredded Swiss
    cheese
2 tbsp. flour
2 eggs, beaten
¾ cup skim milk

½ tsp. dried summer
    savory,
    crumbled
½ tsp. salt
¼ tsp. pepper
2 cups fresh sliced
    mushrooms

Line an 8-inch pie pan with Basic Piecrust. Toss the shredded cheese with the flour in a bowl. Then add the beaten eggs, milk and seasonings. Fold in the sliced mushrooms. Turn this mixture into the pastry-lined pan and bake the pie in a preheated 350° oven for about 1 hour until it is golden brown and a knife inserted off-center comes out clean.
Makes 6 servings

	Calories	Carbo-hydrate (gm)	Protein (gm)	Total Fat (gm)	Saturated Fat (gm)	Choles-terol (mg)
Total	1712.2	79.9	98.0	105.6	38.0	747.8
Per Serving	285.4	13.3	16.3	17.6	6.3	124.6

gm = grams; mg = milligrams. Nutritional figures are approximate. Figures are based on findings of U.S. Department of Agriculture.

Chili Mac

¾ lb. lean ground beef
1 onion, chopped
1 green pepper,
  chopped
2 cups water
8 oz. protein-enriched
  elbow macaroni

16-oz. can kidney
  beans,
  undrained
2 (8-oz.) cans tomato
  sauce
1 tsp. chili powder
1 tsp. salt
½ cup (2 oz.)
  shredded
  cheddar cheese

Brown the ground beef, onion, and green pepper in a large nonstick skillet. Add no oil to the pan; the meat will release enough fat for frying. After the meat and vegetables are brown, add 1 cup water and let it come to a boil. Drain off the liquid from the pan. This will remove the remaining fat from the meat. Add the remaining cup of water to the pan and all of the other ingredients except the cheese. Simmer about 15 minutes, stirring constantly, until most of the liquid has evaporated. Sprinkle the cheese over the top of the meat and continue heating until it has melted. *Makes 8 servings*

	Calories	Carbo-hydrate (gm)	Protein (gm)	Total Fat (gm)	Saturated Fat (gm)	Choles-terol (mg)
Total	1961.3	202.7	154.4	63.1	30.0	376.0
Per Serving	245.2	25.3	19.3	7.9	3.8	47.0

Protein-Packed Pizza

1½ cup soy pancake mix
2 tbsp. corn or safflower
  oil
2 eggs
¼ cup skim milk
¼ tsp. salt
16-oz. can tomatoes in
  purée
1 tsp. (or more) oregano
  or mixed Italian
  seasonings
1 cup shredded part-
  skim mozzarella

4 tbsp. extra-sharp
  grated Romano
½ tsp. garlic salt
¼ tsp. black pepper
¼ tsp. crushed red
  pepper
1 cup sliced
  mushrooms,
  onions, green
  pepper, or
  zucchini
  (optional)

To make the crust, mix together the pancake mix, oil, eggs, milk and salt. Knead them enough so that the dough isn't sticky. Spray a 14-inch nonstick pizza pan with spray-on vegetable coating and press the dough onto the pan until is is completely covered. Bake the crust in a preheated 400° oven for about 8 minutes.

Break up the tomatoes with a fork, and spread them with the purée evenly over the crust. Sprinkle on the oregano, cheeses, salt, peppers, and optional toppings. Return the pizza to the hot oven just until the cheese is melted and bubbly. *Makes 6 servings*

	Calories	Carbo-hydrate (gm)	Protein (gm)	Total Fat (gm)	Saturated Fat (gm)	Choles-terol (mg)
Total	1938.5	186.6	148.1	166.6	22.0	642.0
Per Serving	323.1	31.1	24.7	27.8	3.7	107.0

Broccoli Quiche with High-Fiber Bread Crust

Crust:
6 slices high-fiber or
  diet bread, cut in
  half diagonally
1 tbsp. polyunsaturated
  margarine, melted
⅛ tsp. salt
Dash pepper
Dash paprika

Filling:
Filling:
1 cup chopped
  broccoli (fresh
  or frozen)
1 cube or envelope
  beef bouillon
¼ cup water
2 eggs
¾ cup skim milk

Roll the bread flat with a rolling pin. Assemble the 12 triangles in an 8-inch pie pan, points meeting in the center. Brush lightly with melted margarine and season with salt, pepper, paprika. Bake in a preheated 425° oven until golden, about 6 to 8 minutes.

Combine the broccoli, bouillon and water in a saucepan and simmer, covered, until the broccoli is just tender. Drain and reserve the cooking liquid. Spread the drained broccoli over the crust. Beat the eggs, milk and cooking liquid together and pour over the broccoli. Bake 1 hour in a preheated 350° oven until it is golden brown and a knife inserted off-center comes out clean. *Makes 6 servings*

	Calories	Carbo-hydrate (gm)	Protein (gm)	Total Fat (gm)	Saturated Fat (gm)	Choles-terol (mg)
Total	653.5	65.5	37.2	26.6	6.0	507.8
Per Serving	108.9	10.9	6.2	4.4	1.0	84.6

Swiss Asparagus Quiche

Basic Piecrust (see
  index)
6 tbsp. bacon bits
1 large onion, finely
  chopped
½ cup cubed Swiss
  cheese
2 tbsp. grated
  Parmesan cheese

13-oz. can evaporated
  skim milk
4 eggs
¼ tsp. salt
⅛ tsp. white pepper
¼ tsp. ground
  nutmeg
10-oz. pkg. frozen
  asparagus
  spears,
  defrosted

Line an 8-inch pie pan with Basic Piecrust and bake it for 5 minutes in a preheated 375° oven. Combine the bacon bits, onion, and cheeses. Arrange them in the pastry shell. Mix the milk, eggs, and seasonings together in a bowl and pour this mixture into the pie. Top the pie with the asparagus stalks, arranging them like the spokes of a wheel. Bake the quiche at 375° for 35 to 40 minutes, until it is golden brown, and a knife inserted off-center comes out clean. *Makes 6 servings*

	Calories	Carbo-hydrate (gm)	Protein (gm)	Total Fat (gm)	Saturated Fat (gm)	Choles-terol (mg)
Total	2247.9	127.9	132.2	135.7	49.9	1287.5
Per Serving	374.7	21.3	22.0	22.6	8.3	214.6

gm = grams; mg = milligrams. Nutritional figures are approximate. Figures are based on findings of U.S. Department of Agriculture.

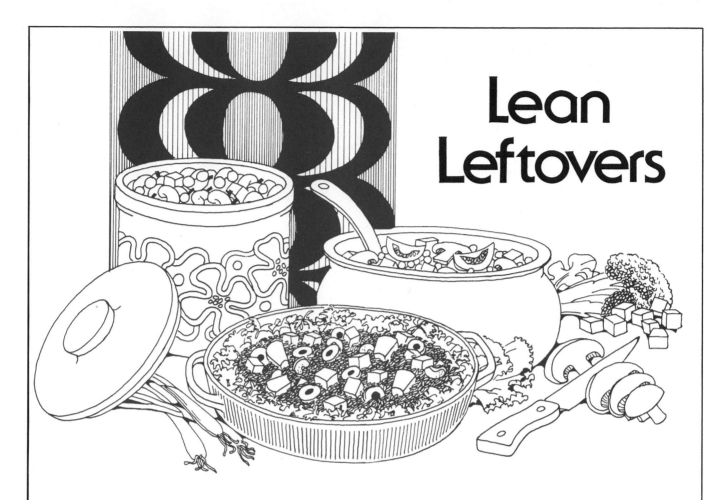

Lean Leftovers

The word leftover has an unpleasant hand-me-down sound to it. Why not think of them as "planned-overs," food purposely prepared in double quantities to simplify meal planning another day? True leftovers should be avoided. The weight-wise cook never, but never, makes more food than needed lest she lead her family into the temptation to overeat. It is better to cook too little than too much when weight is a problem.

Even if your family is small, do not hesitate to cook a large roast, multiple chickens, or a big turkey. The remaining meat can serve as the perfect departure for second-day meals. The advantage of recycled roasts is that most of the fat has already been cooked out, and the remaining fat can be trimmed away before the cooked meat is combined with other ingredients. And if you store the cooked meat in your freezer for a few weeks before it takes another curtain call at the family dinner table, who will be the wiser?

Recipes

Low-Calorie Enchiladas

16 Mexican Enchilada Crepes (recipe follows)

3 cups cooked leftover chicken (turkey, lean roast beef or pork may be substituted)

Sauce
10½-oz. can chicken, turkey or beef broth
1 onion, peeled and chopped
2 cloves garlic, minced, or ¼ tsp. instant garlic
6-oz. can tomato paste
2 tsp. vinegar
1 tsp. cumin seeds (or ¼ tsp. ground cumin)
2 tsp. chili powder (or more, to taste)
Dash tabasco
1½ tsp. salt
¼ tsp. pepper
1 green bell pepper, seeded and chopped

Skim any fat off the broth by chilling until the fat rises to the surface and can be whisked away. Combine all the sauce ingredients in a covered saucepan and simmer 20 minutes. Meanwhile, prepare the crepes. To assemble, spoon some of the chopped meat into each crepe, top with a little of the hot sauce and roll up. Cover with sauce to serve.

Makes 16 enchiladas (2 per serving)

	Calories	Carbo-hydrate (gm)	Protein (gm)	Total Fat (gm)	Saturated Fat (gm)	Choles-terol (mg)
Total	1787.2	101.3	217.7	51.3	16.3	1588.1
Per Serving	223.4	12.7	27.2	6.4	2.0	198.5

gm = grams; mg = milligrams. Nutritional figures are approximate. Figures are based on findings of U.S. Department of Agriculture.

Mexican Enchilada Crepes

4 eggs
4 tbsp. all-purpose flour
4 tbsp. cornmeal
¾ cup skim milk
¼ tsp. salt

Combine all of the ingredients in a blender or mixer and process until smooth. Let the batter rest 20 minutes. Follow the crepe making directions in this book (see index). Use in place of tortillas for enchilada recipes. *Makes 16 crepes (2 per serving)*

	Calories	Carbo-hydrate (gm)	Protein (gm)	Total Fat (gm)	Saturated Fat (gm)	Cholesterol (mg)
Total	598.3	53.7	35.9	25.5	8.3	1011.9
Per Serving	74.8	1.7	4.5	3.2	1.0	126.5

Italian Pepper Steak

1 Bermuda onion, thinly sliced, separated into rings
2 green peppers, seeded and sliced
16-oz. can tomato juice
Pinch red pepper
¼ tsp. basil or oregano
7 oz. sliced leftover rare steak, lean only (about 1 cup)
1 tbsp. grated extra-sharp Romano cheese

Combine onion, sliced pepper, tomato juice, red pepper and basil or oregano in a nonstick skillet. Simmer over low heat, uncovered, until most of the liquid has evaporated and the green pepper is tender-crisp. Add the steak slices and stir over moderate heat until the meat is heated through and coated with sauce. Sprinkle with cheese. *Makes 2 servings*

	Calories	Carbo-hydrate (gm)	Protein (gm)	Total Fat (gm)	Saturated Fat (gm)	Cholesterol (mg)
Total	640.5	36.6	78.2	19.4	10.0	194.7
Per Serving	320.3	18.3	39.1	9.7	5.0	97.4

Salad Stroganoff

1 lb. cold cooked lean beef round, sliced
2 tbsp. dry sherry
3 tbsp. wine vinegar
½ tsp. prepared mustard
1 tbsp. catsup (see index)
¼ cup plain low-fat yogurt
¼ cup sliced fresh mushrooms
2 potatoes

Marinate the beef for 2 hours in a mixture of the sherry, vinegar, mustard, and catsup. In the meantime, peel the potatoes. Boil, dice, and set them aside. After the meat has marinated, mix the yogurt in with the beef and marinade. Toss the mixture with the potatoes and mushrooms. Chill the salad before serving. *Makes 4 servings*

	Calories	Carbo-hydrate (gm)	Protein (gm)	Total Fat (gm)	Saturated Fat (gm)	Cholesterol (mg)
Total	1004.6	53.2	150.3	19.1	6.4	426.0
Per Serving	251.2	13.3	37.8	4.8	1.6	106.5

Spanish Steak Strips

3 cups (about 1 lb.) leftover lean rare roast beef or round steak, cut in ½-in. strips
1-lb. can tomatoes, undrained
1 onion, sliced
1 clove garlic, minced
8 Spanish stuffed olives, sliced
1 green pepper, seeded, sliced in 1-in. squares
1 tsp. salt
¼ tsp. (or more) chili powder
1 tsp. oregano or basil
1 tsp. cumin seed (optional)
1 tbsp. cornstarch
¼ cup water

Combine all ingredients except the cornstarch and water and refrigerate about 1 hour to blend flavors. Place in a 10-inch skillet. Bring to slow boil and simmer approximately 10 minutes over low heat. Mix the cornstarch in the water and add to the meat mixture. Cook and stir until thickened. Serve over rice, if desired. *Makes 6 servings*

	Calories	Carbo-hydrate (gm)	Protein (gm)	Total Fat (gm)	Saturated Fat (gm)	Cholesterol (mg)
Total	1324.2	40.0	131.4	68.3	26.6	408.5
Per Serving	220.7	6.7	21.9	11.4	4.4	68.1

Salade Boeuf

1 lb. leftover lean roast beef, thinly sliced
1 red onion, sliced
2 tbsp. corn or safflower oil
¼ cup wine vinegar
¼ cup chopped parsley
1 tbsp. capers
1 tsp. oregano
2 tsp. prepared mustard
½ tsp. garlic salt
¼ tsp. pepper
1 large or 2 small heads of lettuce

Combine all the ingredients except the lettuce. Cover the mixture and let it marinate in the refrigerator for 3 hours or longer. At serving time, shred the lettuce and toss it with the rest of the salad. *Makes 6 servings*

	Calories	Carbo-hydrate (gm)	Protein (gm)	Total Fat (gm)	Saturated Fat (gm)	Cholesterol (mg)
Total	1716.3	88.3	131.5	90.2	28.7	408.9
Per Serving	286.1	14.7	21.9	15.0	4.8	68.2

Instant Barbecue

2 cups diced cooked leftover lean roast beef or pork, trimmed of fat
2 cups nonalcoholic "Bloody Mary" mix (seasoned tomato juice)
1 tbsp. dried onion flakes
Dash smoke seasoning (optional)

gm = grams; mg = milligrams. Nutritional figures are approximate. Figures are based on findings of U.S. Department of Agriculture.

The Unforbidden Goodies Gallery of Photos

Pies, cream puffs, cheesecake, enchiladas and pizza—you practically can see the pounds accumulating. However, these dishes only look and taste sinfully rich. The calories have been pared back. Pink Strawberry No-Bake Cream Cheese Pie (recipe on page 111) is an impressive dessert to serve on a special occasion.

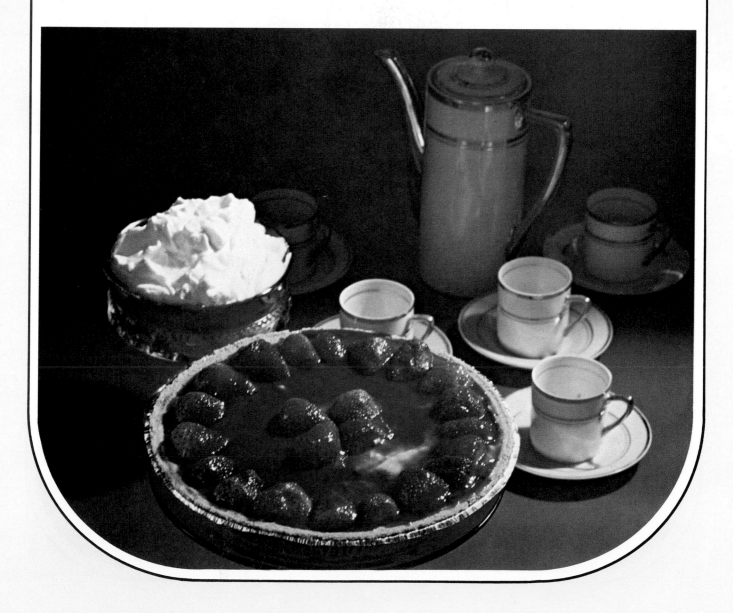

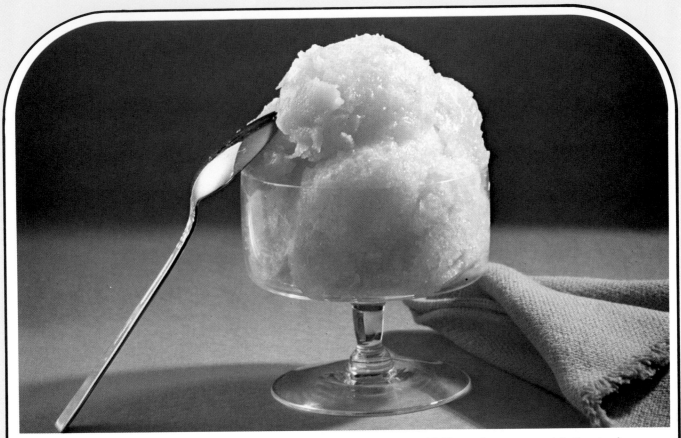

Above, Brandied Peach Sherbet (recipe on page 109) makes a sophisticated dessert. Below, Frosted Cappuchino (page 123), Banana Blueberry Float (page 122), Real Strawberry Milkshake (page 121) and Meal-in-a-Glass Berry Float (page 121) are refreshing beverages you can make without sugar or artificial sweetener.

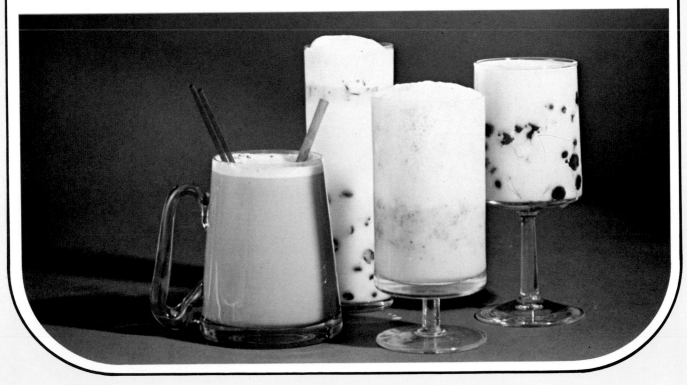

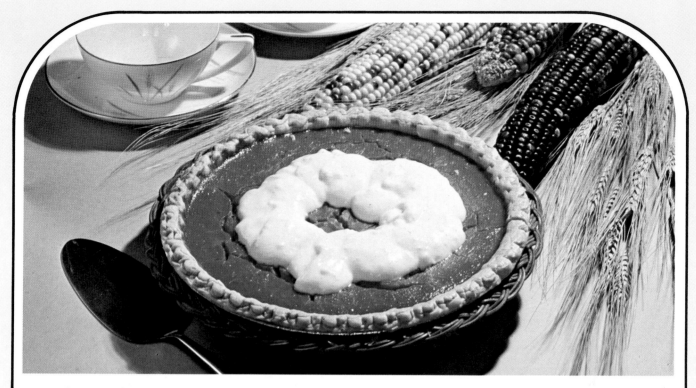

Above, Orange Pumpkin Pie (recipe on page 113) is sweetened with orange juice for only 144 calories a slice. Below, Cream Puffs with Orange Filling (recipe on page 114) is another deliciously low-calorie dessert.

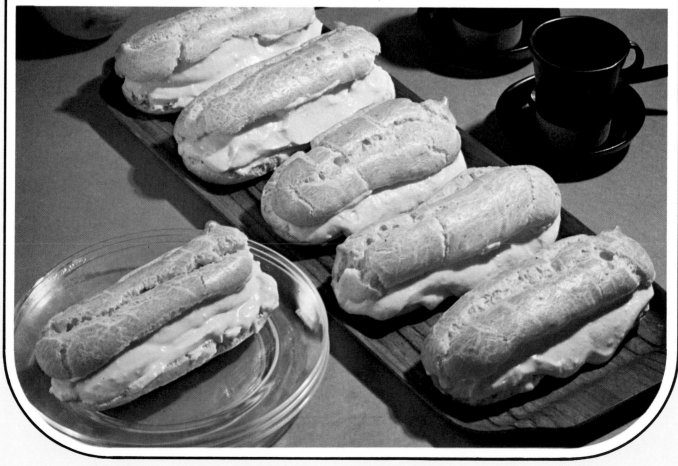

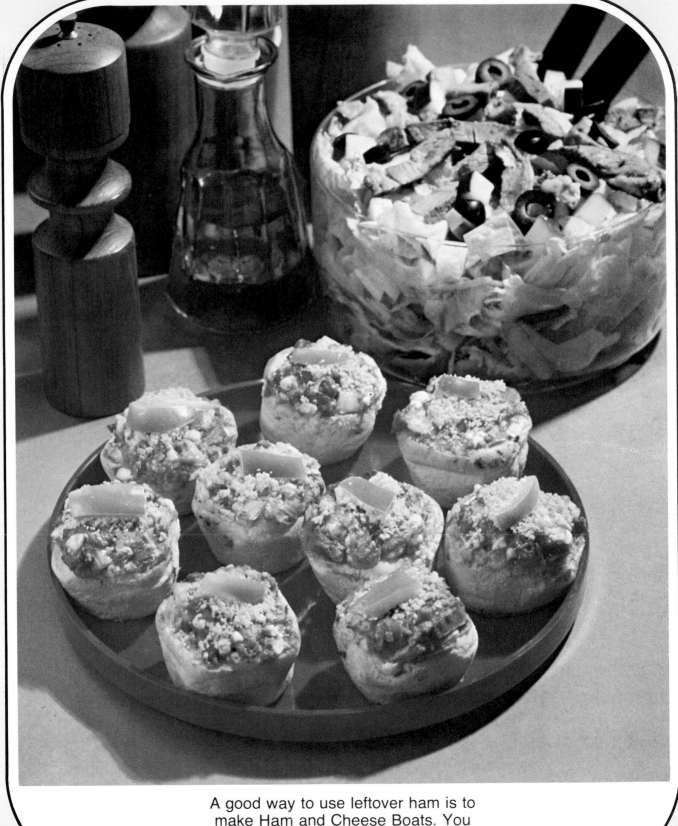

A good way to use leftover ham is to
make Ham and Cheese Boats. You
scoop out brown-and-serve rolls to make
the boats. The recipe is on page 100.

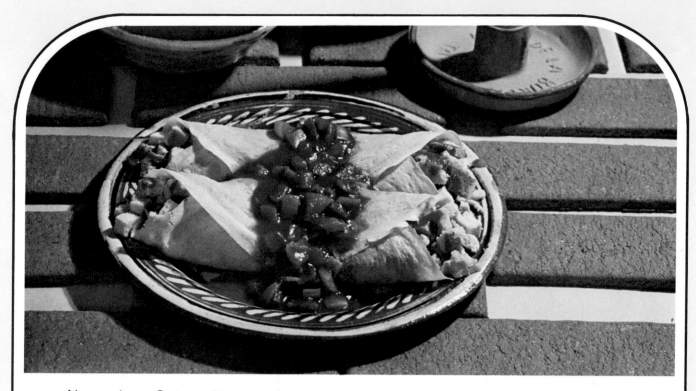

Above, Low-Calorie Enchiladas (recipe on pages 97 and 98) features cornmeal crepes and a spicy hot sauce. Below, Pennsylvania Dutch Cheesecake (recipe on page 115) sinks in the center to make room for fruit.

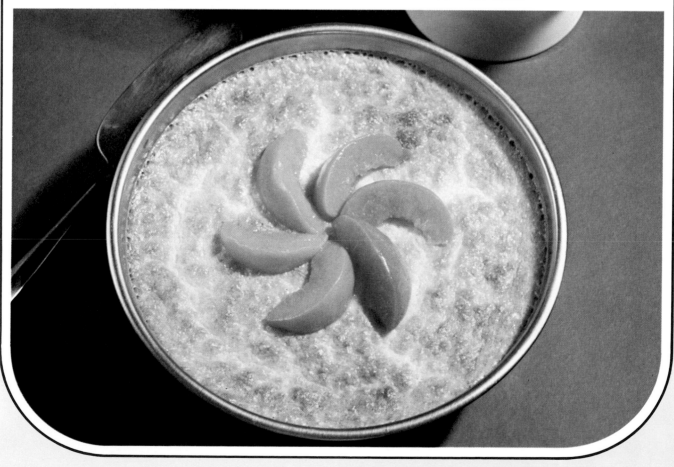

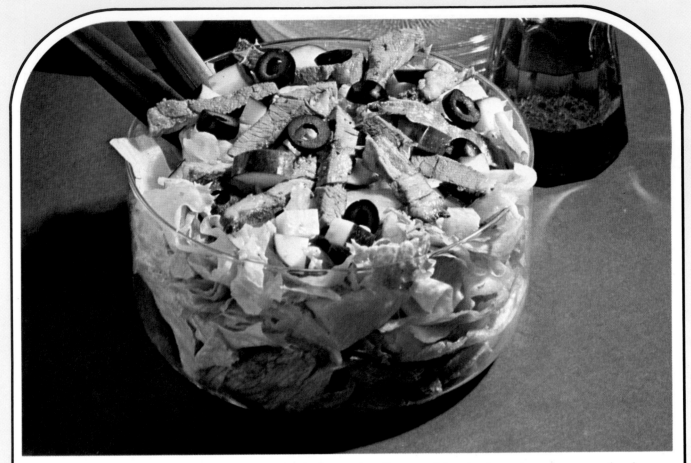

Syrian Salad Julienne, above, includes mint-flavored herb dressing over cooked lamb (recipe on page 99). For Apple Raisin Kuchen (recipe on page 114), you pour a rich tasting custard filling over flaky-style dough.

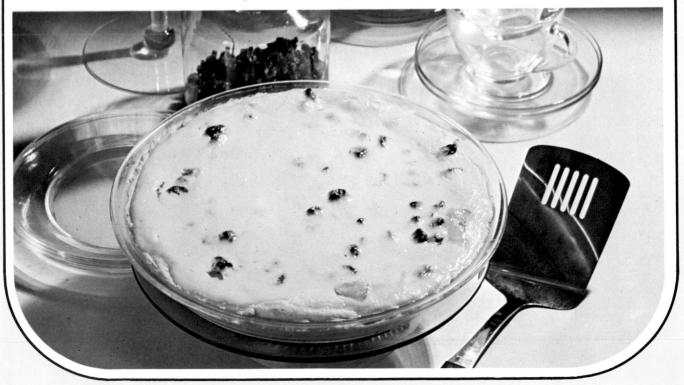

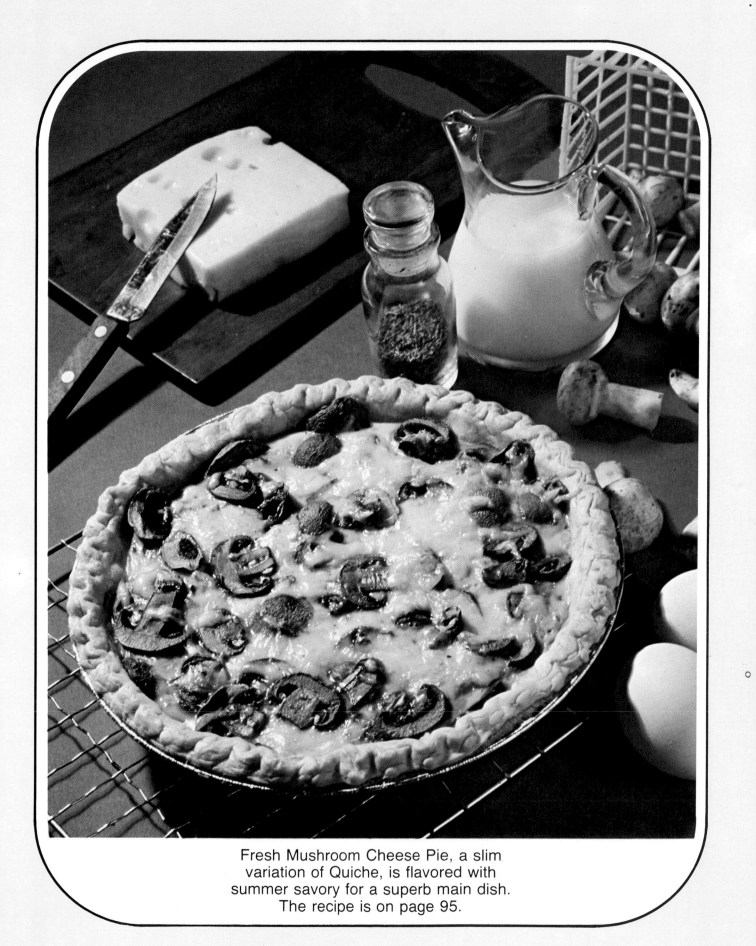

Fresh Mushroom Cheese Pie, a slim
variation of Quiche, is flavored with
summer savory for a superb main dish.
The recipe is on page 95.

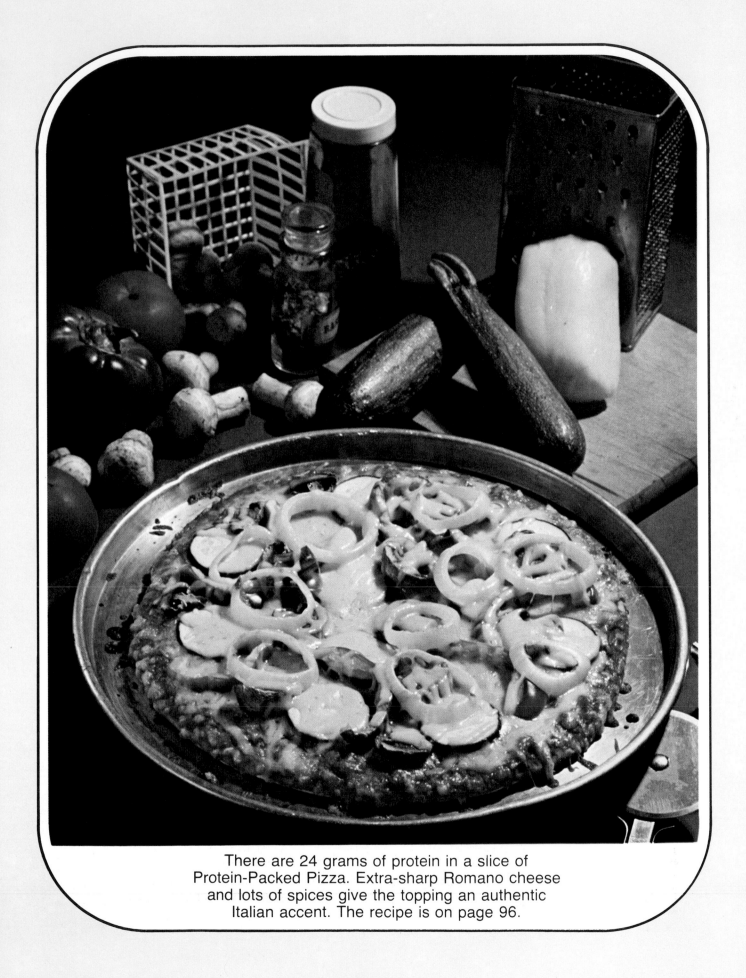

There are 24 grams of protein in a slice of
Protein-Packed Pizza. Extra-sharp Romano cheese
and lots of spices give the topping an authentic
Italian accent. The recipe is on page 96.

Combine all the ingredients in a nonstick skillet. Cook and stir until the liquid evaporates, forming a thick sauce, and meat is hot, tender and well coated. Serve with salad or coleslaw, or as a filling for toasted hamburger buns. *Makes 4 servings*

	Calories	Carbo-hydrate (gm)	Protein (gm)	Total Fat (gm)	Saturated Fat (gm)	Choles-terol (mg)
Total	1077.8	22.5	112.6	54.4	23.3	357.1
Per Serving	269.5	5.6	28.2	13.6	5.8	89.4

Lamb and Broccoli Casserole

2 tbsp. flour
1 cup skim milk
1¼ cups grated processed American diet cheese
½ tsp. Worcestershire sauce
½ tsp. salt
½ tsp. celery seed
¼ tsp. dry mustard
⅛ tsp. pepper
1 lb. cooked sliced leg of lamb, trimmed of fat
10-oz. pkg. frozen broccoli, cooked
1 medium tomato, sliced

Combine the flour with the milk in a saucepan over low heat, stirring until thickened. Add 1 cup of the grated cheese, the Worcestershire sauce, salt, celery seed, mustard, and pepper. Stir and cook until the cheese has melted. Arrange the lamb, broccoli, and tomato slices in layers in a 1½-quart shallow baking dish. Pour the sauce over all and bake in a preheated 350° oven for 15 minutes. Sprinkle the remaining ¼ cup grated cheese over the top and bake 5 minutes longer. *Makes 4 servings*

	Calories	Carbo-hydrate (gm)	Protein (gm)	Total Fat (gm)	Saturated Fat (gm)	Choles-terol (mg)
Total	1706.7	77.0	224.7	61.1	35.4	661.9
Per Serving	426.7	19.3	56.2	15.3	8.9	165.5

Tossed Lamb Salad

2 tbsp. chopped parsley
1 tbsp. instant minced onion
1½ tsp. salt
¼ tsp. pepper
⅓ cup vinegar
2 tbsp. corn or safflower oil
½ tsp. oregano
1 lb. cooked lean leg of lamb, diced
3 cups torn lettuce
2 medium tomatoes, diced
1 cup chopped celery
1 cup cubed cooked potatoes

Combine the parsley, onion, salt, pepper, vinegar, oil, and oregano in a bowl. Add the lamb, and mix well. Chill for 1 hour, turning the lamb occasionally. Meanwhile, combine the rest of the ingredients, toss lightly, and chill them also. Before serving, add the lamb mixture to the salad greens mixture and toss everything lightly but thoroughly. *Makes 6 servings*

	Calories	Carbo-hydrate (gm)	Protein (gm)	Total Fat (gm)	Saturated Fat (gm)	Choles-terol (mg)
Total	1288.0	52.7	135.2	60.0	21.2	454.4
Per Serving	214.7	8.8	22.5	10.0	3.5	75.7

Lamb 'n' Macaroni Salad

2 cups elbow macaroni
3 cups diced cooked lean lamb, loosely packed
1 cup diced celery
½ cup diet mayonnaise
¼ cup drained sweet pickle relish
2 tbsp. chopped onion
1 tsp. salt
⅛ tsp. pepper
8 large lettuce leaves

Cook macaroni according to package directions. Combine all the ingredients except the lettuce. Toss lightly. Chill the entire mixture and serve it on lettuce leaves. *Makes 8 servings*

	Calories	Carbo-hydrate (gm)	Protein (gm)	Total Fat (gm)	Saturated Fat (gm)	Choles-terol (mg)
Total	2125.7	175.3	214.8	60.5	28.8	713.6
Per Serving	265.7	21.9	26.9	7.6	3.6	89.2

Lamb Luncheon Salad

3 cups cold cooked rice
2 cups cubed cooked lamb
1 medium tomato, diced
½ cup chopped red onion
½ cup chopped parsley
½ cup diet Italian salad dressing
3 tbsp. lemon juice
½ tsp. salt
¼ tsp. pepper
Salad greens

Combine all ingredients well and chill before serving on salad greens. *Makes 6 servings*

	Calories	Carbo-hydrate (gm)	Protein (gm)	Total Fat (gm)	Saturated Fat (gm)	Choles-terol (mg)
Total	1412.8	166.6	107.1	31.0	13.8	326.6
Per Serving	235.5	27.8	17.9	5.2	2.3	54.4

Syrian Salad Julienne

2 tbsp. olive oil
2 tbsp. dry red wine
2 tbsp. lemon juice
½ tsp. garlic salt
⅛ tsp. pepper
1 tsp. crushed mint leaves
2 cups cooked lamb, cut in julienne strips, loosely packed
2 medium cucumbers, diced
3 black olives, sliced
4 cups shredded lettuce

Combine the oil, wine, lemon juice, garlic salt, pepper, and mint. Pour the mixture over the lamb strips and let it sit at room temperature for several hours. Add the cucumbers and olives to the meat mixture and toss well. Arrange the meat and vegetables on the shredded lettuce *Makes 4 servings*

	Calories	Carbo-hydrate (gm)	Protein (gm)	Total Fat (gm)	Saturated Fat (gm)	Choles-terol (mg)
Total	1002.6	26.4	82.9	58.6	17.8	294.4
Per Serving	250.7	6.6	20.7	14.7	4.5	73.6

gm = grams; mg = milligrams. Nutritional figures are approximate. Figures are based on findings of U.S. Department of Agriculture.

Quick Barbecued Pork

3 lb. leftover roast pork, trimmed of fat and sliced in 1- to 2-in. pieces
2 tbsp. tomato paste
3 tbsp. cider vinegar

2 tbsp. Worcestershire sauce
1/3 cup unsweetened apple cider
1 tsp. salt
1 tsp. chili powder
1 tsp. paprika

Spread the pork in a baking dish. Combine the remaining ingredients in a saucepan and bring the mixture to boil. Pour the sauce over the pork and heat it in a preheated 325° oven for 15 minutes. Do not allow the pork to dry out. *Makes 12 servings*

	Calories	Carbo-hydrate (gm)	Protein (gm)	Total Fat (gm)	Saturated Fat (gm)	Choles-terol (mg)
Total	5026.0	11.4	336.8	384.0	144.0	1216.0
Per Serving	418.8	0.9	28.1	32.0	12.0	101.3

Ham and Cheese Boats

1 hard-cooked egg
1 cup 99% fat-free cottage cheese, drained
1 cup ground boiled ham
6 tbsp. shredded cheddar cheese

1/2 cup chopped onion
1/4 cup tomato purée
2 tbsp. chopped green pepper
6 brown'n'serve club rolls
6 green pepper strips

Separate the egg white and yolk. Press the yolk through a sieve and chop the egg white. Combine the cottage cheese, ham, cheddar cheese, onion, tomato purée, green pepper, and chopped egg white in a bowl. Cut a thin slice from the top of each roll, scoop out the bready center of the roll, leaving a thin shell. Fill the shells with the cottage cheese mixture, mounding it on top. Place the boats on a baking sheet and bake in a preheated 375° oven for 15 minutes until the roll is golden brown. Sprinkle the tops with egg yolk, and garnish each serving with a green pepper strip. *Makes 6 servings*

	Calories	Carbo-hydrate (gm)	Protein (gm)	Total Fat (gm)	Saturated Fat (gm)	Choles-terol (mg)
Total	1737.0	129.8	111.9	81.0	33.2	523.9
Per Serving	289.5	21.6	18.6	13.5	5.5	87.2

Creamed Ham and Potatoes

1 tbsp. diet margarine
1 cup lean boiled ham, diced
1/2 cup chopped onion
10¾-oz. can condensed cream of celery soup

4 tbsp. imitation sour cream
1/4 tsp. caraway seeds (optional)
2 potatoes, peeled, boiled, cubed

Melt the margarine in a nonstick skillet and sauté the ham and onions for 5 minutes. Add the soup, sour cream, and caraway seeds, and blend well. Then gently mix in the potatoes. Continue cooking until the mixture is heated thoroughly, but do not boil. *Makes 4 servings*

	Calories	Carbo-hydrate (gm)	Protein (gm)	Total Fat (gm)	Saturated Fat (gm)	Choles-terol (mg)
Total	883.0	69.0	58.6	42.9	15.1	151.2
Per Serving	220.8	17.3	14.7	10.7	3.8	37.8

Hawaiian Chicken Salad

2 cups cooked broiler-fryer chicken, cut in chunks, loosely packed
1/4 cup diet mayonnaise
1/4 cup unsweetened juice-packed pineapple tidbits, drained

1/2 cup chopped celery
2 tbsp. slivered almonds
1 tsp. soy sauce
4 crisp lettuce leaves

Combine all the ingredients except the lettuce. Serve the salad on the lettuce leaves. *Makes 4 servings*

	Calories	Carbo-hydrate (gm)	Protein (gm)	Total Fat (gm)	Saturated Fat (gm)	Choles-terol (mg)
Total	898.1	20.7	118.6	35.2	6.5	415.9
Per Serving	224.5	5.2	29.7	8.8	1.6	104.0

Chicken Chop Suey

1/2 cup chicken broth
1 tbsp. diet margarine
1/2 cup sliced onion
1 cup sliced celery
1 green pepper, cut in strips
4-oz. can mushrooms, drained
16-oz. can bean sprouts, drained

1/4 tsp. salt
2 tsp. cornstarch
2 tbsp. soy sauce
2 cups diced cooked broiler-fryer chicken, loosely packed

Skim the fat from the chicken broth by chilling it until the fat rises to the top and can be whisked away. Melt the margarine in a nonstick skillet and sauté the onions, celery, and green pepper. Add the chicken broth, mushrooms, bean sprouts, and salt and bring the mixture to a boil. Blend the cornstarch with the soy sauce in a cup. Add this mixture to the skillet and continue cooking, stirring constantly, until the sauce has thickened slightly. Then add the chicken. Continue cooking just until the chicken is heated through. *Makes 6 servings*

	Calories	Carbo-hydrate (gm)	Protein (gm)	Total Fat (gm)	Saturated Fat (gm)	Choles-terol (mg)
Total	951.1	60.5	129.6	22.5	6.3	364.0
Per Serving	158.5	10.1	21.6	3.8	1.1	60.7

gm = grams; mg = milligrams. Nutritional figures are approximate. Figures are based on findings of U.S. Department of Agriculture.

Chicken Patties

2 cups ground cooked
   broiler-fryer
   chicken, loosely
   packed
1/2 tsp. salt
2 eggs, beaten

2 tsp. instant minced
   onion
1/4 cup tomato purée
1/4 tsp. Tabasco
   sauce
6 hamburger buns

Combine all of the ingredients and shape into 6 patties. Broil the patties about 5 minutes on each side just until they are heated through. Serve on buns.

Makes 6 servings

	Calories	Carbo-hydrate (gm)	Protein (gm)	Total Fat (gm)	Saturated Fat (gm)	Choles-terol (mg)
Total	1297.5	132.8	97.8	34.0	13.3	739.1
Per Serving	216.3	22.3	16.3	5.7	2.2	123.2

Creamy Turkey Curry

1 tbsp. diet margarine
1/2 cup finely chopped
   onion
1 to 2 tbsp. curry
   powder
2/3 cup water

10 1/2-oz. can condensed
   cream of
   chicken soup
3 cups diced cooked
   turkey, loosely
   packed
1 tsp. lemon juice

Melt the margarine in a nonstick skillet and sauté the onions until they are tender. Stir in the curry powder and continue to heat the onions for a few seconds. Add the water and soup. Heat the mixture through, stirring continuously. Add the turkey. Heat the mixture just until the turkey is heated through. Just before serving, add the lemon juice.

Makes 6 servings

	Calories	Carbo-hydrate (gm)	Protein (gm)	Total Fat (gm)	Saturated Fat (gm)	Choles-terol (mg)
Total	1191.8	27.2	155.2	49.2	12.7	433.0
Per Serving	198.6	4.5	25.9	8.2	2.1	72.2

Fruited Turkey Curry Salad

2 1/2 cups diced cooked
   turkey, loosely
   packed
1/3 cup plain low-fat
   yogurt
1/3 cup diet mayonnaise
1 tbsp. lemon juice
1 tsp. salt
1 tsp. curry powder
1 1/2 cups diced celery

2 tbsp. slivered
   almonds
6 large lettuce
   leaves
1/2 cup seedless
   grapes, halved
1 cup canned
   unsweetened
   juice-packed
   pineapple
   chunks, drained

Combine all the ingredients except the almonds, lettuce, and fruit. Chill until serving time. Serve the salad on the lettuce leaves and garnish with the almonds, grapes and pineapple chunks.

Makes 6 servings

	Calories	Carbo-hydrate (gm)	Protein (gm)	Total Fat (gm)	Saturated Fat (gm)	Choles-terol (mg)
Total	1634.6	69.9	204.1	59.3	13.8	595.7
Per Serving	272.4	11.6	34.0	9.9	2.3	99.3

Trim Turkey Hash

2 tbsp. diet margarine
3/4 cup cooked potatoes,
   diced
3 tbsp. chopped onion
3 cups diced cooked
   turkey, loosely
   packed

1/3 cup evaporated
   skim milk
1 1/2 tsp. Worcester-
   shire sauce
1/2 tsp. salt
1/8 tsp. pepper

Melt the margarine in a heavy nonstick skillet and sauté the potatoes and onions until they are brown. Then stir in the remaining ingredients. Cook the mixture over low heat for about 10 minutes, stirring frequently, until the mixture is hot and well combined.

Makes 4 servings

Note: If you do not have leftover potatoes, you may use canned potatoes or frozen slices that have been defrosted.

	Calories	Carbo-hydrate (gm)	Protein (gm)	Total Fat (gm)	Saturated Fat (gm)	Choles-terol (mg)
Total	1149.8	23.3	154.0	46.0	14.7	432.4
Per Serving	287.5	5.8	38.5	11.5	3.7	108.1

Turkey Canton

2 tbsp. diet margarine
1 cup diagonally sliced
   celery
1 cup thinly sliced
   carrots
1 medium onion,
   chopped
2 tbsp. slivered
   almonds
3/4 cup canned
   unsweetened juice-
   packed pineapple
   chunks, drained,
   reserving juice

1/4 tsp. salt
1 tbsp. cornstarch
1/4 tsp. ground ginger
1/4 tsp. nutmeg
1 tbsp. soy sauce
1 tsp. lemon juice
5-oz. can water
   chestnuts, thinly
   sliced
1 cup diced cooked
   turkey, loosely
   packed

Melt the margarine in a large nonstick skillet and sauté the celery, carrots, onion, and almonds until the nuts are lightly browned. Add enough water to the pineapple juice to make 1 1/4 cups, and pour the mixture into the skillet. Add the salt, cornstarch, ginger, nutmeg, soy sauce, and lemon juice to the saucepan. Cook the mixture slowly, stirring constantly, until it has thickened. Then add the pineapple chunks, water chestnuts, and turkey. Continue cooking just until everything is heated through. Serve over rice.

Makes 4 servings

	Calories	Carbo-hydrate (gm)	Protein (gm)	Total Fat (gm)	Saturated Fat (gm)	Choles-terol (mg)
Total	842.4	94.5	56.5	30.6	5.7	127.3
Per Serving	210.6	23.6	14.1	7.7	1.4	31.8

gm = grams; mg = milligrams. Nutritional figures are approximate. Figures are based on findings of U.S. Department of Agriculture.

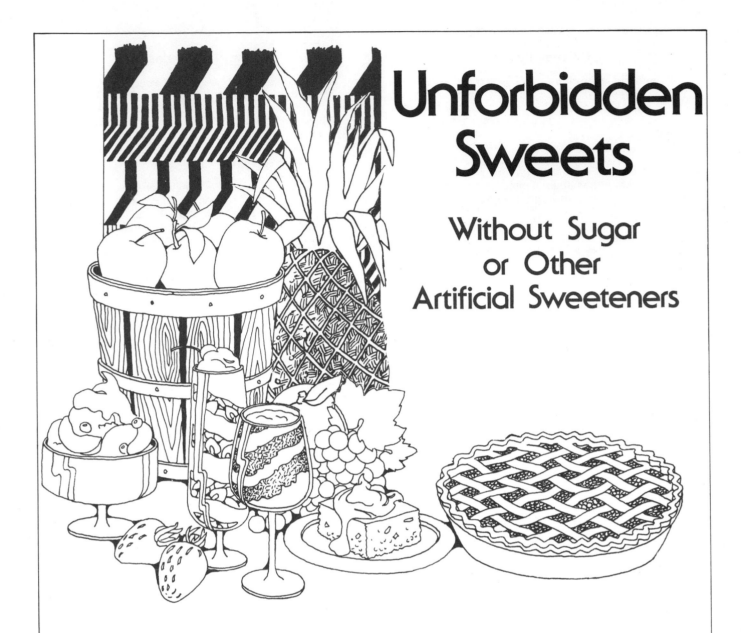

Unforbidden Sweets

Without Sugar or Other Artificial Sweeteners

Yes, sugar is an artificial sweetener, too. It's pure, refined, processed calories with no redeeming nutritional value, perhaps the most abused and overused additive there is. Of all the things we eat that cost us calories, nothing offers less sustained appetite satisfaction or is burned up or turned to fat by the body as quickly as sugar. Mother Nature never created foods as sweet as many of the sweets we eat. There probably is no need for processed sugar in human nutrition. In fact, throughout most of human history, sugar simply did not exist.

In recent years, American sugar consumption has risen as high as 115 pounds per person per year. Much of that sugar is hidden in packaged foods, often in such unlikely places as canned vegetables, salad dressings, and other foods that we do not think of as sweets. If you are the average American, sugar accounts for more than 500 of the calories you consume every day. That is about 200,000 empty calories a year!

Eliminating that many calories a day adds up to 3500 calories per week, or just what it takes to lose — or gain — one pound!

A taste for sweets is something that develops gradually. Critics of the American diet maintain that sugar-rich infant formulas and sweetened baby foods are the start of our national sweet tooth, followed later by sugared cereals and TV-touted snacks, sodas, and junk food. By the time we are adults, our sweet tooth may well be the only tooth left. The taste for excessive sweetness can be reversed by using diminishing amounts of sugar and other artificial sweeteners in the foods we prepare ourselves. But we need not deprive our sweet tooth entirely; we simply need to choose our sweeteners more discriminately. We need to learn how to make better use of the natural, nutritious, low-calorie sweeteners that Mother Nature originally intended for us — the ones that come packaged as oranges, apples, peaches, grapes, and other fruits.

The Bitter Truth about Sweeteners

• **Ordinary white table sugar,** or sucrose, contains 16 calories per level — not rounded or heaping — teaspoon. It is pure, refined carbohydrate, pure calories, with no redeeming nutritional value whatsoever. The carbohydrate in sugar is more quickly turned to fat and more likely to raise blood trigliceride and blood sugar levels associated with heart disease and diabetes than the carbohydrate in starchy foods.

• **Raw sugar, brown sugar, turbinado sugar** and other favorites of the health food set are also refined carbohydrates and like white sugar contain little but calories. Their vitamin and mineral value are infinitesimal compared with their calorie counts.

• **Corn syrup, maple syrup, and molasses** are refined carbohydrates, too, comparable in calorie content to white sugar. Their nutritional value is likewise miniscule. Moreover, they are less sweet than comparable amounts of white sugar. It takes as much as 50 percent more of these to equal the sweetness of white sugar, making them even more fattening than ordinary table sugar!

• **Fructose** is the natural sugar found in fruit and honey. Although its calorie content is about the same as sucrose, it can be as much as 50 percent sweeter than white sugar. The sweetness of fructose is further enhanced when it is used in drinks or desserts containing acid or served chilled. So, because you can use less of it, fructose tends to be less fattening than sucrose. However, it is still purely refined carbohydrate with no appetite-appeasing bulk or fiber, no vitamins, minerals, or other nutritional value. The body does use it more slowly than white sugar, but one marketer ran into trouble over labeling claims suggesting that it could be safely used by diabetics. Fructose is expensive to process from fruit. A technique has been developed to extract it more cheaply from corn products, but it is still expensive and not widely available. Sometimes it can be found in health food stores.

• **Xylitol** is another type of fruit sugar that naturally occurs in plums and stawberries. It can also be extracted from pecan shells and wood. It is very expensive to produce and is not available as a table sweetener. Since it was developed primarily as a sweetener for non-cavity-causing chewing gums, a dieter should not assume that products with xylitol are low in calories.

• **Honey,** wholesome as it may seem, is simply another refined carbohydrate. It is just made by bees instead of man. It contains more fructose than sucrose, so it is sweeter than sugar and you can use less to get the same degree of sweetness provided by white sugar. But like sugar, the nutritional value of honey is very small compared to its high calorie content — about 20 calories per teaspoon.

Synthetic Sweeteners

• **Saccharin** is the only legal noncaloric sweetener now on the market — for the time being at least. Laboratory tests showing its relationship to cancer of the bladder in rats have led to a bitterly debated proposal by the United States Food and Drug Administration to prohibit its use as a commercial food and cosmetic additive. If the FDA's proposed regulation goes into effect, saccharin could be sold as an over-the-counter nonprescription drug. Powder, tablet, and liquid saccharin would have to bear a warning label reading "Saccharin causes bladder cancer in animals. Use of saccharin may increase your risk of cancer."

• **Sorbitol** is a legal artificial sweetener that is approved for use in dietetic foods; however, it is *not* noncaloric. In fact, it is more fattening than sugar because it is not as sweet. It takes more calories' worth of sorbitol to achieve the same degree of sweetness in lesser amounts of sugar. But sorbitol is absorbed more slowly than sugar, and so may be used by diabetics under medical guidance as long as overweight is not a problem. But since diabetes is often related to obesity, avoiding large amounts of empty calories is usually an important part of the treatment. Like sugar, sorbitol is a refined carbohydrate with no nutritional value. Since it has the same calorie content as sugar but is less sweet, sorbitol and sorbitol-sweetened dietetic foods are of no value to the dieter who is not diabetic.

• **Cyclamate** was the most popular synthetic sweetener in this country before it was outlawed in the early 1960s by the United States Food and Drug Administration. Laboratory tests had shown that massive doses of cyclamate fed to animals produced cancer. A better-tasting, more stable, and more versatile sweetener than saccharin, cyclamate continues to be available as an over-the-counter table sweetener in Canada and other foreign countries. Abbott Laboratories, the manufacturer, is seeking permission to remarket cyclamate in this country, claiming that newer scientific studies disprove the test results that brought about the ban.

• **Miracle fruit** is a natural extract from the berries of the miracle fruit tree, a tropical plant whose Latin name is *Synsepalum dulcificum*. These small red cherrylike berries contain a protein that has the unique ability to make sour foods taste sweet. It works by coating the tongue with a substance that changes the way taste buds perceive flavors. After chewing a tablet containing the protein, sour foods like lemon or grapefruit taste as if they had been sprinkled with sugar. The problem is that all other acid-base foods, like salad dressing and dry wine, also taste sweet, whether you want them to or not.

Scientists are working on ways to combine this sweetening agent with foods to make it more useful. At Georgetown University in Washington, D.C., a technique has been developed for combining the sweetener extract with acid ingredients in low-calorie foods in a way that limits the lingering sweetening power. However, it is unlikely that miracle fruit sweeteners will be marketed in the near future, since they still require extensive testing and FDA approval. The sweetener was marketed briefly as fruit drops called Miralin, to be chewed before eating unsweetened food, but was taken off the market by the FDA because approval had never been sought.

• **Aspartame** is a low-calorie sweetener composed of two naturally occurring amino acids (the building blocks of protein). It has the same calories as sugar but many times the sweetness of sugar. So little aspartame is needed to make foods taste sweet that the calories do not even count. Aspartame is also the most sugarlike in taste and texture of all the synthetic sweeteners developed thus far.

In 1974, the FDA approved limited use of aspartame, but then withdrew approval before it reached the marketplace due to questions about the product's safety and the adequacy and accuracy of the data submitted by its developer, G. D. Searle & Company. Searle contends that aspartame is safe and that an independent scientific review of the evidence will support its safety. At the request of the FDA, Searle agreed to pay for a review by a consortium of universities and to submit all findings to a public board of inquiry. Since, at the time of this writing, the details of how this review will be conducted are still being worked out, aspartame seems to be a long way from the marketplace. When, or if, it is ever marketed, aspartame will be known by the trade name Equa.

Soothing Your Sweet Tooth Naturally

Should we add unnatural sweetness to sweets? Is it really smart to extract pure calories in the form of white sugar and sprinkle it all over everything? And what about synthetic sweeteners? Is the noncaloric sweetness we get from them worth the risk of cancer?

Evidence is growing that it may be unwise to fool with Mother Nature. The safety of sugar as well as saccharin is in question. Recent studies seem to link so many typically American ills to the increase in our sugar consumption and the decrease in our consumption of fruit and vegetable fiber. Perhaps it is time we reexamined the way we satisfy our sweet tooth. If we gave up sugar and sugar substitutes in the forms of soda pop, candy, pastries, and other high-calorie junk food, wouldn't we be satisfying our sweet tooth as our ancestors did with oranges, apples, raisins, peaches, and berries?

Mother Nature has provided us with an amply-filled sugar bowl in the form of natural fresh fruits. Natural fruit and treats sweetened with fruits and juices are not only low in calories but also nutritious and appetite-appeasing, full of vitamins, minerals, hunger-delaying bulk, and regularity-producing fiber. All of the desserts, beverages, and treats in this section are naturally sweetened with fresh fruit, fruit juices, or dried, canned, or frozen fruit without sugar, syrup, saccharin, or other unnatural sweeteners. These recipes show you how to satisfy your craving for sweets without sacrificing your health, your diet regimen or your conscience. Discover how exciting and soul-satisfying desserts and treats can be when they are sweetened Mother Nature's way . . . naturally.

Recipes

Apples au Vin Rouge

4 baking apples
½ cup bottled
    unsweetened red or
    purple grape juice
¼ cup red wine
½ tsp. pumpkin pie
    spice

Core apples and remove about one inch of peel from the top. Arrange them in a baking dish just large enough to hold them. Pour on the grape juice and wine. Sprinkle the apples with spice. Bake the apples in a preheated 350° oven about 30 to 45 minutes, basting frequently with the sauce. *Makes 4 servings*

	Calories	Carbo-hydrate (gm)	Protein (gm)	Total Fat (gm)	Saturated Fat (gm)	Choles-terol (mg)
Total	383.8	94.0	0.5	0.0	0.0	0.0
Per Serving	96.0	23.5	0.1	0.0	0.0	0.0

Pink Poached Pears

8 fresh pears, halved
    and cored
1 cup unsweetened
    grape juice
½ cup red wine
5 whole cloves
½ tsp. cinnamon
1 tbsp. arrowroot
½ cup cold water

Set the pear halves cut side up in a shallow skillet and pour the grape juice and wine over them. Add the cloves and cinnamon. Cover and simmer gently until the pears are just tender, about 8 to 10 minutes. Remove the pears with a slotted spoon. Mix the arrowroot and cold water and stir into liquid in the skillet. Cook and stir until the sauce is thick. Pour the sauce over the pears and serve warm or chilled.

Makes 8 servings

	Calories	Carbo-hydrate (gm)	Protein (gm)	Total Fat (gm)	Saturated Fat (gm)	Choles-terol (mg)
Total	1050.0	246.0	9.0	8.0	0.0	0.0
Per Serving	131.3	30.8	1.1	1.0	0.0	0.0

Baked Pears

6 ripe pears
2 tbsp. lemon juice
8¾-oz. can unsweetened
    crushed pineapple,
    drained reserving
    liquid
½ cup water
½ tsp. nutmeg
½ cup unsweetened
    white grape
    juice

Starting with the stem top, peel pears ⅓ of the way down. Brush the cut surface with lemon juice to prevent darkening. Core the bottoms of the pears (up to peeled part) and stuff with the drained crushed pineapple. Stand the pears, stem tops up, in a baking dish. Mix the reserved pineapple juice, water and nutmeg and pour into the dish. Spoon the grape juice over the pears. Cover with foil and bake in a preheated 375° oven, basting occasionally until the pears are tender, about 30 to 40 minutes. Serve warm or cold.

Makes 6 servings

	Calories	Carbo-hydrate (gm)	Protein (gm)	Total Fat (gm)	Saturated Fat (gm)	Choles-terol (mg)
Total	782.5	196.0	7.4	6.3	0.0	0.0
Per Serving	130.4	32.7	1.2	1.1	0.0	0.0

gm = grams; mg = milligrams. Nutritional figures are approximate. Figures are based on findings of U.S. Department of Agriculture.

Fresh Fruit Fondue

2 cups plain low-fat
  yogurt

2 cups fresh fruit
  such as
  strawberries,
  sliced peaches,
  sliced bananas,
  and orange
  sections

Put yogurt in a bowl on a serving tray. Surround the yogurt with the fresh fruit impaled on party picks.

Makes 4 servings

	Calories	Carbo-hydrate (gm)	Protein (gm)	Total Fat (gm)	Saturated Fat (gm)	Choles-terol (mg)
Total	445.0	61.5	16.5	16.5	10.0	40.0
Per Serving	111.3	15.4	4.1	4.1	2.5	10.0

Frosty Fruit Whip

2/3 cup evaporated skim
  milk
8-oz. pkg. low-calorie
  cream cheese,
  softened

16-oz. can
  unsweetened
  fruit cocktail,
  drained
1 banana, sliced
2 tbsp. fresh lemon
  juice

Pour the evaporated skim milk into a mixing bowl and chill in the freezer until ice forms at the edges. In the meantime, beat the cream cheese until it is smooth and creamy. Stir in the fruit cocktail and banana. Using chilled beaters, whip the frosted milk in the chilled bowl with the high speed of your mixer until fluffy. Add the lemon juice and continue whipping until the milk is stiff. Fold the whipped milk into the fruit. Spoon the mixture into a 9-inch square pan and freeze for about 3 hours until it is firm. Cut it into 9 squares for serving.

Makes 9 servings

	Calories	Carbo-hydrate (gm)	Protein (gm)	Total Fat (gm)	Saturated Fat (gm)	Choles-terol (mg)
Total	1210.5	107.4	31.5	61.2	39.3	219.5
Per Serving	134.5	11.9	3.5	6.8	4.4	24.4

Pineapplesauce

4 or 5 cooking apples
  (about 1 lb.), cored,
  peeled, sliced
16-oz. can unsweetened,
  juice-packed
  crushed pineapple

Vanilla, salt or
  cinnamon to
  taste

Combine all of the ingredients in a covered saucepan and simmer until apples are tender, about 20 minutes. Stir sauce until smooth and chill before serving.

Makes 8 servings

	Calories	Carbo-hydrate (gm)	Protein (gm)	Total Fat (gm)	Saturated Fat (gm)	Choles-terol (mg)
Total	547.0	141.4	1.2	0.4	0.0	0.0
Per Serving	68.4	17.7	0.2	0.1	0.0	0.0

Double Applesauce

4 or 5 cooking apples
  (about 1 lb.), cored,
  peeled, sliced
3/4 cup unsweetened
  apple juice

Pinch salt
  (optional)
1/4 tsp. cinnamon or
  nutmeg
  (optional)

Spread the apples in a saucepan. Add the juice and sprinkle with salt and cinnamon. Cover and cook until the apples are soft, about 20 minutes. Stir the applesauce until smooth. Serve warm or chilled.

Makes 4 servings

	Calories	Carbo-hydrate (gm)	Protein (gm)	Total Fat (gm)	Saturated Fat (gm)	Choles-terol (mg)
Total	370.0	114.5	0.0	0.0	0.0	0.0
Per Serving	92.5	28.6	0.0	0.0	0.0	0.0

Easy No-Peel Applesauce I

4 or 5 cooking apples
  (about 1 lb.), cored
  and quartered
3/4 cup water

Pinch salt
  (optional)
1/4 tsp. cinnamon or
  apple pie spice
  (optional)
Few drops vanilla

Combine all of the ingredients in a covered saucepan. Cook over low heat until the apple quarters are tender, about 20 minutes. Remove from heat and allow to cool. When the apples are cool, simply lift off the peels (scrape with a spoon) and discard them. Stir the applesauce until smooth and chill before serving.

Makes 4 servings

	Calories	Carbo-hydrate (gm)	Protein (gm)	Total Fat (gm)	Saturated Fat (gm)	Choles-terol (mg)
Total	315.0	81.0	0.0	0.0	0.0	0.0
Per Serving	78.4	20.3	0.0	0.0	0.0	0.0

Easy No-Peel Applesauce II

20-oz. can unsweetened
  pie-sliced apples
  (not apple pie
  filling)

Pinch salt
Few drops vanilla
1/3 cup water or
  unsweetened
  white grape
  juice

Combine all of the ingredients in covered saucepan over low heat and simmer 15 to 20 minutes, until apples are soft. Stir the applesauce until smooth and chill before serving. *Makes 5 servings*

	Calories	Carbo-hydrate (gm)	Protein (gm)	Total Fat (gm)	Saturated Fat (gm)	Choles-terol (mg)
Total	180.0	44.0	1.3	0.5	0.0	0.0
Per Serving	36.0	8.8	0.3	0.1	0.0	0.0

gm = grams; mg = milligrams. Nutritional figures are approximate. Figures are based on findings of U.S. Department of Agriculture.

Fresh Applesauce

4 or 5 McIntosh apples
(about 1 lb.), peeled,
cored, and chunked
3 or 4 tbsp. lemon juice
(or ¼ of a 100-mg.
ascorbic acid
tablet, crushed)

Pinch salt
Few drops vanilla
¼ tsp. cinnamon
(optional)

Process the apple chunks in covered blender with lemon juice or crushed ascorbic acid tablet (these will keep applesauce from turning brown). Blend in the salt, vanilla and cinnamon. Pour into a serving bowl and chill. *Makes 4 servings*

	Calories	Carbo-hydrate (gm)	Protein (gm)	Total Fat (gm)	Saturated Fat (gm)	Choles-terol (mg)
Total	331.0	84.6	0.4	0.0	0.0	0.0
Per Serving	82.8	21.2	0.1	0.0	0.0	0.0

Easy No-Fat Crepe Making

A special crepe pan is nice to have around but not really necessary for making crepes at home. Excellent crepes can be made easily in an ordinary skillet or omelet pan — with no added fat. Choose a small 6- or 7-inch pan with a nonstick surface. Apply cooking spray to the pan until the surface is slick and wet. Preheat the pan over a moderate flame until a slight vapor rises from the surface. When the surface is hot enough, a drop of water will bounce on it. Make 1 crepe at a time. Pour about 2 tablespoons of batter into the pan. Rotate the pan quickly to spread the batter as thinly as possible. Cook about 30 to 40 seconds, until the surface of the crepe is dry. Flip the pan over onto a clean towel and let the crepe drop out. Continue making crepes, one at a time, until all the batter is used. Apply cooking spray to the skillet before pouring the batter for each new crepe.

High-Protein Egg Crepes

3 eggs
6 tbsp. all-purpose flour
½ cup skim milk

2 tbsp. diet
margarine, at
room
temperature
Few drops vanilla
(optional)

Combine all of the ingredients in a blender or mixing bowl and beat smooth. Let the batter rest 20 minutes. Follow crepe making directions on this page. Fill with fruit, and top with one of the sauces in this book. Or use as a base for any crepe recipe.
Makes 12 crepes (1 per serving)

	Calories	Carbo-hydrate (gm)	Protein (gm)	Total Fat (gm)	Saturated Fat (gm)	Choles-terol (mg)
Total	438.0	39.3	25.8	18.3	6.0	758.5
Per Serving	36.5	3.3	2.2	1.5	0.5	63.2

Eggless High-Protein Crepes

½ cup frozen (defrosted)
or liquid no-
cholesterol egg
substitute

4 tbsp. all-purpose
flour
6 tbsp. skim milk

Combine all of the ingredients and beat smooth. Let the batter rest 20 minutes. Follow the crepe making directions in this section. Use as a base for any crepe recipe. *Makes 8 crepes (1 per serving)*

	Calories	Carbo-hydrate (gm)	Protein (gm)	Total Fat (gm)	Saturated Fat (gm)	Choles-terol (mg)
Total	332.0	26.2	18.4	15.2	0.0	2.2
Per Serving	41.5	3.3	2.3	1.9	0.0	0.3

Soy Egg Crepes

2 eggs
4 tbsp. soy-enriched
high-protein
pancake mix

6 tbsp. skim milk

Combine all of the ingredients in a blender or mixing bowl and beat smooth. Let the batter rest 20 minutes. Follow crepe-making directions in this section and use as base in any crepe recipe.
Makes 8 crepes (1 per serving)

	Calories	Carbo-hydrate (gm)	Protein (gm)	Total Fat (gm)	Saturated Fat (gm)	Choles-terol (mg)
Total	287.5	23.5	18.8	12.8	4.0	505.7
Per Serving	35.9	2.9	2.4	1.6	0.5	63.2

Dessert Blintzes

2 cups 99% fat-free pot-
style cottage
cheese
2 tsp. vanilla
¼ tsp. butter-flavored
salt
2 eggs

12 High-Protein Egg
Crepes (recipe in
this section)
16-oz. can crushed
unsweetened
juice-packed
pineapple,
undrained
1 tsp. arrowroot

Combine cottage cheese, vanilla, salt and eggs. Beat until smooth. Spoon the cheese filling into the crepes and roll up. Arrange the rolled crepes in a nonstick pan that has been sprayed with a vegetable coating. Cover lightly with foil. Bake in a preheated 300° oven 20 minutes. Meanwhile, combine undrained pineapple and arrowroot in a saucepan. Cook and stir until the sauce is thick and bubbling. To serve, spoon the pineapple sauce over the hot blintzes. *Makes 12 servings*

	Calories	Carbo-hydrate (gm)	Protein (gm)	Total Fat (gm)	Saturated Fat (gm)	Choles-terol (mg)
Total	1190.0	111.7	99.0	34.7	12.4	1301.3
Per Serving	99.2	9.3	8.3	2.9	1.0	108.4

gm = grams; mg = milligrams. Nutritional figures are approximate. Figures are based on findings of U.S. Department of Agriculture.

Peachy Strawberry Dessert Crepes

1 pt. fresh strawberries, hulled and sliced
2 ripe soft peaches, peeled and sliced
¼ cup orange juice
1 cup plain low-fat yogurt
½ cup sour cream or low-fat sour cream dressing
1 tsp. vanilla
12 High-Protein Egg Crepes (recipe in this section)

Combine the strawberries, peaches and orange juice. Chill several hours to blend the flavors. In a separate bowl, blend the yogurt, sour cream and vanilla. Chill. Fill the crepes with fruit mixture and a little of the yogurt-cream mixture. Roll up and top with additional yogurt-cream. *Makes 12 servings*

	Calories	Carbo-hydrate (gm)	Protein (gm)	Total Fat (gm)	Saturated Fat (gm)	Choles-terol (mg)
Total	1113.5	115.3	41.3	47.8	21.0	854.5
Per Serving	92.8	9.6	3.4	4.0	1.8	71.2

Fruit-Jeweled Gelatin

16-oz. can unsweetened juice-packed fruit cocktail, drained reserving juice
1 cup unsweetened bottled white grape juice
1 tbsp. unflavored gelatin

Combine the juice from the fruit cocktail and the grape juice, adding cold water if necessary to make 1¾ cups. In a small saucepan, combine the gelatin granules with ½ cup of the juice mixture. Wait 1 minute, then heat gently until granules are dissolved. Remove from heat and stir in the remaining juice. Pour into a bowl and chill until syrupy. Fold in the reserved canned fruit. Chill until set. *Makes 6 servings*

	Calories	Carbo-hydrate (gm)	Protein (gm)	Total Fat (gm)	Saturated Fat (gm)	Choles-terol (mg)
Total	338.0	80.8	3.2	0.4	0.0	0.0
Per Serving	56.3	13.3	0.5	0.1	0.0	0.0

True Fruit Gelatin

1 cup cold water
1 envelope plain gelatin
Dash salt
1 cup unsweetened red grape juice
1 cup sliced ripe strawberries, raspberries, or pitted sweet cherries

Combine water, gelatin and salt in a saucepan. Wait 1 minute to soften the gelatin, then heat to boiling. When the gelatin dissolves, stir in the grape juice. Pour into a bowl and refrigerate until syrupy. Stir in the fruit. Chill until set. *Makes 4 servings*

	Calories	Carbo-hydrate (gm)	Protein (gm)	Total Fat (gm)	Saturated Fat (gm)	Choles-terol (mg)
Total	245.0	55.0	8.0	1.0	0.0	0.0
Per Serving	61.3	13.8	2.0	0.3	0.0	0.0

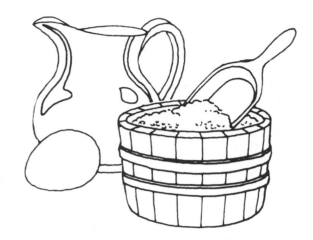

Real Orange Gelatin I

1 tbsp. or 1 envelope unflavored gelatin
2 cups fresh orange juice, unsweetened

Combine the gelatin with ¼ cup of the orange juice in a small saucepan. Wait 1 minute, then heat gently until the granules are dissolved. Stir in the remaining juice. Pour the gelatin into 4 dessert cups and chill until set. *Makes 4 servings*

	Calories	Carbo-hydrate (gm)	Protein (gm)	Total Fat (gm)	Saturated Fat (gm)	Choles-terol (mg)
Total	245.0	52.0	10.0	2.0	0.0	0.0
Per Serving	61.3	13.0	2.5	0.5	0.0	0.0

Real Orange Gelatin II

1 tbsp. unflavored gelatin
¼ cup cold water
1 cup boiling water
6-oz. can unsweetened frozen orange juice concentrate, partly defrosted but undiluted

Combine the gelatin and cold water in a blender. Wait 1 minute, until gelatin is soft, then add the boiling water, cover and blend on high speed until all granules are dissolved. Scrape down sides frequently. Add the orange juice, cover and blend until smooth. Pour into dessert cups and chill until set. *Makes 4 servings*

Hint: For a delightful variation on this recipe, fold some thin sliced banana into each cup when the gelatin has chilled enough to become syrupy. Then chill until set.

	Calories	Carbo-hydrate (gm)	Protein (gm)	Total Fat (gm)	Saturated Fat (gm)	Choles-terol (mg)
Total	385.0	87.0	11.0	0.0	0.0	0.0
Per Serving	96.2	21.8	2.8	0.0	0.0	0.0

gm = grams; mg = milligrams. Nutritional figures are approximate. Figures are based on findings of U.S. Department of Agriculture.

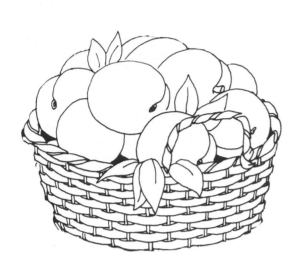

	Calories	Carbohydrate (gm)	Protein (gm)	Total Fat (gm)	Saturated Fat (gm)	Cholesterol (mg)
Total	790.5	164.6	47.1	25.8	8.0	1018.9
Per Serving	131.8	27.4	7.9	4.3	1.3	169.8

Crepes Melba (cover photo)

1 pt. fresh raspberries	12 regular or 6
3 ripe soft peaches, peeled and thinly sliced	double-size High-Protein Egg Crepes (see dessert chapter)
1/3 cup peach or apricot liqueur	1 cup plain low-fat yogurt
	1 cup part-skim ricotta cheese

Combine the raspberries, peaches, and liqueur in a covered bowl. Chill thoroughly to blend the flavors. Meanwhile, prepare crepes as explained in Easy No-Fat Crepe Making (see dessert chapter). If you want to make a party crepe stack as shown on the cover, rather than individual rolled crepes, use a larger skillet and pour 4 tablespoons of batter for each crepe.

Drain the liqueur from the fruit. Combine the liqueur with the yogurt and the ricotta in a blender or mixing bowl and blend until fluffy. For rolled crepes, spoon some of the fruit mixture and about 1 tablespoon of the yogurt mixture onto each crepe. Roll and top with the remaining yogurt. To make a party stack, lay 1 crepe on a pretty platter. Pinwheel peach slices on top. Add another crepe. Spread this with raspberries and then yogurt mixture. Continue layering the crepes fruit and topping. Cut into wedges to serve.   *Makes 6 servings*

	Calories	Carbohydrate (gm)	Protein (gm)	Total Fat (gm)	Saturated Fat (gm)	Cholesterol (mg)
Total	1228.7	141.7	83.8	25.4	8.6	775.8
Per Serving	204.8	23.6	14.0	4.2	1.4	129.3

Fresh Peach Melba Compote

1/2 pt. fresh raspberries	1/4 cup frozen
8 ripe sweet peaches, peeled and sliced	unsweetened apple juice concentrate, defrosted but not diluted
	Few drops vanilla or brandy flavoring

Combine all of the ingredients in a glass bowl and chill. Spoon the fruit into parfait glasses to serve. Top each parfait with a tablespoon of plain low-fat yogurt, if desired.   *Makes 6 servings*

	Calories	Carbohydrate (gm)	Protein (gm)	Total Fat (gm)	Saturated Fat (gm)	Cholesterol (mg)
Total	440.0	119.0	9.0	1.0	0.0	0.0
Per Serving	73.3	19.8	1.5	0.2	0.0	0.0

gm = grams; mg = milligrams. Nutritional figures are approximate. Figures are based on findings of U.S. Department of Agriculture.

Sangria Gelatin

8-oz. can unsweetened juice-packed fruit cocktail, drained reserving juice	1/2 cup port wine
1 tbsp. unflavored gelatin	6-oz. can frozen unsweetened orange juice concentrate, partially thawed, undiluted
1 cup boiling water	

Measure the juice from the fruit cocktail, adding water if necessary to equal 1/4 cup. Combine the gelatin with juice-water in a blender container. Wait 1 minute, until the gelatin granules are soft. Add the boiling water, cover, and blend on high speed until the granules are dissolved. Add the wine and juice concentrate; blend again. Pour into a serving bowl and chill until syrupy. Fold in the reserved fruit and chill until set.
Makes 6 servings

	Calories	Carbohydrate (gm)	Protein (gm)	Total Fat (gm)	Saturated Fat (gm)	Cholesterol (mg)
Total	599.0	114.4	11.8	0.2	0.0	0.0
Per Serving	99.8	19.1	2.0	0.1	0.0	0.0

High-Fiber Bread and Apple Pudding

4 slices white high-fiber bread, toasted, cubed	1/2 tsp. apple pie spice
1 1/2 cup skim milk, scalded	Pinch salt
4 eggs	1 apple, peeled and diced
	1/2 cup raisins

Put the toast cubes into an ovenproof casserole. Add the scalded milk and let stand for 15 minutes. Beat the eggs, spice and salt together. Add the apple and raisins and stir into bread mixture. Bake in a preheated 325° oven until the custard mixture is set, about 35 minutes. Chill the pudding before serving.
Makes 6 servings

Fluffy Grape Dessert

1 envelope unflavored gelatin	1¼ cups bottled unsweetened grape juice
½ cup cold water	⅛ tsp. salt

Sprinkle the gelatin over the water in a saucepan and let it stand until the gelatin softens. Place the pan over low heat for about 3 minutes, stirring constantly until the gelatin dissolves. Remove the pan from the heat and stir in the grape juice and salt. Chill the mixture, stirring occasionally, until it has thickened slightly. Pour it into a chilled bowl and beat it with your electric mixer or rotary beater until it is light and fluffy and doubled in volume. Spoon the whipped mixture into dessert dishes and chill until firm.   *Makes 4 servings*

	Calories	Carbo-hydrate (gm)	Protein (gm)	Total Fat (gm)	Saturated Fat (gm)	Choles-terol (mg)
Total	231.3	52.5	7.3	0.0	0.0	0.0
Per Serving	57.8	13.1	1.8	0.0	0.0	0.0

Brandied Peach Sherbet

3 tbsp. peach brandy	16-oz. can unsweetened juice-packed peaches, drained reserving juice
1 envelope unflavored gelatin	Pinch salt (or butter-flavored salt)

Put the brandy in a blender container. Sprinkle on the gelatin and wait 1 minute until the granules soften. Measure the peach juice and add cold water if necessary to equal 1½ cups. Heat the juice and water to boiling. Pour into the blender, cover, and blend until all the gelatin granules are dissolved. Add the peaches and salt; cover and blend smooth. Pour the mixture into a shallow metal dish and freeze only until slushy. Break up into a mixing bowl and beat until fluffy. Freeze firm. Soften briefly before serving.   *Makes 8 servings*

	Calories	Carbo-hydrate (gm)	Protein (gm)	Total Fat (gm)	Saturated Fat (gm)	Choles-terol (mg)
Total	255.0	42.4	2.2	0.4	0.0	0.0
Per Serving	32.0	5.3	0.3	0.1	0.0	0.0

Easy Blender Frozen Yogurt

½ envelope unflavored gelatin	⅔ cup instant nonfat dry milk powder (or ½ cup non-instant dry milk)
¼ cup cold water	¼ tsp. salt
1 cup boiling water	6-oz. can unsweetened frozen orange juice concentrate, partially thawed
8 oz. low-fat vanilla yogurt	

In a blender container, combine the gelatin and cold water. Wait 1 minute for the gelatin to soften, then add the boiling water. Cover and blend on high speed until all the gelatin granules are dissolved. Add the yogurt, milk powder, salt and orange juice and blend smooth. Pour the mixture into a shallow metal dish and freeze until slushy. Remove from the freezer and quickly beat smooth. Return to the freezer and freeze firm. Allow the frozen yogurt to soften briefly at room temperature before serving.   *Makes 12 servings*

	Calories	Carbo-hydrate (gm)	Protein (gm)	Total Fat (gm)	Saturated Fat (gm)	Choles-terol (mg)
Total	660.9	123.4	32.0	4.0	2.0	30.0
Per Serving	55.1	10.3	2.7	0.3	0.2	2.5

Peach Sugarless Jelly

3 cups canned unsweetened peach nectar (available in health food stores)	1 tbsp. cornstarch
	1 envelope unflavored gelatin

Combine the nectar and cornstarch in a saucepan. Sprinkle the gelatin on the nectar mixture. Stir until the gelatin and cornstarch are dissolved. Wait 1 minute, then heat to boiling, stirring frequently. Boil 1 minute. Cool, then pour into airtight containers and refrigerate.   *Makes 3 cups (48 servings)*

	Calories	Carbo-hydrate (gm)	Protein (gm)	Total Fat (gm)	Saturated Fat (gm)	Choles-terol (mg)
Total	385.0	93.0	7.5	0.0	0.0	0.0
Per Serving	8.0	1.9	0.2	0.0	0.0	0.0

Jiffy Marmalade

1 envelope unflavored gelatin	6-oz. can frozen unsweetened orange juice concentrate, partly defrosted but not diluted
¼ cup cold water	1 orange, peeled, seeded and diced
1 cup boiling water	¼ of the orange peel

Sprinkle the gelatin on the cold water in a blender container. Wait 1 minute, then add the boiling water. Cover and blend on high speed until the gelatin is dissolved, scraping sides of container. Add the orange concentrate and blend smooth. Add the orange chunks and orange peel; blend until coarsely chopped. Cool, then pour into an airtight container and refrigerate.   *Makes about 1½ cups (24 servings)*

	Calories	Carbo-hydrate (gm)	Protein (gm)	Total Fat (gm)	Saturated Fat (gm)	Choles-terol (mg)
Total	400.0	103.0	12.0	0.0	0.0	0.0
Per Serving	16.7	4.3	0.5	0.0	0.0	0.0

gm = grams; mg = milligrams. Nutritional figures are approximate. Figures are based on findings of U.S. Department of Agriculture.

Pineapple Preserves

1 tbsp. unflavored
    gelatin
¾ cup unsweetened
    white grape juice

20-oz. can
    unsweetened,
    juice-packed
    crushed
    pineapple,
    undrained

Sprinkle the gelatin on the grape juice in a small saucepan. When the granules have softened, add the pineapple. Cook and stir until boiling. Simmer gently 1 minute. Cool, then pour into airtight containers and refrigerate. *Makes about 2 cups (32 servings)*

	Calories	Carbo-hydrate (gm)	Protein (gm)	Total Fat (gm)	Saturated Fat (gm)	Choles-terol (mg)
Total	438.9	107.5	8.3	0.4	0.0	0.0
Per Serving	13.7	3.4	0.3	0.0	0.0	0.0

Raspberry Preserves

3 cups fresh
    raspberries,
    crushed
1½ tsp. (½ envelope)
    unflavored gelatin

4 tbsp. unsweetened
    grape juice
    concentrate,
    defrosted but
    undiluted

Combine all of the ingredients in a saucepan. Wait 1 minute until the gelatin is softened, then cook 2 minutes, stirring constantly and crushing the berries. Cool, then pour the preserves into airtight containers and chill until set. Store in the refrigerator. *Makes 2 cups (32 servings)*

	Calories	Carbo-hydrate (gm)	Protein (gm)	Total Fat (gm)	Saturated Fat (gm)	Choles-terol (mg)
Total	337.1	77.4	6.4	3.0	0.0	0.0
Per Serving	10.5	2.4	0.2	0.1	0.0	0.0

Low-Calorie Jam with Fresh Fruit

1 envelope unflavored
    gelatin
1½ tsp. cornstarch
½ cup unsweetened
    white grape juice,
    undiluted

1 tbsp. lemon juice
2 cups chopped,
    pitted, peeled
    fresh fruit (any
    fruit except fresh
    pineapple)

Combine the gelatin, cornstarch, grape juice and lemon juice in a saucepan. Wait 1 minute, then heat gently until the gelatin dissolves, stirring constantly. Add the chopped fruit and heat to boiling. Simmer, stirring constantly, for 3 minutes. Cool, pour into airtight containers and store in refrigerator. *Makes 2¼ cups (36 servings)*

	Calories	Carbo-hydrate (gm)	Protein (gm)	Total Fat (gm)	Saturated Fat (gm)	Choles-terol (mg)
Total	196.5	48.2	2.6	2.0	0.0	0.0
Per Serving	5.5	1.3	0.1	0.1	0.0	0.0

Jam from Frozen Berries

2½ cups frozen
    unsweetened
    berries
    (strawberries,
    blueberries,
    raspberries),
    defrosted

¼ cup unsweetened
    frozen grape
    juice
    concentrate,
    defrosted but
    undiluted
1 envelope
    unflavored
    gelatin
1½ tsp. cornstarch

Combine all of the ingredients in a saucepan. Wait 1 minute for the gelatin granules to soften, then cook and stir until the mixture thickens. Cool, then pour into airtight containers and chill until set. Store in the refrigerator. *Makes 2 cups (32 servings)*

	Calories	Carbo-hydrate (gm)	Protein (gm)	Total Fat (gm)	Saturated Fat (gm)	Choles-terol (mg)
Total	267.1	58.9	8.9	2.5	0.0	0.0
Per Serving	8.3	1.8	0.3	0.1	0.0	0.0

Apricot Butter

16-oz. can unsweetened
    juice-packed
    apricots, drained
    reserving liquid

1 tbsp. unflavored
    gelatin
½ cup boiling
    unsweetened
    apple juice

Measure 2 tablespoons of apricot juice into blender container. Sprinkle the gelatin on the juice. When the gelatin has softened, pour on the boiling apple juice and blend on high speed, covered, until all gelatin granules are dissolved. Add the canned apricots and remaining juice. Cover and blend until smooth and fluffy. Chill until set. *Makes 2½ cups (40 servings)*

	Calories	Carbo-hydrate (gm)	Protein (gm)	Total Fat (gm)	Saturated Fat (gm)	Choles-terol (mg)
Total	237.0	53.4	8.8	0.4	0.0	0.0
Per Serving	5.9	1.3	0.2	0.0	0.0	0.0

Basic Piecrust

½ cup all-purpose flour
Pinch salt

2 tbsp. salad oil
1 tbsp. ice water

Stir all of the ingredients together in a bowl with a fork. Then knead the mixture lightly until the pastry forms a ball. Flatten out the dough; wrap it in waxed paper and chill thoroughly. Roll the dough out on a lightly floured board. This will line an 8-inch pie plate. For a two-crust pie, double the recipe. *Makes 8 servings*

	Calories	Carbo-hydrate (gm)	Protein (gm)	Total Fat (gm)	Saturated Fat (gm)	Choles-terol (mg)
Total	477.5	47.5	6.5	28.5	2.0	0.0
Per Serving	59.7	5.9	0.8	3.6	0.3	0.0

gm = grams; mg = milligrams. Nutritional figures are approximate. Figures are based on findings of U.S. Department of Agriculture.

Buttery Pastry Shell

1 cup flour
1½ tsp. butter-flavored
 salt

2 tbsp. diet
 margarine
2 tbsp. butter

Sift the flour and butter-flavored salt into a bowl. Cut in the margarine and butter. Knead the mixture just long enough for the dough to form a ball. Roll the dough out thinly on a well-floured board. This makes enough for an 8-inch double-crust pie. *Makes 8 servings*

	Calories	Carbo-hydrate (gm)	Protein (gm)	Total Fat (gm)	Saturated Fat (gm)	Choles-terol (mg)
Total	757.5	95.3	13.3	36.0	14.8	70.8
Per Serving	94.7	11.9	1.7	4.5	1.9	8.9

Graham Cracker Crust

⅔ cup graham cracker
 crumbs

2 tbsp. diet
 margarine

Lightly combine the graham cracker crumbs and diet margarine. Press them firmly into the bottom of an 8- or 9-inch nonstick pie pan. This crust is quite tender. For a sturdier crust, quick-bake it in a preheated 425° oven for 6 to 8 minutes. Watch the crust — it burns easily. Cool before filling. *Makes 8 servings*

	Calories	Carbo-hydrate (gm)	Protein (gm)	Total Fat (gm)	Saturated Fat (gm)	Choles-terol (mg)
Total	390.4	55.4	5.3	19.9	2.0	0.0
Per Serving	48.8	6.9	0.7	2.5	0.3	0.0

Apple-Raisin Pie

Buttery Pastry Shell
 (the recipe is on this
 page)
1 cup golden raisins
1 tbsp. cornstarch
1 tsp. ground
 cinnamon

½ tsp. ground
 nutmeg
¼ tsp. butter-flavored
 salt
5 cups cooking apples,
 pared, cored, and
 sliced

Roll out half the pastry and place it in an 8-inch pie plate. In a bowl combine the raisins, cornstarch, cinnamon, nutmeg, butter-flavored salt, and apple slices. Spoon this mixture into the pastry-lined pie plate. Roll out the remaining pastry and place it on top for the top crust. Press the edges of the top and bottom crust together and flute them. Cut vents in the top crust to allow steam to escape. Bake the pie for 40 minutes in a preheated 425° oven until golden brown.
Makes 8 servings

	Calories	Carbo-hydrate (gm)	Protein (gm)	Total Fat (gm)	Saturated Fat (gm)	Choles-terol (mg)
Total	1621.8	321.7	16.9	360.3	14.8	70.8
Per Serving	202.7	40.2	2.1	45.0	1.9	8.9

Orange Cheese Pie

Graham Cracker
 Crust (recipe on this
 page)
2 egg whites
 Pinch salt
8-oz. pkg. diet cream
 cheese or
 Neufchatel cheese
2 whole eggs

6-oz. can
 unsweetened
 frozen orange
 juice
 concentrate,
 defrosted but not
 diluted
1 tbsp. arrowroot
1 tsp. vanilla
½ tsp. pumpkin pie
 spice

Prepare Graham Cracker Crust. In a mixing bowl, beat the egg whites and salt until stiff peaks form. Combine the remaining ingredients in a blender. Cover and blend smooth. Gently but thoroughly fold the blender mixture into egg whites. Spoon into the crust. Bake in a preheated 300° oven until the filling is set. Cool at room temperature, then chill. *Makes 8 servings*

	Calories	Carbo-hydrate (gm)	Protein (gm)	Total Fat (gm)	Saturated Fat (gm)	Choles-terol (mg)
Total	1500.4	150.4	46.3	79.9	38.0	672.0
Per Serving	187.6	18.8	5.8	10.0	4.8	84.0

Pink Strawberry No-Bake Cream Cheese Pie

Graham Cracker
 Crust (recipe on this
 page)
2 tsp. vanilla
1 tbsp. lemon juice
1 cup unsweetened
 bottled red grape
 juice, undiluted
1 envelope unflavored
 gelatin

8-oz. pkg. low-
 calorie cream
 cheese or
 Neufchatel
 cheese
¼ tsp. salt or butter-
 flavored salt
¼ tsp. grated lemon
 peel
1 cup ice cubes
 Jellied Berry
 Topping (recipe
 in this section)

Prepare Graham Cracker Crust. Combine the vanilla, lemon juice and 1 tablespoon of the grape juice in a blender. Sprinkle on the gelatin and wait 1 minute. Meanwhile, heat the remaining grape juice to boiling. Pour it into the blender. Cover and blend on high speed until the gelatin is dissolved (scrape sides of container frequently.) Add the cream cheese, salt and lemon peel. Cover and blend smooth. Add the ice cubes, a few at a time, and continue to blend until the ice is thoroughly dissolved. Spoon the filling into the crust and chill. (Mixture will be thick and partly set already.) Prepare the topping. When the filling is thoroughly set, arrange the topping on it. Chill again until topping is set. *Makes 8 servings*

	Calories	Carbo-hydrate (gm)	Protein (gm)	Total Fat (gm)	Saturated Fat (gm)	Choles-terol (mg)
Total	1335.8	151.1	33.3	68.9	34.0	168.0
Per Serving	167.0	18.9	4.2	8.6	4.3	21.0

gm = grams; mg = milligrams. Nutritional figures are approximate. Figures are based on findings of U.S. Department of Agriculture.

Spiced Harvest Pie

Basic Piecrust (recipe in this section)
20-oz. can unsweetened pie-sliced apples (not apple pie filling), undrained
1/2 cup raisins
4 soft prunes, chopped
1 eating orange, peeled and chopped

1 tbsp. minced orange peel
1/4 cup orange liqueur
3 tbsp. arrowroot
1 tsp. mixed pumpkin pie spice, or: 1/2 tsp. cinnamon, 1/4 tsp. nutmeg, 1/8 tsp. ground cloves and 1/8 tsp. ginger
1/8 tsp. salt

Line an 8-inch pie plate with Basic Piecrust. Combine the filling ingredients and mix well. Spoon the filling into the crust. Invert another piepan over the filling to protect it from burning. Bake in a preheated 425° oven for 30 to 40 minutes.   *Makes 8 servings*

	Calories	Carbo-hydrate (gm)	Protein (gm)	Total Fat (gm)	Saturated Fat (gm)	Choles-terol (mg)
Total	1151.1	185.1	11.9	29.0	2.0	0.0
Per Serving	143.9	23.1	1.5	3.6	0.3	0.0

Spicy Spiked Apple Pie

Basic Piecrust (recipe in this section)
20-oz. can unsweetened pie-sliced apples (not pie filling), undrained
1/2 cup raisins

1 sweet eating orange, seeded, peeled and diced
1 tsp. vanilla
2 tbsp. brandy (optional)
2 tbsp. arrowroot
Pinch salt
1 1/2 tsp. pumpkin pie spice

Line an 8-inch pie plate with Basic Piecrust. Combine all of the filling ingredients thoroughly and spoon into the crust. Trim a sheet of aluminum foil to cover only the filling, so the crust will brown but the filling will not dry out. Bake in a preheated 425° oven for 30 to 40 minutes. Serve warm or chilled.   *Makes 8 servings*

	Calories	Carbo-hydrate (gm)	Protein (gm)	Total Fat (gm)	Saturated Fat (gm)	Choles-terol (mg)
Total	1026.1	155.1	10.9	29.0	2.0	0.0
Per Serving	128.3	19.4	1.4	3.6	0.3	0.0

Spiked Apricot Cheese Pie

1 tbsp. diet margarine
1/2 cup graham cracker crumbs
1 lb. 99% fat-free pot-style cottage cheese
1/3 cup peach or apricot liqueur

3 eggs
Pinch salt
1/2 cup golden raisins
1/2 cup dried apricot halves, finely chopped
Cinnamon

Spread the margarine over the bottom of a nonstick 8-inch pie pan. Sprinkle on the graham cracker crumbs and press firmly into the bottom. In a blender container, combine the cheese, liqueur, eggs and salt. Cover and blend smooth, scraping down sides well. Pour half of the mixture into the pie pan. Sprinkle the raisins and apricots evenly over the filling. Pour on remaining filling, covering all the fruit. Sprinkle with cinnamon. Bake in a preheated 325° oven about 45 to 55 minutes until the filling is set. Cool before serving.   *Makes 10 servings*

	Calories	Carbo-hydrate (gm)	Protein (gm)	Total Fat (gm)	Saturated Fat (gm)	Choles-terol (mg)
Total	1301.4	138.8	84.4	31.0	9.4	794.8
Per Serving	130.1	13.9	8.4	3.1	1.0	79.5

Easy Yogurt Pie

Basic Piecrust (the recipe is in this section)
2 eggs, well beaten
1 tbsp. flour
1/2 tsp. cinnamon

1 cup low-fat fruit yogurt, any flavor
1 tsp. grated lemon peel
Pinch butter-flavored salt

Line an 8-inch pie plate with Basic Piecrust. Blend the filling ingredients thoroughly. Pour them into the pie shell. Bake the pie in a preheated 400° oven for 50 minutes until set. Chill before serving. Garnish with fresh fruit, if desired.   *Makes 8 servings*

	Calories	Carbo-hydrate (gm)	Protein (gm)	Total Fat (gm)	Saturated Fat (gm)	Choles-terol (mg)
Total	925.4	532.4	27.1	43.3	7.0	524.0
Per Serving	115.7	66.6	3.4	5.4	0.9	65.5

South Seas Pineapple Pie

Basic Piecrust (recipe in this section)
1 eating orange, peeled, seeded and diced
20-oz. can unsweetened juice-packed crushed pineapple, undrained

2 tbsp. granulated tapioca
4 tbsp. golden raisins
2 tbsp. grated orange peel (optional)
Pinch salt

Line an 8-inch pie plate with Basic Piecrust. Combine all of the filling ingredients thoroughly and spoon into the crust. Trim a sheet of aluminum foil to fit over the filling, so the crust will brown but the filling won't dry out. Bake in a preheated 425° oven for 30 to 45 minutes, until the crust is brown. Serve warm or chilled.   *Makes 8 servings*

	Calories	Carbo-hydrate (gm)	Protein (gm)	Total Fat (gm)	Saturated Fat (gm)	Choles-terol (mg)
Total	1047.3	187.5	10.3	28.9	2.0	0.0
Per Serving	130.9	23.4	1.3	3.6	0.3	0.0

gm = grams; mg = milligrams. Nutritional figures are approximate. Figures are based on findings of U.S. Department of Agriculture.

Orange Pumpkin Pie

Basic Piecrust (the recipe is in this section)
1 cup canned pumpkin (not sweetened pie filling)

2 eggs
¾ cup skim milk
6-oz. can frozen orange juice concentrate, defrosted and undiluted
½ tbsp. cornstarch
¼ tsp. salt
2 tsp. pumpkin pie spice

Line an 8-inch pie plate with Basic Piecrust. Combine the rest of the ingredients in a bowl and beat them thoroughly. Pour the mixture into the prepared pastry shell. Bake the pie for 1 hour in a preheated 350° oven.

Makes 8 servings

	Calories	Carbo-hydrate (gm)	Protein (gm)	Total Fat (gm)	Saturated Fat (gm)	Choles-terol (mg)
Total	1155.3	165.0	36.9	41.6	6.0	510.3
Per Serving	144.4	20.6	4.6	5.2	0.8	63.8

Deep-Dish Apple Pie

Basic Piecrust (the recipe is in this section)
4 cups sliced apples
½ cup honey

2 tsp. fresh lemon juice
1 tbsp. arrowroot
¼ tsp. butter-flavored salt
1 tsp. apple pie spice

Prepare a double batch of Basic Piecrust. Line an 8-inch pie plate with half the pastry dough. Mix the apples with all the remaining ingredients and arrange them in the crust. Roll out the second half of the pastry dough and lay it over the top of the pie, pressing the edges of the crust to the rim of the plate with a fork. Make slits in the crust for steam to escape. Bake the pie in a preheated 425° oven about 45 minutes until the crust is golden brown.

Makes 8 servings

	Calories	Carbo-hydrate (gm)	Protein (gm)	Total Fat (gm)	Saturated Fat (gm)	Choles-terol (mg)
Total	1297.8	261.5	6.5	28.5	2.0	0.0
Per Serving	162.2	32.7	0.8	3.6	0.3	0.0

Cheese Pie

Graham Cracker Crust (the recipe is in this section)
1 cup evaporated skim milk
4 eggs
¼ tsp. butter-flavored salt

1 tbsp. fresh lemon juice
2 tsp. vanilla extract
2 tbsp. arrowroot or cornstarch
2 cups (1 lb.) 99% fat-free cottage cheese

Prepare Graham Cracker Crust. In a blender, combine all the filling ingredients. Blend the mixture until it is completely smooth and pour it into the crust. Bake the pie in a preheated 250° oven for 1 hour. Turn the oven off and leave the pie in the oven 1 more hour. Remove the pie from the oven and chill it. If you wish, prepare one of the fruit glazes in this section and spread it on top of the pie after it is cool. Chill for several hours before serving.

Makes 8 servings

Special hint: This recipe calls for 1 cup of evaporated skim milk from a 12-ounce can. The remaining canned milk can be chilled and whipped and served as a low-fat whipped cream with the pie.

	Calories	Carbo-hydrate (gm)	Protein (gm)	Total Fat (gm)	Saturated Fat (gm)	Choles-terol (mg)
Total	1512.4	112.6	84.4	124.0	25.8	1116.2
Per Serving	189.1	14.1	10.6	15.5	3.2	139.5

Apple Tart

Basic Piecrust (recipe in this section)
20-oz. can unsweetened pie-sliced apples (not apple pie filling), undrained

1½-oz. box raisins
1 egg
½ cup skim milk
¼ tsp. butter-flavored salt
½ tsp. apple pie spice

Line an 8-inch pie plate with Basic Piecrust. Combine the apples and raisins in the crust. Beat the egg, milk and salt together, and pour over the fruit. Sprinkle with the spice. Bake in a preheated 450° oven for 10 minutes. Lower the heat to 350° and bake 30 minutes more until the filling is set. Chill before serving.

Makes 8 servings

	Calories	Carbo-hydrate (gm)	Protein (gm)	Total Fat (gm)	Saturated Fat (gm)	Choles-terol (mg)
Total	767.5	94.5	18.0	35.0	2.2	254.5
Per Serving	96.0	11.8	2.3	4.4	0.3	31.8

Apple Oven Pancake

1 cup canned unsweetened apple slices (not apple pie filling)
2 tbsp. raisins

¼ tsp. cinnamon
⅛ tsp. nutmeg
⅛ tsp. cloves
Pinch salt
½ cup pancake mix

Mix the apples, raisins, spices and salt in a saucepan; let the mixture stand while preparing the pancake. Prepare the pancake mix according to package directions, adjusting the proportion of liquid for ½ cup mix. Spray a 9-inch pie plate with vegetable coating. Pour the batter evenly over the bottom of the pan and bake 10 minutes in a preheated 425° oven. Heat the fruit mixture and pour it over the pancake. Serve immediately.

Makes 4 servings

	Calories	Carbo-hydrate (gm)	Protein (gm)	Total Fat (gm)	Saturated Fat (gm)	Choles-terol (mg)
Total	320.0	72.4	6.6	1.8	0.0	0.0
Per Serving	80.0	18.1	1.7	0.5	0.0	0.0

gm = grams; mg = milligrams. Nutritional figures are approximate. Figures are based on findings of U.S. Department of Agriculture.

Apple-Raisin Kuchen

1 pkg. flaky-style
biscuit dough (10
biscuits)
21-oz. can unsweetened
pie-sliced apples
(not pie filling),
undrained

6 tbsp. raisins
1/2 tsp. apple pie
spice
1 egg, beaten
1 cup plain or
vanilla low-fat
yogurt

Lay the biscuits out in a 9-inch pie pan and flatten them, sealing the edges together and pressing the dough around the edges of the pan. Bake the dough in a preheated 350° oven for 5 minutes. Combine the apple slices, raisins, and apple pie spice in a bowl. Toss the ingredients together and spoon the mixture over the baked biscuit dough. Combine beaten egg with the yogurt and pour over the fruit. Bake the kuchen at 350° for 20 minutes. *Makes 10 servings*

	Calories	Carbo-hydrate (gm)	Protein (gm)	Total Fat (gm)	Saturated Fat (gm)	Choles-terol (mg)
Total	1213.0	133.1	33.2	20.0	4.0	292.0
Per Serving	121.3	13.3	3.3	2.0	0.4	29.2

Slim-Down Shortcake

Sugar-Free
Strawberries for
Shortcake
3 cups sifted all-
purpose flour

3 tsp. baking powder
1 tsp. salt
1/2 cup diet margarine
1 1/4 cups skim milk

Prepare Sugar-Free Strawberries for Shortcake. Sift the flour, baking powder and salt together into a bowl. Cut in the margarine until the mixture resembles corn-meal. Add the milk and stir quickly with a fork until the dry ingredients are moistened. Divide the dough in half and press each half into an 8-inch nonstick layer cake pan that has been sprayed with vegetable coating. Bake the dough in a preheated 350° oven for about 15 minutes until it is golden brown. Remove the cakes from the pans and spoon half the sliced berries over 1 layer. Place the second layer of cake over the berries and then spoon the remaining berries on top. *Makes 8 servings*

	Calories	Carbo-hydrate (gm)	Protein (gm)	Total Fat (gm)	Saturated Fat (gm)	Choles-terol (mg)
Total	1940.2	296.9	64.1	70.7	0.0	0.0
Per Serving	242.5	37.1	8.0	8.8	0.0	0.0

Sugar-Free Strawberries for Shortcake

1 qt. fresh strawberries,
hulled and sliced
1 cup unsweetened
bottled red
grape juice

Combine the 2 ingredients and chill until serving time. Spoon the strawberries over Slim-Down Shortcake. *Makes 8 servings*

	Calories	Carbo-hydrate (gm)	Protein (gm)	Total Fat (gm)	Saturated Fat (gm)	Choles-terol (mg)
Total	383.2	93.5	5.0	4.0	0.0	0.0
Per Serving	47.9	11.7	0.6	0.5	0.0	0.0

Cream Puffs or Eclairs

1/2 cup diet margarine
1/2 cup water
1/2 tsp. salt

1 cup sifted all-
purpose flour
4 eggs

Heat the margarine with the water in a medium sauce-pan over high heat, stirring occasionally, until the margarine melts and the mixture boils. Turn the heat down to low. Add the salt and flour all at once. Stir vigorously until the mixture leaves the sides of the pan in a smooth compact ball. Remove the pan from the heat. Quickly add the eggs — one at a time — beating well after each addition until the mixture is smooth and shiny. Drop the mixture by spoonfuls, 3 inches apart, on an ungreased cookie sheet, shaping each into a mound (or 4×1-inch strip for eclairs). Bake in a preheated 400° oven for 50 minutes. Remove from the cookie sheet and cool on a wire rack. To serve, slice the tops off and fill with Orange Cream Puff Filling; replace the tops. *Makes 18 servings*

	Calories	Carbo-hydrate (gm)	Protein (gm)	Total Fat (gm)	Saturated Fat (gm)	Choles-terol (mg)
Total	1175.0	95.0	37.0	73.0	16.0	1008.0
Per Serving	65.3	5.3	2.1	4.1	0.9	56.0

Orange Cream Puff Filling

6-oz. can frozen
unsweetened
orange juice
concentrate,
defrosted

15 oz. part-skim
ricotta cheese
1/8 tsp. salt

Combine all of the ingredients in a bowl and beat until smooth. Spoon the filling into the Cream Puffs and serve. *Makes 18 servings*

	Calories	Carbo-hydrate (gm)	Protein (gm)	Total Fat (gm)	Saturated Fat (gm)	Choles-terol (mg)
Total	744.0	3.2	84.4	66.0	1.2	32.0
Per Serving	41.3	0.2	4.7	3.7	0.1	1.8

Orange Coconut Drops

1 1/4 cups all-purpose flour
1 tsp. baking powder
1/4 tsp. baking soda
1/4 tsp. salt
1/3 cup diet margarine
1/3 cup flaked coconut

Juice of one
orange
2 tsp. grated fresh
orange peel
1 tsp. vanilla extract
1 egg, beaten

Combine the flour with the baking powder, soda and salt. Cut in the diet margarine. Stir in the remaining ingredients. Drop by teaspoon 2 inches apart on non-stick cookie sheets. Bake in a preheated 400° oven for 10 to 12 minutes until light golden brown.
(36 servings) Makes 3 dozen

	Calories	Carbo-hydrate (gm)	Protein (gm)	Total Fat (gm)	Saturated Fat (gm)	Choles-terol (mg)
Total	1136.9	140.3	25.1	55.1	20.3	252.0
Per Serving	31.6	3.4	0.7	1.5	0.6	7.0

gm = grams; mg = milligrams. Nutritional figures are approximate. Figures are based on findings of U.S. Department of Agriculture.

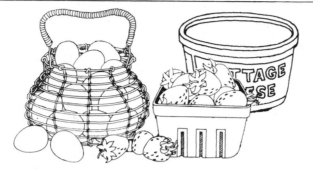

Rum 'n' Honey Fruitcake

1 egg, separated
1⅓ cups graham cracker
  crumbs
3 tbsp. honey
2 tbsp. rum
½ tsp. pumpkin pie spice
½ tsp. bottled orange
  peel (optional)
¾ tsp. baking powder

16-oz. can
  unsweetened
  juice-packed
  fruit cocktail,
  drained
  reserving liquid
½ tsp. salt
3 tbsp. seedless
  raisins
3 tbsp. chopped nuts
  (optional)

Combine the egg yolk, crumbs, honey, rum, pumpkin pie spice, orange peel, and baking powder in a large bowl. Add the juice from the canned fruit cocktail and stir until smooth. Combine the salt and egg white in a separate bowl and whip the egg white until it is stiff. Gently but thoroughly fold the egg white into the batter. Fold in the fruit cocktail, raisins and nuts. Spoon the batter into an 8-inch nonstick cake pan that has been sprayed with vegetable coating. Bake the cake in a preheated 350° oven for 35 to 40 minutes. Allow it to cool thoroughly before slicing.   *Makes 8 servings*

	Calories	Carbo-hydrate (gm)	Protein (gm)	Total Fat (gm)	Saturated Fat (gm)	Choles-terol (mg)
Total	1053.3	175.5	18.1	28.3	2.8	252.0
Per Serving	131.7	21.9	2.3	3.5	0.4	31.5

Orange Cheesecake

2 tbsp. diet margarine
½ cup graham cracker
  crumbs
2 cups 99% fat-free
  cottage cheese
2 tbsp. flour
¼ tsp. butter-flavored
  salt

4 eggs, separated
½ cup evaporated
  skim milk
2 tsp. vanilla
6-oz. can frozen
  orange juice
  concentrate,
  defrosted,
  undiluted

Coat the bottom of a 9-inch spring pan with the diet margarine. Sprinkle the cracker crumbs over the margarine. In a bowl, whip the cottage cheese, flour, and butter-flavored salt until smooth. Add the egg yolks one at a time, mixing well after each addition. Stir in the milk, vanilla, and orange juice. In another bowl, beat the egg whites until stiff, and fold them into the cheese batter. Pour the batter over the crumbs. Bake

the cheesecake in a preheated 325° oven for 1 hour. Allow it to cool before removing the rim of the pan. Do not invert the cake.   *Makes 12 servings*

	Calories	Carbo-hydrate (gm)	Protein (gm)	Total Fat (gm)	Saturated Fat (gm)	Choles-terol (mg)
Total	1632.8	156.5	110.7	63.1	23.4	1122.3
Per Serving	136.1	13.0	9.2	5.3	2.0	93.5

Pennsylvania Dutch Cheesecake

Pinch salt
4 egg whites
3 egg yolks
1½ cups 99% fat-free
  cottage cheese

¼ cup buttermilk
1 tbsp. fresh lemon
  juice
1½ tsp. vanilla

Beat the salt and the egg whites with an electric mixer until stiff peaks form. Set aside. Put all the remaining ingredients in a blender and blend until smooth and creamy. Pour the cheese mixture into the egg whites. Gently but thoroughly fold together. Spoon the mixture into a 9-inch nonstick square or round cake pan. Bake in a preheated 350° oven for 40 to 50 minutes, until a knife inserted in the center comes out clean. Chill thoroughly. The cake sinks in the center as it cools, making a depression for fruit. Fill with berries or sliced unsweetened peaches to serve.   *Makes 8 servings*

	Calories	Carbo-hydrate (gm)	Protein (gm)	Total Fat (gm)	Saturated Fat (gm)	Choles-terol (mg)
Total	553.0	16.0	70.1	18.0	7.8	786.4
Per Serving	69.1	2.0	8.8	2.3	1.0	98.3

Peach or Apricot Sauce

4 tsp. cornstarch
1 cup unsweetened
  apricot or peach
  nectar

2 tsp. brandy extract

Combine all of the ingredients in a medium saucepan. Heat the mixture, stirring constantly, until it bubbles and thickens.   *Makes 8 servings*

	Calories	Carbo-hydrate (gm)	Protein (gm)	Total Fat (gm)	Saturated Fat (gm)	Choles-terol (mg)
Total	211.3	52.1	0.0	0.0	0.0	0.0
Per Serving	26.4	6.5	0.0	0.0	0.0	0.0

gm = grams; mg = milligrams. Nutritional figures are approximate. Figures are based on findings of U.S. Department of Agriculture.

Pineapple Sauce II

3 cups unsweetened
juice-packed
crushed pineapple

1 tbsp. plain gelatin

Drain the juice from the pineapple into a saucepan. Stir in the gelatin and let it stand until it has softened. Then heat the juice slowly until the gelatin has melted. Remove the pan from the heat and stir in the pineapple. Chill the topping until it is of spreading consistency. Spread it on pound cake or angel food cake.

Makes 16 servings

	Calories	Carbo-hydrate (gm)	Protein (gm)	Total Fat (gm)	Saturated Fat (gm)	Choles-terol (mg)
Total	478.0	117.0	9.0	0.0	0.0	0.0
Per Serving	29.9	7.3	0.6	0.0	0.0	0.0

Strawberry Romanoff Sauce

1 pt. fresh ripe
strawberries, hulled

¼ cup frozen,
unsweetened
orange juice
concentrate,
defrosted but not
diluted

Combine strawberries and juice concentrate in a blender. Cover and process by repeatedly turning blender on and off, just until berries are chopped chunky. (Don't overblend or you'll have a purée.) Serve over sliced bananas or other fruit desserts, on low-fat yogurt or cottage cheese.

Makes about 1 cup (4 servings)

	Calories	Carbo-hydrate (gm)	Protein (gm)	Total Fat (gm)	Saturated Fat (gm)	Choles-terol (mg)
Total	200.0	47.8	3.8	2.0	0.0	0.0
Per Serving	50.0	12.0	1.0	0.5	0.0	0.0

Polynesian Fruit Sauce

1 eating orange, peeled
and diced
¼ of the orange peel,
sliced
16-oz. can unsweetened
juice-packed
crushed pineapple

2 tbsp. frozen
unsweetened
orange juice
concentrate,
defrosted but not
diluted
6 tsp. dried shredded
coconut
(optional)

Combine all of the ingredients except coconut in blender. Cover and process, on and off, until chunky. Use as a topping and sprinkle with coconut.

Makes 6 servings

	Calories	Carbo-hydrate (gm)	Protein (gm)	Total Fat (gm)	Saturated Fat (gm)	Choles-terol (mg)
Total	426.3	89.7	2.7	9.1	7.2	0.0
Per Serving	71.0	15.0	0.5	1.5	1.2	0.0

Calorie Counter's Whipped Cream

1 cup evaporated skim
milk

2 tsp. fresh lemon
juice

Pour the evaporated skim milk into a mixing bowl and chill in your freezer until ice crystals begin to form on the milk. Also chill the beaters of your electric mixer. Whip the milk at the high speed of your mixer until it triples in volume. To speed the whipping, add 1 or 2 teaspoons lemon juice for each cup of milk.

Makes 3 cups

	Calories	Carbo-hydrate (gm)	Protein (gm)	Total Fat (gm)	Saturated Fat (gm)	Choles-terol (mg)
Total	352.8	26.6	18.1	20.0	11.0	78.0

Hot Rum Raisin Sauce

1 apple, peeled and
diced
4 tbsp. raisins
¼ tsp. apple pie spice

¼ cup unsweetened
apple juice
¼ cup rum, warmed

Combine all of the ingredients in a saucepan except rum and simmer 1 minute. Pour the rum on the sauce. Ignite with a long match. Spoon flaming sauce over sliced bananas.

Makes 4 servings

	Calories	Carbo-hydrate (gm)	Protein (gm)	Total Fat (gm)	Saturated Fat (gm)	Choles-terol (mg)
Total	342.8	56.3	1.2	0.0	0.0	0.0
Per Serving	85.7	14.1	0.3	0.0	0.0	0.0

Jellied Berry Topping

¾ cup ice-cold bottled
unsweetened red
grape juice
(purple or white
grape juice may
be substituted)

1½ tsp. (½ envelope)
unflavored
gelatin
1 cup sliced
strawberries (or
other fresh fruit
such as
peaches,
blueberries, or
raspberries)

Put 2 tablespoons of the grape juice in a small saucepan and sprinkle with the gelatin. Wait 1 minute, until the gelatin is soft, then heat gently until the gelatin melts. Remove from heat and stir in the remaining cold fruit juice. Refrigerate until syrupy. Arrange the berries on top of chilled filling (filling must be set), then spoon the gelatin mixture to cover the fruit with a jellied glaze. Chill until set.

Makes about 1½ cups (8 servings)

	Calories	Carbo-hydrate (gm)	Protein (gm)	Total Fat (gm)	Saturated Fat (gm)	Choles-terol (mg)
Total	191.4	44.5	4.9	1.0	0.0	0.0
Per Serving	23.9	5.6	0.6	0.1	0.0	0.0

gm = grams; mg = milligrams. Nutritional figures are approximate. Figures are based on findings of U.S. Department of Agriculture.

Whipped Cheese Topping for Fruit

4 oz. low-calorie "imitation" cream cheese, or Neufchatel cheese, softened

¾ cup plain or vanilla low-fat yogurt

Combine the ingredients and beat until fluffy. Chill before serving. *Makes 1¼ cup (20 servings)*

	Calories	Carbo-hydrate (gm)	Protein (gm)	Total Fat (gm)	Saturated Fat (gm)	Choles-terol (mg)
Total	373.8	13.8	14.0	27.0	17.5	99.9
Per Serving	18.7	0.7	0.7	1.4	0.9	5.0

White Chocolate Cream Topping

15-oz. container part-skim ricotta cheese
½ cup white crème de cacao

2 eggs
1 oz. unsweetened chocolate, shaved

Combine the ricotta, crème de cacao and eggs in a blender or electric mixer and blend well. Chill and serve sprinkled with the shaved chocolate as a topping on crepes or other desserts.

Makes about 2½ cups (12 servings)

	Calories	Carbo-hydrate (gm)	Protein (gm)	Total Fat (gm)	Saturated Fat (gm)	Choles-terol (mg)
Total	882.0	35.5	98.0	29.0	5.2	536.0
Per Serving	73.5	3.0	8.2	2.4	0.4	44.7

Strawberry Topping

8-oz. pkg. frozen unsweetened strawberries, thawed

2 tbsp. arrowroot or cornstarch
1 cup undiluted, unsweetened red grape juice

Combine all of the ingredients in a saucepan. Cook and stir the mixture over moderate heat until it simmers and thickens. Serve the topping warm or cold.

Makes 12 servings

	Calories	Carbo-hydrate (gm)	Protein (gm)	Total Fat (gm)	Saturated Fat (gm)	Choles-terol (mg)
Total	706.3	181.8	1.9	0.8	0.0	0.0
Per Serving	58.9	15.2	0.2	0.1	0.0	0.0

Glazed Fresh Fruit for Cheese Pie

2 cups hulled fresh strawberries or fresh blueberries
1 tbsp. arrowroot or cornstarch

1 cup unsweetened white or red grape juice

If you are using strawberries, leave the small ones whole and slice the large ones in half lengthwise. Arrange the strawberries cut side down on top of a cooled cheese pie. If you are using blueberries, spread them in a single layer over the surface of a cheese pie.

Stir the arrowroot and grape juice together in a saucepan over medium heat until the mixture clears and thickens. Set the pan aside for 10 minutes to cool. Using a spoon, drip the glaze over the fresh fruit. Use only as much as needed to completely coat the fruit. Discard the rest. *Makes 8 servings.*

Hint: If fresh fruit is not available, a 20-ounce can of unsweetened red pitted cherries may be used instead. Use the canned juice in place of the grape juice. If there is not enough juice to make 1 cup, add water. If additional sweetness is desired for either of these glazes, add honey to taste.

	Calories	Carbo-hydrate (gm)	Protein (gm)	Total Fat (gm)	Saturated Fat (gm)	Choles-terol (mg)
Total	300.3	74.2	3.0	2.0	0.0	0.0
Per Serving	37.5	9.3	0.4	0.3	0.0	0.0

gm = grams; mg = milligrams. Nutritional figures are approximate. Figures are based on findings of U.S. Department of Agriculture.

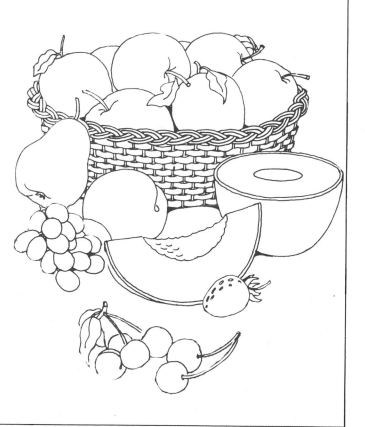

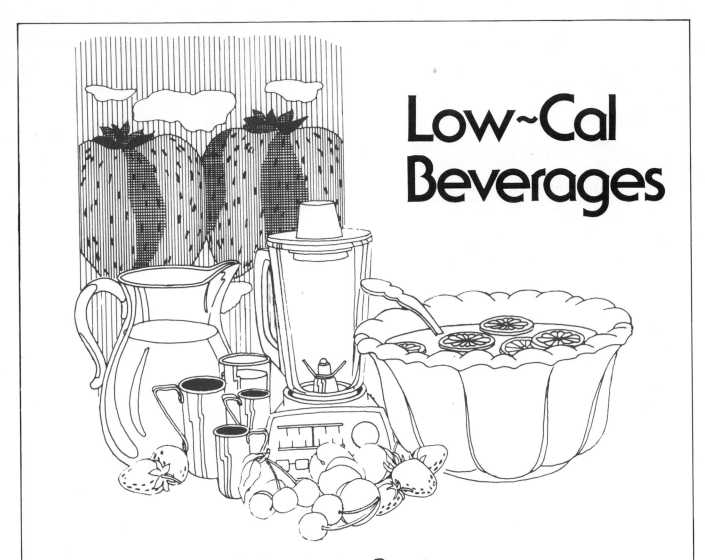

Low~Cal Beverages

For years, dieters have relied on artificially sweetened diet drinks to quench their thirst. If saccharin is banned as a food additive, diet drinks as we know them will disappear from grocery store shelves. Here is what will happen to your calorie consumption if you go back to drinking sugar-sweetened beverages.

- If you replace one 12-ounce can of diet cola with sugar-sweetened Coke or Pepsi: 144 calories per day times 365 days equals 52,560 calories divided by 3500 equals 15 pounds gained in one year!
- If you replace one 12-ounce can of diet lemon or other fruit flavored soda with sugar-sweetened 7-Up: 177 calories per day times 365 days equals 62,050 calories divided by 3500 equals 17 pounds gained in one year!
- If you replace *two* cans of diet cola with regular cola: 228 calories a day times 365 days equals 105,120 calories divided by 3500 equals 30 pounds gained in one year.

The beverage recipes in this chapter are designed to quench your thirst without putting on pounds. Many of these refreshing drinks rely on natural fruit juices mixed with club soda. You will also find delicious fruit-flavored milkshakes, meal-in-a-glass floats, and some tasty new treatments for coffee and tea.

Recipes

Cucumber Cooler

2 cups chopped seeded cucumber	1 tsp. lemon juice
1 tsp. salt	1/4 tsp. Tabasco sauce
1 cup chicken broth	6 ice cubes
1/2 cup plain low-fat yogurt	3 cucumber slices for garnish

Sprinkle the chopped cucumber with salt and let it stand 15 minutes. Skim the fat from the broth by chilling until the fat rises and can be whisked away. Place the cucumbers and all remaining ingredients in a blender and process until smooth. Serve in tall glasses garnished with cucumber slices.   *Makes 3 servings*

	Calories	Carbo-hydrate (gm)	Protein (gm)	Total Fat (gm)	Saturated Fat (gm)	Choles-terol (mg)
Total	108.8	14.1	7.6	2.2	1.0	10.0
Per Serving	36.3	4.7	2.5	0.7	0.3	3.3

gm = grams; mg = milligrams. Nutritional figures are approximate. Figures are based on findings of U.S. Department of Agriculture.

Spicy Tomato Cooler

¾ cup tomato juice
Dash Worcester-
shire sauce

Dash hot pepper
sauce
1 tbsp. lemon juice
1 celery stalk for
stirrer (optional)

Combine all of the ingredients and pour over ice cubes in a tall glass. Use a celery stalk as stirrer, if desired.
Makes 1 serving

	Calories	Carbo-hydrate (gm)	Protein (gm)	Total Fat (gm)	Saturated Fat (gm)	Choles-terol (mg)
Total	37.6	8.7	2.6	0.0	0.0	0.0

B-T Cooler

2 cans (10½ oz.)
condensed beef
bouillon, undiluted

2½ cups tomato juice
1 tbsp. lemon juice
½ tsp. Tabasco sauce
5 lemon wedges

Combine all the ingredients well. Pour over ice and serve with lemon wedges. *Makes 5 servings*

	Calories	Carbo-hydrate (gm)	Protein (gm)	Total Fat (gm)	Saturated Fat (gm)	Choles-terol (mg)
Total	200.5	33.6	19.8	0.0	0.0	69.4
Per Serving	40.1	6.7	4.0	0.0	0.0	13.9

Strawberry Pink Lemonade Syrup

1 cup fresh
lemon juice

2 cups unsweetened
red grape juice,
undiluted

Combine ingredients in a small covered jar and shake well. Store in the refrigerator and shake before using. To make a glass of lemonade, combine ⅓ cup of the syrup with cold water and ice cubes in a tall glass.
Makes 9 servings

	Calories	Carbo-hydrate (gm)	Protein (gm)	Total Fat (gm)	Saturated Fat (gm)	Choles-terol (mg)
Total	390.0	104.0	3.0	0.0	0.0	0.0
Per Serving	43.3	11.6	0.3	0.0	0.0	0.0

Apple Lemonade Syrup

½ cup fresh lemon juice
¼ cup water

6-oz. can frozen
unsweetened
apple juice
concentrate,
defrosted,
undiluted

Combine the lemon juice, water and apple juice. To prepare a glass of lemonade, put 3 tablespoons of syrup in a tall glass. Add ice cubes and water.
Makes 8 servings

	Calories	Carbo-hydrate (gm)	Protein (gm)	Total Fat (gm)	Saturated Fat (gm)	Choles-terol (mg)
Total	300.0	76.0	0.5	0.0	0.0	0.0
Per Serving	37.5	9.5	0.1	0.0	0.0	0.0

Lemonade Syrup

1 cup fresh lemon juice
2 cups unsweetened
white grape
juice, undiluted

2 tsp. grated lemon
rind (optional)

Combine all of the ingredients in a small covered jar and shake well. Store in the refrigerator and shake before using. To make a glass of lemonade, combine ⅓ cup of the syrup with cold water and ice cubes in a tall glass.
Makes 9 servings

	Calories	Carbo-hydrate (gm)	Protein (gm)	Total Fat (gm)	Saturated Fat (gm)	Choles-terol (mg)
Total	390.0	104.0	3.0	0.0	0.0	0.0
Per Serving	43.3	11.6	0.3	0.0	0.0	0.0

Port Wine Lemonade

1½ tbsp. fresh lemon
juice

3 tbsp. port wine

Combine the lemon juice and wine in a tall glass. Fill with water and ice, stir and serve. *Makes 1 serving*

	Calories	Carbo-hydrate (gm)	Protein (gm)	Total Fat (gm)	Saturated Fat (gm)	Choles-terol (mg)
Total	58.5	4.8	0.8	0.0	0.0	0.0

Spiced Orange Cider

1 cup unsweetened
apple cider
⅓ cup unsweetened
orange juice

½ tsp. ground
cinnamon
¼ tsp. ground cloves
1 cup crushed ice
¼ tsp. Tabasco sauce

In a blender, combine all the ingredients at high speed for 1 minute. *Makes 2 servings*

	Calories	Carbo-hydrate (gm)	Protein (gm)	Total Fat (gm)	Saturated Fat (gm)	Choles-terol (mg)
Total	160.0	39.0	0.8	0.0	0.0	0.0
Per Serving	80.0	19.5	0.4	0.0	0.0	0.0

Tropical Fruit Punch Syrup

1 cup unsweetened
orange juice
¾ cup unsweetened
grape juice

¼ cup unsweetened
pineapple juice

Combine the juices in a covered refrigerator container. To serve, mix ¼ cup of the punch syrup with club soda or water and ice cubes in a tall glass. *Makes 8 servings*

	Calories	Carbo-hydrate (gm)	Protein (gm)	Total Fat (gm)	Saturated Fat (gm)	Choles-terol (mg)
Total	377.7	68.0	2.9	0.0	0.0	0.0
Per Serving	47.2	8.5	0.4	0.0	0.0	0.0

gm = grams; mg = milligrams. Nutritional figures are approximate. Figures are based on findings of U.S. Department of Agriculture.

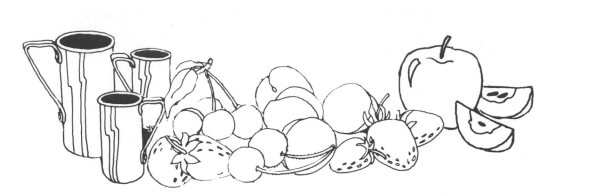

Berry Crush

1 cup fresh	1 cup ice cubes and
strawberries, hulled	water
1 cup unsweetened	
pineapple juice	

Combine all of the ingredients in a covered blender. Blend until the ice melts. Serve in tall glasses with straws. *Makes 2 servings*

	Calories	Carbo-hydrate (gm)	Protein (gm)	Total Fat (gm)	Saturated Fat (gm)	Choles-terol (mg)
Total	206.0	52.0	2.0	1.0	0.0	0.0
Per Serving	103.0	26.0	1.0	0.5	0.0	0.0

Grapefruit Fizz

1/4 cup unsweetened	8 oz. club soda or
grapefruit juice	carbonated
2 tbsp. bottled	water
unsweetened white	
grape juice	

Combine the ingredients well and serve over ice cubes. *Makes 1 serving*

	Calories	Carbo-hydrate (gm)	Protein (gm)	Total Fat (gm)	Saturated Fat (gm)	Choles-terol (mg)
Total	45.6	11.2	0.5	0.0	0.0	0.0

Grapefruit Grape Freeze

16-oz. can unsweetened	6-oz. can frozen
grapefruit sections,	unsweetened
frozen	grape juice
	concentrate,
	undiluted
	2 cups cold water
	48 oz. club soda

Scoop the frozen grapefruit into a blender. Add the grape concentrate and water and blend. Pour into 8 chilled glasses and fill with club soda. *Makes 8 servings*

	Calories	Carbo-hydrate (gm)	Protein (gm)	Total Fat (gm)	Saturated Fat (gm)	Choles-terol (mg)
Total	433.8	109.6	3.6	0.4	0.0	0.0
Per Serving	54.2	13.7	0.5	0.1	0.0	0.0

Orchard Fizz

1 3/4 cups unsweetened	1 cup unsweetened
orange juice	apple juuce
	16 oz. club soda

Combine juices and stir well. Divide among 4 tall glasses. Add cracked ice and club soda. *Makes 4 servings*

	Calories	Carbo-hydrate (gm)	Protein (gm)	Total Fat (gm)	Saturated Fat (gm)	Choles-terol (mg)
Total	204.5	48.5	3.5	0.0	0.0	0.0
Per Serving	51.1	12.1	0.9	0.0	0.0	0.0

Tropical Fizz

2 cups unsweetened	1/2 cup unsweetened
grapefruit juice	pineapple juice
1 cup unsweetened	16 oz. club soda
tangerine juice	6 mint sprigs

Combine the juices and pour over ice cubes in 6 tall glasses. Fill with club soda, and garnish with mint. *Makes 6 servings*

	Calories	Carbo-hydrate (gm)	Protein (gm)	Total Fat (gm)	Saturated Fat (gm)	Choles-terol (mg)
Total	400.0	90.5	4.0	0.0	0.0	0.0
Per Serving	66.7	15.1	0.7	0.0	0.0	0.0

Real Orange Soda

2 tbsp. frozen	8 oz. club soda or
unsweetened	carbonated
orange juice	water
concentrate,	
defrosted but not	
diluted	

Stir the juice concentrate and soda (or water) together in a tall glass and add ice cubes. *Makes 1 serving*

	Calories	Carbo-hydrate (gm)	Protein (gm)	Total Fat (gm)	Saturated Fat (gm)	Choles-terol (mg)
Total	51.4	1.8	0.8	0.0	0.0	0.0

gm = grams; mg = milligrams. Nutritional figures are approximate. Figures are based on findings of U.S. Department of Agriculture.

Real Grape Soda

4 tbsp. unsweetened bottled purple grape juice	8 oz. club soda or carbonated water

Stir the juice and soda together in a tall glass. Add ice cubes and serve. *Makes 1 serving*

	Calories	Carbo-hydrate (gm)	Protein (gm)	Total Fat (gm)	Saturated Fat (gm)	Choles-terol (mg)
Total	41.2	10.4	0.4	0.0	0.0	0.0

Lemon Twist Soda

2 tbsp. frozen unsweetened apple juice concentrate, defrosted, undiluted	1 tbsp. lemon juice 8 oz. club soda or carbonated water

Combine the ingredients thoroughly and serve over ice. *Makes 1 serving*

	Calories	Carbo-hydrate (gm)	Protein (gm)	Total Fat (gm)	Saturated Fat (gm)	Choles-terol (mg)
Total	42.6	10.6	0.1	0.0	0.0	0.0

Orange Cow

6-oz. can frozen unsweetened orange juice concentrate, defrosted, undiluted	3 cups ice cubes 1½ cups cold water 1½ cups instant nonfat milk powder ⅛ tsp. vanilla

Combine all of the ingredients in a covered blender. Blend until frothy. Pour into 6 chilled tall glasses to serve. *Makes 6 servings*

	Calories	Carbo-hydrate (gm)	Protein (gm)	Total Fat (gm)	Saturated Fat (gm)	Choles-terol (mg)
Total	727.5	139.5	41.0	0.0	0.0	22.5
Per Serving	121.3	23.3	6.8	0.0	0.0	3.8

Meal-in-a-Glass Berry Float

1 single-serving envelope vanilla diet meal powder (Such as Metrecal or Slender) ¾ cup skim milk	1 cup ice cubes ½ cup fresh, sliced strawberries or blueberries, chilled

Combine the meal powder, skim milk and ice cubes in a blender. Cover and blend until smooth. Pour over chilled berries in a tall glass. *Makes 1 serving*

	Calories	Carbo-hydrate (gm)	Protein (gm)	Total Fat (gm)	Saturated Fat (gm)	Choles-terol (mg)
Total	320.0	43.0	24.9	5.5	0.0	39.0

Pineapple Yogurt Cooler

½ cup unsweetened crushed juice-packed pineapple, chilled	½ cup low-fat plain yogurt Dash vanilla ½ cup ice cubes

Blend all of the ingredients in a covered blender until smooth. *Makes 1 serving*

	Calories	Carbo-hydrate (gm)	Protein (gm)	Total Fat (gm)	Saturated Fat (gm)	Choles-terol (mg)
Total	111.5	18.2	4.4	2.1	1.0	10.0

Peach or Nectarine Milkshake

1 large ripe peach or nectarine, peeled, pitted and cut in chunks ⅓ cup instant nonfat milk powder	Dash salt Few drops vanilla (optional) 1 cup ice cubes and water

Combine all of the ingredients in a covered blender and blend until the ice melts. Serve in a tall glass with a straw. *Makes 1 serving*

	Calories	Carbo-hydrate (gm)	Protein (gm)	Total Fat (gm)	Saturated Fat (gm)	Choles-terol (mg)
Total	85.2	21.7	9.0	0.0	0.0	5.0

Real Strawberry Milkshake I

4 or 5 frozen whole unsweetened strawberries	1 cup ice-cold skim milk ½ tsp. vanilla

Combine all of the ingredients in a blender. Cover and blend smooth. Serve in a tall glass with a straw. *Makes 1 serving*

	Calories	Carbo-hydrate (gm)	Protein (gm)	Total Fat (gm)	Saturated Fat (gm)	Choles-terol (mg)
Total	117.5	7.7	9.5	0.5	0.0	5.0

Real Strawberry Milkshake II

4 or 5 large fresh strawberries, hulled ⅓ cup instant nonfat milk powder	½ tsp. vanilla Dash salt 1 cup ice cubes and water

Combine all of the ingredients in a covered blender and blend until the ice melts. Serve in tall glass with a straw. *Makes 1 serving*

	Calories	Carbo-hydrate (gm)	Protein (gm)	Total Fat (gm)	Saturated Fat (gm)	Choles-terol (mg)
Total	150.0	24.0	21.0	0.0	0.0	12.5

gm = grams; mg = milligrams. Nutritional figures are approximate Figures are based on findings of U.S. Department of Agriculture.

Raspberry Flip

½ cup fresh or
    unsweetened frozen
    whole raspberries
5 tbsp. instant nonfat
    milk powder

5 ice cubes
½ cup cold water or
    carbonated
    water

Combine all of the ingredients in a covered blender and blend until the ice is melted. Serve in a tall glass.

Makes 1 serving

	Calories	Carbo-hydrate (gm)	Protein (gm)	Total Fat (gm)	Saturated Fat (gm)	Choles-terol (mg)
Total	163.5	26.7	13.0	0.8	0.0	0.0

Banana Blueberry Float

1 cup ice-cold
    skim milk
1 small banana, peeled
    and sliced

2 tbsp. fresh blueberries

Blend the milk and half the banana in a covered blender until smooth. Place the remaining banana slices and the berries in a tall glass. Add the milk and banana mixture.

Makes 1 serving

	Calories	Carbo-hydrate (gm)	Protein (gm)	Total Fat (gm)	Saturated Fat (gm)	Choles-terol (mg)
Total	200.6	17.2	10.0	0.2	0.0	5.0

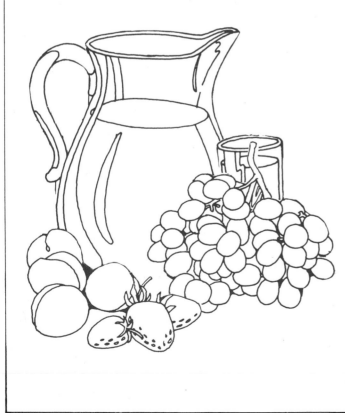

Breakfast in a Glass

1 cup ice-cold skim
    milk
1 egg
¼ cup 99% fat-free
    cottage cheese

8-oz. can juice-
    packed
    unsweetened
    peach pieces,
    chilled or partly
    frozen
¼ tsp. vanilla

Combine all of the ingredients in a blender, cover and blend. If desired, 1 or 2 ice cubes may be added to chill the drink.

Makes 2 servings

	Calories	Carbo-hydrate (gm)	Protein (gm)	Total Fat (gm)	Saturated Fat (gm)	Choles-terol (mg)
Total	281.4	28.7	23.3	6.7	2.3	261.9
Per Serving	140.7	14.4	11.7	3.4	1.2	131.0

Orange Instant Breakfast

1 tbsp. unsweetened
    orange juice
    concentrate,
    defrosted, undiluted

1 egg
1 cup ice-cold skim
    milk
½ cup ice cubes

Pour all the ingredients in a covered blender and blend until smooth.

Makes 1 serving

	Calories	Carbo-hydrate (gm)	Protein (gm)	Total Fat (gm)	Saturated Fat (gm)	Choles-terol (mg)
Total	195.7	12.9	15.4	6.0	2.0	257.0

Eggless Nog

⅓ cup instant nonfat
    milk powder
½ tsp. rum extract
¼ tsp. vanilla extract

1 cup ice cubes and
    water
Dash nutmeg or
    cinnamon
    (optional)

In a covered blender, blend all of the ingredients until the ice melts. Pour into a tall glass and add a dash of spice.

Makes 1 serving

	Calories	Carbo-hydrate (gm)	Protein (gm)	Total Fat (gm)	Saturated Fat (gm)	Choles-terol (mg)
Total	129.0	18.5	12.8	0.4	0.0	0.0

Jamaican Iced Coffee

4 cups fresh strong
    coffee

2 tsp. rum flavoring

Combine the coffee and rum flavoring and chill. Pour over ice cubes in 4 tall glasses.

Makes 4 servings

	Calories	Carbo-hydrate (gm)	Protein (gm)	Total Fat (gm)	Saturated Fat (gm)	Choles-terol (mg)
Total	5.0	0.8	0.3	0.1	0.0	0.0
Per Serving	1.3	0.2	0.1	0.0	0.0	0.0

gm = grams; mg = milligrams. Nutritional figures are approximate. Figures are based on findings of U.S. Department of Agriculture.

Iced Cafe au Lait

1 rounded tsp. instant coffee
¼ cup boiling water

Few drops vanilla (optional)
¾ cup chilled skim milk

Dissolve the instant coffee in the boiling water and combine it with the remaining ingredients. Serve over ice. *Makes 1 serving*

	Calories	Carbo-hydrate (gm)	Protein (gm)	Total Fat (gm)	Saturated Fat (gm)	Choles-terol (mg)
Total	72.5	9.8	7.2	0.1	0.0	3.9

Frosted Cappuchino

1 rounded tsp. instant espresso
⅓ cup instant nonfat milk powder

Pinch cinnamon
1 cup ice cubes and water

Combine the instant expresso, milk powder and cinnamon in a blender. Add the ice cubes and water. Cover and blend until all the ice melts. Serve in a tall glass with straws. *Makes 1 serving*

	Calories	Carbo-hydrate (gm)	Protein (gm)	Total Fat (gm)	Saturated Fat (gm)	Choles-terol (mg)
Total	35.0	4.8	3.3	0.0	0.0	1.7

Spiced Iced Coffee

1 rounded tsp. instant coffee
Pinch bottled orange peel

Pinch allspice
Pinch cinnamon
¼ cup boiling water

Stir the instant coffee, orange peel and spices into boiling water. Combine in a tall glass with ice cubes and add cold water to fill. *Makes 1 serving*

	Calories	Carbo-hydrate (gm)	Protein (gm)	Total Fat (gm)	Saturated Fat (gm)	Choles-terol (mg)
Total	5.0	0.8	0.3	0.1	0.0	0.0

Iced Cuban Coffee

1 rounded tsp. instant coffee (or instant espresso)
¼ cup boiling water

Few drops rum flavoring
¾ cup ice-cold skim milk
Dash cinnamon (optional)

Dissolve the coffee in the boiling water. Combine it with all the remaining ingredients and serve over ice in a tall glass. *Makes 1 serving*

	Calories	Carbo-hydrate (gm)	Protein (gm)	Total Fat (gm)	Saturated Fat (gm)	Choles-terol (mg)
Total	72.5	9.8	7.2	0.1	0.0	3.9

Fruity Spiced Tea

1 cup boiling water
1 tea bag
⅛ tsp. each cinnamon, ginger, allspice, and nutmeg

1¼ cups fresh orange juice, unsweetened
4 tbsp. unsweetened pineapple juice
12-oz. can club soda
Orange peel for garnish (optional)

Combine the boiling water, tea bag, and spices and let stand 4 to 5 minutes. Remove the tea bag and let the tea cool. Add the fruit juices and chill. To serve, stir in the club soda and pour over cracked ice in tall iced tea glasses. Garnish with orange peel if you like. *Makes 4 servings*

	Calories	Carbo-hydrate (gm)	Protein (gm)	Total Fat (gm)	Saturated Fat (gm)	Choles-terol (mg)
Total	170.6	41.3	3.0	0.0	0.0	0.0
Per Serving	42.7	10.3	0.8	0.0	0.0	0.0

Perfect Iced Tea

1 qt. cold water

8 tea bags
6 lemon wedges

Combine the ingredients in a pitcher and store overnight. Remove tea bags, squeezing out liquid. To serve, pour into ice-filled tall glasses. Garnish with lemon wedges. *Makes 6 servings*

	Calories	Carbo-hydrate (gm)	Protein (gm)	Total Fat (gm)	Saturated Fat (gm)	Choles-terol (mg)
Total	32.0	8.4	1.6	0.0	0.0	0.0
Per Serving	5.3	1.4	0.3	0.0	0.0	0.0

Orange Iced Tea

1 cup boiling water
3 tea bags
5 cups water

6-oz. can frozen unsweetened orange juice concentrate, defrosted, undiluted

Pour the boiling water over the tea. Wait 5 minutes while the tea steeps. Remove the tea bags and stir in the remaining water and orange juice concentrate. Pour over ice in tall glasses. *Makes 8 servings*

	Calories	Carbo-hydrate (gm)	Protein (gm)	Total Fat (gm)	Saturated Fat (gm)	Choles-terol (mg)
Total	366.0	88.2	5.3	0.0	0.0	0.0
Per Serving	45.8	11.0	0.7	0.0	0.0	0.0

gm = grams; mg = milligrams. Nutritional figures are approximate. Figures are based on findings of U.S. Department of Agriculture.

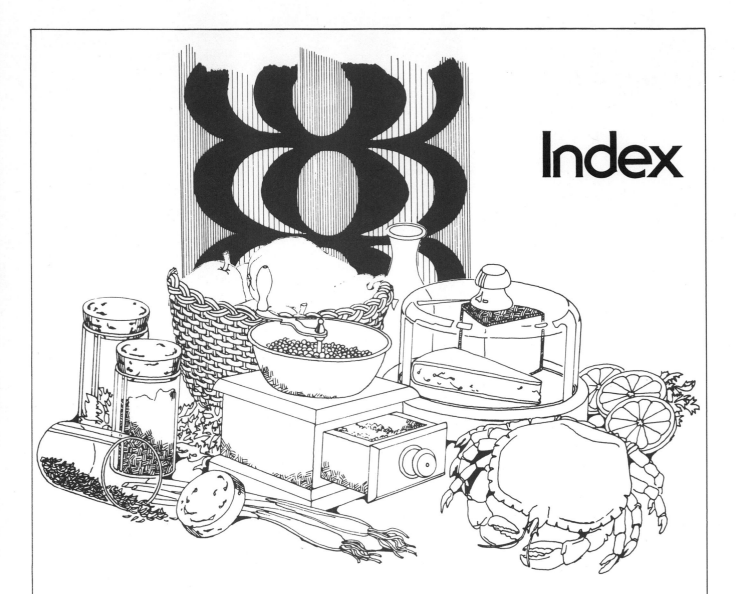

Index

M

Macaroni,
    and cheese salad 42
    and lamb salad 99
    salad, simple 41
    shell salad 42
Mandarin marinade 83
Manicotti 63
Marinades (see also, Dressings and
        Sauces),
    French tenderizing 83
    Italian wine 83
    Mandarin 83
    pineapple 83
    seasoned tenderizing 83
    yogurt 83
Marmalade (see, Jams and jellies)
Meal-in-a-glass berry float 120
Meat (see, individual listings)
Meatballs,
    and spaghetti 42
    casserole 63
    goulash 95
    Swedish 93
Meatloaf for diet-watchers 62
Mediterranean chicken 67
Melon boats with seafood 21
Mexican enchiladas 98
Milkshakes,
    nectarine 121
    peach 121
Mini-calorie veal Marengo 52
Mini-caloried marinated vegetables 37
Minute steaks alla Parmigiana 50
Moroccan salad 24
Mozzarella cheese, with sole 77
Muffins, blueberry cornmeal 15
Mushrooms,
    and cheese pie 95
    and Chinese broccoli 31
    and wild rice 43
    curried, and rice 43
    medley 25
    pickled 86
    poultry stuffing 68
    steak-stuffed 86
Mustard sauce 82

N

Nectarine milkshake 121
Neopolitan peppers 34
New Delhi dip 86
Nog, eggless 122

O

Olive dip 85
Omelette pommes de terre 40
Onion,
    and French steak soup 20
    and rutabaga casserole 37
Orange,
    and cheese pie 111
    and coconut drops 114
    and pumpkin pie 113
    and raisin and carrot slaw 23

cheesecake 115
cider 119
cream puff filling 114
harvest pie 112
iced tea 123
instant breakfast 122
Polynesian fruit sauce 116
real gelatin I 107
real gelatin II 107
sauce, for beets 30
soda 120
spiced tea 123
Oven French fries au naturel 40
Oven-fried chicken 68
Oven-fried fish fillets I 76
Oven-fried fish fillets II 76

P

Pancakes,
    apple 113
    blueberry 16
    cornmeal 16
    hotcakes 16
Parsley potatoes en casserole 39
Pasta (see also, individual listings),
    calorie chart 38
    soup 43
Peach,
    and strawberry dessert crepes 107
    breakfast-in-a-glass 122
    crepes Melba 108
    jelly, sugarless 109
    luau sauce 82
    Melba compote 108
    milkshake 121
    sauce 115
    sherbet, brandied 109
Peachy strawberry dessert crepes 107
Pears,
    baked 104
    pink poached 104
Peas,
    and cauliflower 37
    and chicken 89
    minted 34
Peppers,
    crab-filled 78
    Neopolitan 34
Perfect iced tea 123
Pickled beets 30
Pickled mushrooms 86
Pie,
    apple and raisin 111
    cheese 113
    deep-dish apple 113
    mushroom and cheese 95
    orange and cheese 111
    orange and pumpkin 113
    South Seas pineapple 112
    spiced harvest 112
    spiked apple 112
    spiked apricot 112
    strawberry cream cheese 111
    yogurt 112
Piecrust,
    basic 110
    buttery pastry shell 110
    graham cracker 111
Pineapple,

and carrots 32
and ham stir-fry 61
cheese Danish squares 17
ham patties aloha 60
marinade 83
pancake sauce 17
Polynesian fruit sauce 116
Polynesian Waldorf salad 23
sauce I 105
sauce II 116
South Seas pie 112
yogurt cooler 121
Pink lemonade syrup 119
Pink poached pears 104
Pizza,
    chicken 68
    protein-packed 96
Polynesian fruit sauce 116
Polynesian Waldorf salad 23
Pork (see also, Ground meats) 58-61,
    and kraut 60
    calorie chart 47
    Chinese 60
    chop barbecue 59
    chop surprise 59
    country sausage 17
    pepper steak 59
    savory sausage 17
    steak Viennese 60
    tomato and rice chops 59
Potatoes,
    and creamed ham 100
    au gratin 41
    calorie chart 38
    cheesy creamed 39
    cottage cheese salad 41
    decalorized salad 41
    omelette 40
    oven-fried 40
    pancakes 39
    parsley, en casserole 39
    savory bacon 39
    scalloped 40
    stuffed 39
    tangy apple salad 41
    twice-baked 40
Pot roast,
    Burgundy 48
    cider-spicy 48
    olé 47
    slim-but-saucy 48
Poultry (see, Chicken and Turkey)
Poultry stuffing,
    apple and bacon 71
    high-fiber 71
    mushroom 68
Preserves (see, Jams and jellies)
Protein-enriched potato pancakes 39
Protein-packed pizza 96
Pudding, apple and bread 108
Pumpkin and orange pie 113

Q

Quiche,
    asparagus 96
    broccoli 96
Quick barbecued pork 100
Quick hot curry sauce 82
Quick pickled beets 30